THE KAMA SUTRA

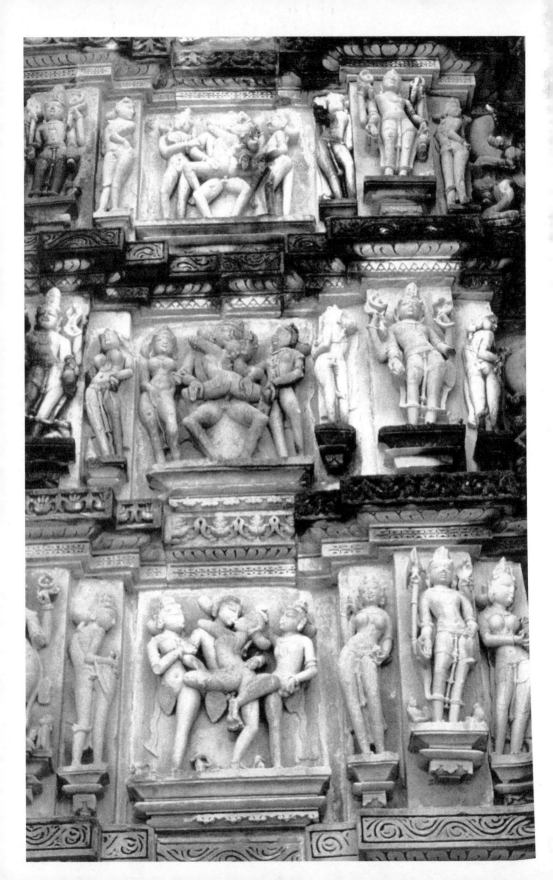

THE KAMA SUTRA

THE HINDU ART OF LOVE

VATSYAYANA

COMPLETE TRANSLATION FROM THE
ORIGINAL SANSKRIT BY

S.C. UPADHYAYA

FOREWORD BY
MOTI CHANDRA

WATKINS PUBLISHING
LONDON

This edition published in the UK 2004 by
Watkins Publishing,
Sixth Floor, Castle House, 75-76 Wells Street, London W1T 3QH

Originally published by Dr R. J. Mehta for
D. B. Taraporevala Sons & Co. Pvt. Ltd.
210 Dr. D. N. Road, Mumbai – 400 001

Designed and typeset by Jerry Goldie

Printed and bound in Great Britain

British Library Cataloguing in Publication data available

Library of Congress Cataloging in Publication data available

ISBN 1 84293 065 6

www.watkinspublishing.com

CONTENTS

Contents

Contents

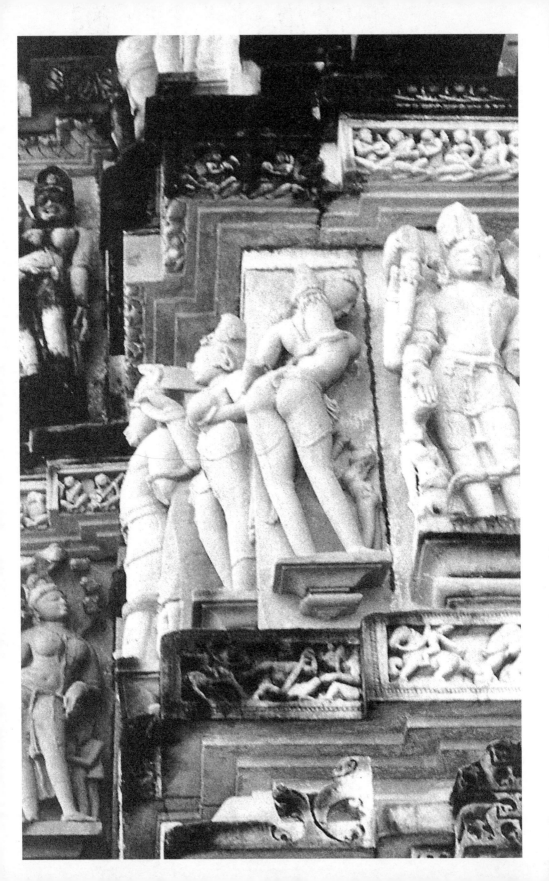

OPINIONS ON THE KAMA SUTRA AND ON LOVE

India's most famous and presumably the oldest breviary of love (is) the Kama Sutra. The composer of this work Mallanaga Vatsyayana was no light-hearted Don Juan; his repute was that of an exceptionally sage and pious man and this is entirely borne out by the pedantic accuracy with which he introduces his readers to the secrets of eroticism ... Even sexual intercourse, for all the excitement attendant on it, is an art which must be studied scientifically to get the full pleasure of it ...

It is noteworthy, however, that the art of love is not designed solely to give pleasure to the man: the woman, too, must get the maximum pleasure ... Vatsyayana claims to write not only as a scientist but also as a moralist. His whole purpose, he says, is to strengthen married life by perfecting its technique and thus make men more virtuous.

Richard Lewinsohn, *A History of Sexual Customs*

The third of the aims of man is Kama, love, and this is taken as seriously by Indian writers as Dharma or Artha. As Arthacastra is intended for kings and ministers, so the Kamacastra is to be studied by men of taste, Nagarakas who desire to practise refinement and profit to the most by their knowledge of all that is meant by love ... The sociological and medical importance of the treatise is admittedly considerable.

A. Berriedale Keith, *A History of Sanskrit Literature*

The principal surviving classic of India's Kama teachings is Vatsyayana's celebrated Kama sutra. The justly celebrated Kamasutra of Brahman Vatsyayana ... is a masterly yet very much condensed and all too abbreviated version of the materials of the earlier tradition.

Heinrich Zimmer, *Philosophies of India*

Vatsyayana's Kamasutra also, by its wealth and accuracy of varied content, affords considerable material to history, psychology, sociology and even medicine. It is not a lightly written tract on sexology merely for the pleasure of the voluptuary or the virtuoso in love, but a serious and scientific composition which approaches the generally forbidden subject as a part of humanity ... but it is certainly not a pedantic and superficial production of scholasticism, written that it is with considerable objectivity of observation, understanding and balanced thinking.

S. K. De, *Ancient Indian Erotics and Erotic Literature*

This is a scientific treatise on erotics, the only early treatise in the world on the subject, which gives us a thoroughly accurate and wonderfully effective solution of the problem of procreation. The spirit and the method in which the author attacks the problem is astonishingly modern.

G. P. Majumdar, 'Plants in Erotics', *Ind. Cul.*, XV, P. 74

Vatsyayana draws a picture of the good wife which may be taken as usual to be a faithful reflection of real life.

U. N. Ghoshal, *The Classical Age*

The book (Kama Sutra) deals with the subject in a comprehensive manner and throws much revealing light on the manners and customs of society.

G. V. Devasthali, *The Classical Age*

Vatsyayana, one of the greatest authorities ...

Havelock Ellis, *Sex in Relation to Society*

The most characteristic product of the Indian mind is the formal exposition of a particular science in dogmatic enunciations accompanied by a discussion (bhashya). Such are the grammatical works of Patanjali, the Arthashastra of Chanakya, the Kamashastra of Vatsyayana.

F. W. Thomas, *Cambridge History of India*

The East from the immemorial past has handed down invaluable instruction in the Art of Love. This their wise men have taught as the most important branch of education. In consequence of this complex study of the body of men and women Easterners scientifically learnt how to rise to heights of pleasure rarely attained by the comparatively ignorant Westerners. The Hindus have a rich treasure of classical works on erotology that gives detailed and scientific instruction in the Art of Love: they tell of an infinite variety of refinements of physical love; how to increase pleasure and virility, and caution against pitfalls of sex.

Paolo Mantegazza, Former Professor of Anthropology,
University of Florence

The works of men of genius do follow them and remain as a lasting treasure. And though there may be disputes and discussions about the immortality of the body or the soul, nobody can deny the immortality of genius, which ever remains as a bright and guiding star to the struggling humanities of the succeeding ages. This work (the Kama Sutra), then, which has stood the test of centuries, has placed Vatsyayana among the immortals, and on this, and on him no better elegy or eulogy can be written than the following lines:

So long as lips shall kiss, and eyes shall see,

So long lives this, and This gives life to Thee.

Sir Richard Burton

The Kamasutra ... is the most famous in a long list of works revealing a certain pre-occupation with the physical and mental techniques of sex ... Vatsyayana gives a delightful picture of a girl in love, but his wisdom is lavished chiefly upon the parental art of getting her married away, and the husbandly art of keeping her physically content.

Will Durant, *Our Oriental Heritage*

There is a prevalent idea that the Hindu view concedes no reality of life, that it despises vital aims and satisfactions, that it gives no inspiring motive to human effort. If spirit and life were unrelated, spiritual freedom would become an unattainable ideal, a remote passion of a few visionaries. There is little in Hindu thought to support the view that one has to attain spiritual freedom by means of a violent rupture with ordinary life. On the other hand, it lays down that we must pass through the normal life conscientiously and with knowledge, work out its values, and accept its enjoyments. Spiritual life is an integration of man's being, in its depth and breadth, in its capacity for deep meditation as well as reckless transport. *Kama* refers to the emotional being of man, his feelings and desires. If a man is denied his emotional life, he becomes a prey to repressive introspection and lives under a continual strain of moral torture. When the reaction sets in, he will give way to a wildness of ecstasy which is ruinous to his sanity and health.

S. Radhakrishnan, *Eastern Religions and Western Thought*

Kama is of the essence of magic, magic of the essence of love; for among nature's own spells and charms that of love and sex is preeminent. This is the witchcraft that compels life to progress from one generation to the next, the spell that binds all creatures to the cycle of existences, through deaths and births.

Heinrich Zimmer, *Philosophies of India*

It is my firm belief that it is love that sustains the earth. There only is life where there is love. Life without love is death.

Mahatma Gandhi

What in common language we call beauty, which is in harmony of lines, colours, sounds, or in grouping of words or thoughts, delights us only because we cannot help admitting a truth in it that is ultimate. 'Love is enough,' the poet has said; it carries its own explanation, the joy of which can only be expressed in a form of art which also has that finality. Love gives evidence to something which is outside us but which intensely exists and thus stimulates the sense of our own existence. It radiantly reveals the reality of its objects, though these may lack qualities that are valuable or brilliant.

Rabindranath Tagore

Love that is based on the goodness of those whom you love is a mercenary affair, whereas true love is self-suffering and demands no consideration. It is like that of a model Hindu wife, Sita, for instance, who loved her Rama even whilst he bid her pass through a raging fire. It was well with Sita, for she knew what she was doing. She sacrificed herself out of her strength, not out of her weakness. Love is the strongest force the world possesses and yet it is the humblest imaginable.

Mahatma Gandhi

I love as the rudder in the water might love the sail in the sky, answering its rhythm of wind in the rhythm of waves.

The heart's laws are not the laws of scripture. Eyes cannot see with their own light,—the light must come from the outside.

Two hearts beat in unison, immersing themselves in the waves of melody. Nothing now seemed common or unclean and the whole world swam in a rosy mist. It was as though all the passion that had ever throbbed in human hearts were gathered up and showered on these two lovers, and that it now pulsated within them in all its super-abundance of bliss and anguish, longing and distress.

Rabindranath Tagore

What barrier is there that love cannot break?

True love is boundless like the ocean and rising and swelling within one spreads itself out and crossing all boundaries and frontiers envelops the whole world.

The more efficient a force is, the more silent and the more subtle it is. Love is the subtlest force in the world.

Mahatma Gandhi

ABBREVIATIONS

A.R.	Anangaranga	R.R.	Ratirahasya
G.G.	Gitagovinda	R.R.P.	Ratiratnapradipika
K.C.	Kandarpachudamani	R.S.D.	Rudrakrita Smaradipika
K.M.	Kuttanimata		
K.S.	Kama Sutra	S.D.	Shringaradipika (Harihara)
N.S.	Nagarasarvasva		
P.S.	Panchasayaka	S.M.	Shringaramanjari
R.K.K.	Ratikelikutuhala	M.	Male
R.M.	Ratimanjari	F.	Female

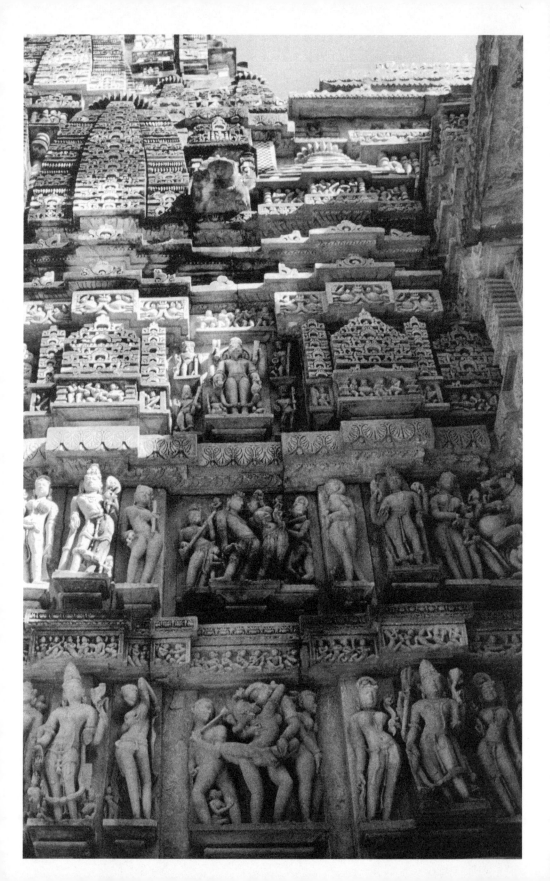

FOREWORD

Dr S. C. Upadhyaya is an erudite scholar of Sanskrit whose knowledge of the ancient Indian art of love requires no commendation. In this work he has produced a literal translation of Vatsyayana's *Kama Sutra* which is, without any doubt, the most important treatise on the subject.

Vatsyayana not only incorporated various schools of thought on the science of love but also arranged his material in such a way that it was handy to poets, artists and above all to those lovers for whom the *Kama Sutra* was the very life-breath of existence. The entire range of topics on love is set out with a scientific thoroughness unparalleled in Sanskrit literature. Vatsyayana's aphorisms are models of brevity. From his observant eyes nothing seems to have escaped. The art of love-making in various phases, the instruments of love-making, the psychology of sex, the courtesans and their victims, the routine of accomplished lovers – all have been treated with precision and a scientific viewpoint.

In such a treatment of love, courtesans and uninhibited sex, one could imagine the writer soaring to fanciful heights, but this expectation is belied in the face of a scientific work arranged topic-wise which reveals the analytic mind of a great thinker. Vatsyayana no doubt acknowledges the debt of past masters on the science of sex, but his critical mind refuses to accept views with which he could not agree.

The *Kama Sutra* is not a dry catalogue of love acts. Its wider canvas touches many aspects of social manners and customs – the luxurious life of the city, the sports and pastimes of the elite and the common folk, the sacredness of the home, the cultivated wiles of the courtesans, the *goshthis* or club houses and other institutions which served as convivial gatherings accompanied by drinking, gambling, dancing and music.

To ancient Indians prudery had no meaning. While delighting in spiritual speculation, and forever in the quest of final emancipation, Indian thinkers also realised the value of money as a necessary adjunct for piety and comfortable living. Sex had no vulgar connotation for them. Indian poets sang the charms of love and sex and went into ecstasies over the beauties of the human body. Even dry-as-dust books on religion touched upon love and beauty in the anecdotes they related for the edification of the pious and the god-fearing. This feeling for sex and beauty became a guiding spirit of Indian art and there is little doubt that Vatsyayana played no mean part in evolving and sustaining a warmth for love and sex in art and literature.

No attempt has yet been made to trace and analyse the influences of the *Kama Sutra* on Indian literature, art and religion. Sex in ancient Indian religion was not looked upon with abhorrence, but its functions were clearly recognised. The nude figures of the mother goddesses, the fertility figures of the Mithunas, Yakshas and Yakshis engaged discreetly in love gestures, but becoming more erotic in the medieval period, show an intimate knowledge of sex impulses.

It cannot be said that religious sensuality as reflected in the Tantras was in any way inspired by the *Kama Sutra,* the feeling of sex being natural to all primitive religions. But there is no doubt that in mystic Tantrism, which enjoined sexual union as one of its essential features, there was a definite understanding of the principles of the *Kama Sutra,* perhaps elated to mystic heights, but nevertheless revealing a worldliness which could not be mistaken easily. In medieval Indian sculptures of Khajuraho and Orissa which fully reflect the *Kaula-kapalika* practices, sex relations under the garb of religious practice presuppose the knowledge of the *Kama Sutra*. In the ancient bas-reliefs and terracotta plaques as well as in the representations of Mithuna figures, dancing, drinking and revelry presuppose the existence of such forms of enjoyment which fully support the state of society as depicted in the *Kama Sutra*.

Study of the *Kama Sutra*, which was considered as a necessary part of the liberal education and culture of a man of the world in ancient India, is looked upon suspiciously by some present-day reformers and prudes for whom the very mention of sex connotes profanity, obscenity and pornography. The *Kama Sutra*, however, could easily disprove the charges made against it. Vatsyayana has treated sex in a scientific spirit and if the modern killjoys do not like his descriptions of the acts of love he is not to be blamed. Moreover, the study of the *Kama Sutra* points to one of the earliest attempts at sanity in sex life. Within recent years sane sex life as a happy mode of existence has been treated scientifically by renowned authors. As one of the earliest in the chain of thinkers on sex and love, Vatsyayana deserves our fullest approbation.

The *Kama Sutra* has been translated into English many times, but Dr Upadhyaya's translation has tried to keep up the spirit of the original as far as possible. He has followed the commentary of Yashodhara to clarify certain points, but the emphasis is mostly on the *sutra*.

Moti Chandra
Director, Prince of Wales Museum of Western India, Bombay

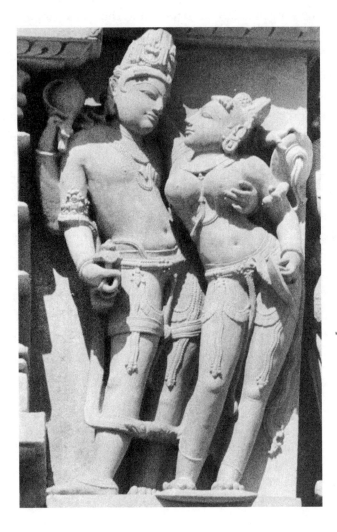

INTRODUCTION

CHAPTER I

DEVELOPMENT OF THE SCIENCE OF EROTICS IN THE VEDIC AND POST-VEDIC PERIODS

During the Vedic period, schools of different sciences developed. We know of the schools of etymology, grammar, law, geometry, astronomy and medicine. The science of love – Kama – had a similar beginning during that period. This science of erotics occupied a prominent place along with other sciences that developed in this country and shaped its civilization and culture.

Erotics in India means the science of human creation with its antecedents and consequents. It has for its object the enunciation, elucidation and enforcement of the laws governing the antecedents to that necessary act, the creation of the species, the control of the foetus throughout all the stages of its growth and development within the womb together with the essential preliminaries.[1]

The science is mainly concerned with fulfilling the desires of the flesh. It aims to teach a person the best method to control and properly guide the desires, particularly the sexual urge, so that the person may be a useful member of the family, society and his country and contribute to their welfare by his way of life.

If we look into the old texts, both of the Vedic and post-Vedic periods, we find that every aspect is elaborately dealt with. The life of a person as Nagaraka (an expert in the affairs of love), his food, recreations, amusements and garments are prescribed. Various charms are mentioned for health and wealth. There are even prayers for virility. The use of aphrodisiacs is minutely dealt with.

In the Hymn to Creation[2] the poet describes the time prior to creation. He then imagines that the primordial substance arose through the power of Tapas. The first product of the Mind was Kama, sexual desire, love, the bond between the non-existent and existent. As this desire leads to the procreation and birth of beings, the s

ages considered it as the primal source of all existence. Kama appears here for the first time as an abstract personification, but the description shows a connection with sex symbolism. The symbolism of the act of human procreation is applied to the act of cosmic creation. Here we have the earliest acknowledgment, in literature, of sex desire as the prime source of existence.[3]

In the Rig Veda[4] we hear Lopamudra complaining to the sage Agastya that she was tired of serving him night and day, year after year. She tells him that old age withers physical beauty and that every male endowed with virility should cohabit with the female. Agastya then consoles her, saying that together they would win the battle of amorous dalliance. The narratives of Romasha, the daughter of Brihaspati, and Ghosha, the daughter of Kakshivan, point to the development of this science of erotics. In the Atharva Veda particularly we find charms to cure diseases, prayers for long life, health and virility; charms pertaining to women; charms for obtaining a husband, a wife, a son, ensuring conception, making a woman sterile, preventing miscarriage, having easy parturition, securing love of a woman, and allaying jealousy. To quote only one concrete instance, these charms in the Atharva Veda,[5] in language not at all veiled, profess to promote virility. In the Shatapatha Brahmana, even though eroticism is subservient to religious theory and practice, we can perceive the underlying idea.[6]

The Garbhopanishad[7] describes how the Pancha-bhutas (five elements) act, how the Shadrasas help to produce semen, and how the Garbha (embryo) develops. It also says how twins are born. In the Brihadaranyaka Upanishad[8] we come across the Mantha doctrine of Uddalaka, the son of Aruna. This knowledge was passed on from teacher to pupil – to Madhuka, Chula, Ayasthuna and Satyakama. This doctrine in short is: 'If the initiated person pours the Mantha on a dried trunk of a tree, the latter gets sprouts and branches too.'

The Mahabharata contains the earliest reference to Linga-worship.[9] In the Grihyasutras[10] we find that the blessings of wealth, stout sons and the cordial life of husband and wife are mentioned. At the time of the marriage,[11] the father of the daughter says that the daughter is given away in marriage for continuation of the family and happiness of the forefathers. Both the bride and the bridegroom solemnly declare that their marriage is meant for the purpose mentioned above.

Ancient authorities on medicine[12] such as Charaka and Sushruta say that a person who is normally quite healthy should have a son as laid down in the sacred texts. They give elaborate prescriptions for food and recreation for the woman who desires to have a child. Ancient Smriti texts[13] openly declare that if a person sees the face of his son during his own lifetime, his debt towards his forefathers is passed on to his son and he himself acquires immortality. There are innumerable places for the parents of a son; but those without a son have no place anywhere.

Manu[14] declares that because the son saves the parents from going to Hell, otherwise named 'Pum', he is called Putra. For the wife[15] it is said that she is really a wife, 'bharya', if she has given birth to children. A married lady is really like the goddess of wealth if, along with other feminine virtues, she has given birth to children. The Smritis and Puranas[16] go further and say that if a person dies child-less he becomes an evil spirit. The story of Atmadeva and

4

Dhundhuli[17] brings out the feelings of a childless couple very vividly. Atmadeva laments that life, home, wealth and family all are disgusting to him as he is childless.

Ancient texts are full of instances of kings performing sacrifices in order to obtain a son. We know that King Para Atnara[18] got a son after performing a sacrifice. The Ramayana[19] describes how king Dasharatha performed a sacrifice and got four sons even in his old age. From the Mahabharata[20] we learn that King Drupada approached the sage Yaja and asked him how he could get a son that would kill Drona. A sacrifice was then performed and a powerful son was born.

Innumerable anecdotes are found in the Mahabharata, all of which describe the cherished desire for having a son whose birth would ensure happiness of the father and forefathers. Once Jaratkaru,[21] while wandering, found his forefathers hanging head downwards as they could not attain final emancipation, because Jaratkaru had no son to continue the family line. They asked him to marry and have a son for their emancipation which he did by marrying the sister of Vasuki.

Once upon a time the sage Agastya[22] saw his forefathers hanging head downwards as Agastya had no son. He then created a maiden with beautiful limbs and placed her under the care of the King of the Vidarbha country who was also practising penance to get a son. The sage Agastya married that Vaidarbhi princess who was named Lopamudra. Once the sage desired to co-habit with her, but she refused, saying that she would consent only if she had jewels, ornaments, beautiful garments, and a fine bed. The sage, being poor, approached King Shrutarvana but the latter could not give him anything as he had nothing to share. The sage then approached King Bradhnashva accompanied by King Shrutarvana. This second king also could not give the sage anything for the same reason. The sage next approached King Purukutsa accompanied by the two kings. But this third king also could not give the sage anything. At last the sage approached the demon King Ilvala accompanied by the three kings.

The sage killed Vatapi, the brother of Ilvala, by his yogic powers and consequently the demon king gave Agastya as much wealth as he desired. The sage returned to his hermitage and having pleased Lopamudra, cohabited with her. Lopamudra delivered a powerful and learned son after seven years and was named Idhmavaha.

King Bali[23] saved the blind sage Dirghatamas from a drifting canoe and requested him to beget sons through his queens. The sage having agreed to it, the king sent his Queen Sudeshna. The queen on seeing the blind sage, did not go herself but sent her maidservant to him. The sage produced eleven shudra sons, Kakshivat and others. The king once more propitiated the sage and directed Queen Sudeshna to go to him who had five sons – Anga, Vanga, Kalinga, Pundra and Suhma.

The sage Galava[24] wanted to give a present to his teacher Vishvamitra as his guru dakshina, but he had nothing with him. He therefore approached King Yayati on the advice of his friend Suparna. King Yayati at the time had already given away his wealth in charity. He therefore asked Galava to take away his beautiful princess named Madhavi and told him that other kings would gladly offer even their kingdoms in exchange for the princess and that he (Yayati) would also be a grandfather. Galava then approached King Haryashva of Ayodhya who agreed to accept the princess in order to have a son, in return for two hundred horses of excellent breed, having one ear black and white in colour. In the course of time King Haryashva got a son (Vasu). The sage then approached King Divodasa of Kasi. This king also agreed to accept the princess in exchange for an equal number of horses. King Divodasa got one son (Pratardana) from the Princess. The sage then approached King Aushinara of Bhoganagara who also agreed to accept the princess for a similar number of horses. The king got a son (Shibi) from the princess. As there was no king who could offer the sage Galava two hundred horses more (as required by Vishvamitra), Vainateya, the friend of Galava, advised him to go to Vishvamitra and narrate to him all the facts. Galava accordingly approached Vishvamitra and requested him to accept the princess to have a fourth son in exchange for the remaining two hundred horses. The sage, on seeing the beautiful princess, rebuked his pupil Galava saying that he should have shown her first to him and that he (Vishvamitra) would have had all four sons by her. He then accepted her to have a son in exchange for a similar gift. The sage got a son named Ashtaka. Galava, being now pleased, told Madhavi that by her four sons she had ensured the final emancipation of her father (Yayati) and then he returned the princess to King Yayati.

It was Vyasa who told Yudhishthira that if a pupil cohabited with the wife of the teacher, for the latter's benefit, the pupil was said to have committed no sin.[25] He gave him the instance of Uddalaka for whom one of the pupils had a son named Shvetaketu from his (Uddalaka's) wife.

Rathitara, the son of Prishadashva,[26] got a son from his wife through Angiras. The later generations were therefore a mixture of Brahmana and Kshatriya. We also know that women were equally anxious, like men, to have children. Once the sage Dhaumya[27] was away from his hermitage and one of his wives was in the monthly period. At this, other co-wives asked Uttanka, a pupil of Dhaumya, to see that she did not pass it away fruitlessly.

We also know that persons suffering from certain handicaps also tried to satisfy their desires for obtaining a son. Once King Pandu[28] narrated to Kunti the misfortunes of a childless person, the story of Sharadandayini whose queen selected a Brahman after bathing on the expiry of the monthly period, and after worshipping fire. She delivered three sons, Durjaya and others. The queen of King Sharadandayini of Kekaya was Shrutasena, the sister of Kunti, and King Pandu exhorted her to select a Brahmana, better than him, to produce sons as he had lost the power of procreation due to the curse of a sage.

This desire for having sons was so deep-rooted in the minds of the people that even law books[29] ordered getting children by proxy. On the death of King Vichitravirya,[30] without a child, Satyavati told Bhishma to fetch Vyasa for the purpose of getting sons by the widows

7

of (his brother) Vichitravirya. After the lapse of a year, duly purified, the first Queen Kaushalya got a son who was blind from birth as she had closed her eyes due to the fearful sight of the sage Vyasa who had shining eyes, a large tuft of hair on the head and a long beard. He was prevailed upon by Satyavati to have another son by Ambalika. This second queen gave birth to a son who was pale (Pandu) as she had turned pale at the sight of the sage at the time of the union. Once more the sage was requested to get a son by the elder queen. She did not go to bed but sent her maidservant after bedecking her with ornaments and fine garments. This son became later known as Vidura.

We know from the ancient texts that every person has to pursue the aims of life, Dharma, Artha, Kama and Moksha. This order does not mean that they should follow one after the other.

In the Mahabharata[31] we read that once Yudhishthira asked his brothers and Vidura about the order of these aims of life. In Vidura's opinion Dharma was first, then Artha and then Kama. Arjuna said that without Artha, Dharma and Kama could not be pursued satisfactorily. Then Sahadeva and Nakula said that Dharma should be practised first and then Artha and Kama. Bhima said that Kama should be first and then Dharma and Artha; but later he reconsidered and said that they should be pursued simultaneously.

We also come across in the same epic,[32] a discussion between Yudhishthira and Bhishma. Bhishma replied that Artha was dependent on Dharma and that Kama followed Artha. He cited the story of the sage Kamandaka and King Angarishta. The sage told the king that a person who pursues Kama leaving aside Dharma and Artha loses his intellect, and his acts give rise to atheism and practices which are censured by the sacred texts. Therefore all the three should be pursued simultaneously.

Kautilya[33] has said that the pursuit of Kama should be such as would not interfere with those of Dharma and Artha. Even Vatsyayana[34] has modified his own order (Artha in young age, Kama after maturity, Dharma and Moksha in old age) and said, like

Kautilya, that as the duration of a man's life is uncertain, the order is not unchangeable, but a person may pursue these aims of his life as and when the opportunity arises. Vatsyayana's attitude shows a definite advance[35] on the more ancient outlook on the sexual impulse. He firmly states that sexual satisfaction is essential for the upkeep of bodily health and consequently is equally important like wealth and religion.

A perusal of literary sources has enabled Barua[36] to remark that the Mantha doctrine of Uddalaka is the 'canonical basis of the rules regarding practical amplification of the principles of eugenics and it is not improbable that the erotics science developed on the lines of Uddalaka's Mantha doctrine.' References cited in this chapter go to uphold Keith's[37] opinion, that the science of genetics occupied the attention of the Rishis – founders of the various schools of sciences. To quote Baruas[38] once more, 'its primary object as set forth in the closing chapter of the Brihadaranyaka Upanishad is to teach a way of life which is essential to the preservation and betterment of the race and as such the system forms an integral part of the Brahmanic Ethics ... None should fight shy of claiming ancient Indian treatises of erotic science as a rich heritage.'

NOTES

[1] Majumdar. G. P., 'Plants in Erotics', *Indian Culture*, XV, 1, p. 66.
[2] Rigveda, X, 129, 1 to 7.
[3] (i) Macdonell, (i)*Vedic Mythology*, p. 13; (ii) Winternitz, *History of Indian Literature*, I, p. 99, n. 2; (iii) De, *Ancient Indian Erotics and Erotic Literature*, pp. 85-86.
[4] The Rigveda, I, 23–179; 1-19-127: 1-17-117, 122.
[5] (i) The Atharva Veda, IV 4; VI 72, 101; (ii) Bloomfield, *Atharvaveda*, pp. 57, 62; (iii) Max Muller, S.B.E. XLII, p. 31.
[6] Shatapatha Brahmana, 1-2-5, 15-16; (1) Sechizig Upanishads des Veda.
[7] Deussen: (i) Garbhopanishad, p. 650; (ii) *The Philosophy of Upanishads*, pp. 283-295.
[8] (1) Brihadaranyaka Upanishad VI–3; (ii) Majumdar, G. P., *Some Aspects of Indian Civilization*, Ch. X (ii).

9   Mahabharata: (*i*) Drona Parva, 172-173 (critical); (*ii*) Anushasana Parva, 161 (Poona).

10   Meyer, *Sexual Life in Ancient India,* p. 139.

11   Brahmakarmasamuchchaya, pp. 448-459.

12   (*i*) Charaka Samhita, II, VIII, etc; (*ii*) Sushruta, II, etc.

13   (*i*) Vasishtha Smriti, 17-22; (*ii*) Atri Samhita, 53-54.

14   Manu Smriti, IX, 138.

15   Shamkha Smriti, IV, 5; (*ii*) Daksha Smriti, IV, 11; (*iii*) Mahabharata, 1, 74-40.

16   (*i*) Garuda P*urana*, Pretakalpa, IX, 56-62; 11-4, 20-4; (*ii*) Devi Bhagavata, 1-14; (*iii*) Prajapati Smriti, 188.

17   Bhagavata Purana, Mahatmya, 4-29, 38.

18   (*i*) Taittiriya Samhita, 5-6-5-3; (*ii*) Katha Samhita, 22-3.

19   Ramayana, Balakanda, 8/9, 12/9, 13/1, 14/60.

20   Mahabharata, I, 167 (Poona).

21   Mahabharata, I. 45; Devi Bhagavata, II, 42.

22   Mahabharata, III. 96-99.

23   Mahabharata, I, 104.

24   Mahabharata. V, 114-119.

25   Mahabharata, XII, 34-22.

26   Bhagavata Purana, IX, 6-3.

27   Mahabharata, I, 3.

28   Mahabharata, I, 120.

29   Naradasrnriti, XII, 80; Manusmriti, IX; Yagnavalkyasmriti, I, 3.

30   Mahabharata, I, 105-106.

31   Mahabharata, XII, 167.

32   Mahabharata, XII, 123.

33   Kautilya, Arthashastra, I, 7-3.

34   Vatsyayana, Kamasutra, I, 1-2 to 5.

35   Ghosh, *Urban Morals in Ancient India,* pp. 13–14.

36   Barua, *A History of Pre-Buddhistic Indian Philosophy,* p. 127.

37   Keith, *A History of Sanskrit Literature,* pp. 403–405, 450, 467.

38   Barua, ibid. p. 341.

CHAPTER II

TUMESCENCE IN SANSKRIT LITERATURE

Textbooks on the psychology of sex tell us that the skin not only protects the delicate vessels, nerves, viscera and muscles, but also brings us into sensitive contact with the external world. As the organ of touch, it is the seat of the most widely diffused sense. Touch sensations are the first of all the sensory impressions to prove pleasurable. The pleasurable sensation of the lips causes a child to respond to the contact of its mother's nipple while being breast-fed. Animals like cows and buffaloes lick their young ones. The tonic value of cutaneous stimulation is quite well known. It can allay painful sensations and has powerful reverberations in the emotional sexual sphere.

Sanskrit literature abounds in the examples of love at first sight or touch. We have two famous instances in Dushyanta and Pururava. Shakuntala fell in love with Dushyanta at first sight, and Urvashi became quite enamoured of Pururava when his shoulder touched her. Ancient Indian writers on erotics, such as Kokkoka and others, have elaborately discussed this subject as it is very important for tumescence. It was known to them from their observations and perhaps from personal experience that the sexual orgasm is founded on a special adaptation and intensification of touch sensations and hence they laid down that *Alingana* and *Chumbana* are essential components of *Bahyarata*. Hence they propounded the theory of erogenous zones and cutaneous excitations – Kamasthanas, Chandrakala, Ratitithis, Ratikalas and Chandrakala Prabodhanavidhis in case of females of all the four types. Kokkoka (II, 1 to 6) refers to two previous schools of the science of erotics, headed by Nandikeshvara and Gonikaputra. According to the school of Nandikeshvara, Anangasthiti is observed, starting from the first Tithi of the Sukiapaksha up to Purnima, in the right side of the body of a female and beginning with the right toe, upwards, to the head. Then it takes the downwards course from the left side of the head, down to the left toe, beginning with the first Tithi of Krishnapaksha up to Amavasya.

The anatomical parts listed are toe, sole, knee, thigh, jaghana, navel, chest, breast, side, neck, cheek, lips, eyes, forehead and head. He then goes on to say that the lovers indulge in catching locks of hair; kissing the forehead and eyes; biting the lips and cheeks; scratching with the fingernails, the sides, the neck, the breasts; fisting the chest; thumping the navel; manipulating the sexual organ with the fingers; dashing with the thighs, the knees and the toes. This results in the woman reaching the climax just as rays of the moon falling on a moon-stone cause it to ooze.

According to Gonikaputra, Anangasthiti is observed in the different anatomical parts (sixteen according to Kanchinatha) and on each Tithi, and the male, concentrating on one vowel, indulges in love-play. In the next eleven verses (II, 7 to 17) he describes the love-play during the fifteen Tithis of each Paksha. He also gives Ratitithis for all the four types. But he gives Ratikala for Chitrini and others excluding Padmini.

Padmashri (XVII-XIX) gives a list of parts of Komodaya, but differs and says that Ananga is found going up in these parts, starting from the first Tithi of the Krishnapaksha up to Amavasya, and descending from the head downward to the left toe, starting from the first Tithi of the Shuklapaksha up to Purnima. He gives in four verses the Svaramatrika Nayasa and goes on to describe *Nadikshobhana* and its benefits.

Jyotirisha refers to Nandikeshvara and follows Kokkoka but mentions the parts of Chandrakala and its waxing and waning. He gives (I, 10, 15 to 27) Ratitithis, Ratikalas and Chandrakala Pradipanavidhis. There is, however, some difference in these Kalas and Tithis from those given by Kokkoka.

Praudhadevaraya (I, 26-27) does not give the list but says that Kama is observed going up from the left toe upwards to the head in Shuklapaksha and descending from the head to the right toe, in the Krishnapaksha. He refers to Nandisha (I, 4) and to Gonikaputra (I, 40 to 68) for the four kinds of females and mentions Svaramatrika Nyasa. He also gives, like Jyotirisha, the Tithis, Kala and Pradipanavidhis. He gives additional information regarding the posture for congress liked by each of the four types of females. Kalyanamulla (I, 7 to 17, II, 1 to 18) gives the list of parts for Manasijasthiti, the four types of females, Tithis, Kalas and Chandrakala Pradipanavidhis. As regards the beginning and the end of the Kamasthiti the extant text is not exact, as other editions have contradictory readings.

Harihara is the only writer on erotics who says in his Samaradipika that Shuklapaksha begins from the first day of menstruation and Krishnapaksha from the sixteenth to the thirtieth day. This is perhaps based on sound observations on the part of the author.

Now let us deal with tumescence and its various components. It was Mall who first said that the sexual impulse is made up of two separate components, 1) the impulse of detumescence and 2) the impulse of contrectation. Under the second he included not only the tendency to general physical contact; but also the psychic inclination to become generally interested in a person of the opposite sex. Mall did not regard these two impulses as intimately related to each other. As against this, Numa Proetorius, Robert Miller, Max Kate and Havelock Ellis considered them to be much more associated. Heape distinguished between the pro-estrum or preliminary period of congestion and the estrus or the period of desire. These writers agree that tumescence must be obtained before desire can become acute, and courtship runs *pari passu* with physiological processes. Contrectation, according to Ellis, is an extremely primitive and fundamental part of tumescence and detumescence. The last two are alike fundamental, primitive and essential. Tumescence which comes first is the most important and nearly the whole of sexual psychology is rooted in it. It takes an active form in the male and brings him into the condition in which discharge becomes imperative and at the same time arouses, in the female, a similar state of emotional excitement and sexual turgescence.[1]

Now let us see how this has been treated in Sanskrit literature. Vatsyayana uses one technical term – *Samprayoga* – which includes Bahya and Abhyantara Ratas. The chapter, therefore, in his Kama Sutra, bears the title Samprayogika Adhikarana. Yashodhara, the commentator, explains that *Avapa* is the technical term for the art of wooing a female (Strisadhanam cha avapah), and for deriving the maximum pleasure out of courtship and the final consummation a male must necessarily know the various components of that art called Tantra alias *Samprayoga*.[2]

Ancient writers do not agree in the exact total number of the component parts of *Samprayoga*. According to the school of Babhravya, it is made up of eight parts and each is divided into eight varieties, and the general term of Chatuhshashti[3] is given to it. Vatsyayana, after quoting the school of Babhravya, adds that there are some additions according to others.[4] Shankara Mishra has clearly mentioned that the school of Vatsyayana[5] favours the eightfold *Samprayoga*. But there is no clear reference to this order in the present text of Kama Sutra. Yashodhara,[6] on the other hand, quotes a certain school favouring the tenfold *Samprayoga*. But Damodara[7] is the only author who clearly mentions the eightfold *Bahyarata*.

Thus it is certain that the number is eight or more but not less. Vatsyayana,[8] however, clearly states that lovers may indulge in any number of modifications of these components provided they add to the pleasures resulting from such amorous dalliance. He further states that there is no order of priority as such. The authority of the scientific texts holds good as long as the lovers are not excited to the higher pitch of sexual turgescence. But as soon as the battle of love has once commenced, there is neither any authority of the texts nor any order of priority for the various components. However, he makes an exception saying that the components such as *Alingana, Chumbana, Nakhachchhedya, Dantachchhedya* are indulged in by lovers prior to the union as they tend to heighten the passion; while *Prahanana* and *Sitkrita* are generally indulged in during the actual union.[9]

Several of these *Alingana*s and other components are described in classical Sanskrit literature. Readers who are interested may read with profit the same mentioned above. Now it is possible to identify their representations, in stone, in the temples at Khajuraho, Bhubaneshwar, Konarak and other places. Works such as *The Hindu Temple* and *The Art of India,* both by Stella Kramrisch, *Indian Sculpture in Bronze and Stone, Madanjeet Collection* and *Hindu Mediaeval Sculpture* by Raymond Burnier, will help a lot in understanding the ancient sculptures and their background of the science of erotics as developed in India.

Let us now see how the ancient writers of Kamashastra texts have treated this subject. I have already dealt with detumescence separately and hence it is omitted here.

UPAGUHANA [9A] – THE EMBRACE

According to Vatsyayana, lovers may indulge in the four kinds of *Alingana* - *Sprishtaka, Viddhaka, Udghrishtaka* and *Piditaka* - as they are expressive of mutual love. Another four - *Lataveshtitaka, Vrikshadhirudha, Tilatandula* and *Kshiranira* - are to be indulged in at the time of the union. The first two are to be done when both the partners are standing. The third one is to be done while lying in the bed, the fourth one, while sitting. Both of these (the third and the fourth) are to be done when passion is fully roused. These eight are according to the school of Babhravya.[10]

Vatsyayana mentions that according to Suvarnanabha there are four *Alingana*s in which one particular part touches a similar one of the other person. Thus *Urupaguhana* gives much pleasure as the thighs of the active partner are fleshy. In the second one, *Jaghanopaguhana*, the female being the active partner, it is equally pleasing. In the third one, *Stanalingana*, the male derives much pleasure as he feels as if crushed by the impact of heavy and big breasts. The fourth, *Lalatika*, is equally pleasing as the male is able to see fully and appreciate the beauty of the female form. Some writers consider *Samvahana* (*Angamardana, Tvacha, Mansa, Asthi*) as an *Alingana*, but Vatsyayana does not include it in his list of *Alingana*s.[11] Kokkoka[12] classifies *Alingana* into two parts, *Ajatasmara* and *Jatasmara*. The first class includes four kinds of *Alingana*s for Abhukta and the second one consists of eight ones for Upabhukta. Out of these eight, *Lataveshtitaka* and *Vrikshadhirudha* are practised while standing; the remaining six are done while lying down or sitting. Padmashri[13] gives ten kinds of *Alingana*s without much difference from those given by the previous writers. Jyotirisha[14] gives eight kinds of *Alingana*s without much difference from those given by previous writers. Praudhadevaraya[15] classifies *Alingana*s into twelve kinds, just like Kokkoka., Kalyanamalla[16] gives eight kinds of *Alingana*s without much difference from those given by the previous writers.

Thus we see that the maximum number of *Alingana*s given by Kokkoka and Praudhadevaraya is twelve, but the subject is treated in greater detail by Vatsyayana and fully commented on by Yashodhara in his Jayamangala on Kamasutra.

CHUMBANA[16A] – THE KISS

Vatsyayana gives twenty-six types of *Chumbana*s: three to be indulged in by maidens, five *Sama* and others for *Adharagrahana*, one for the upper lip, one for both the lips, four for the inside of the mouth, three for different Avasthas for arousing greater excitement, two for pleasure (vilasa), two for showing respect (mana), one for showing feeling (bhava) and four more like *Sama* and others.

Vatsyayana clearly warns the man not to indulge in *Chumbana*, *Nakhachchhedya* and *Dantachchhedya* rashly at the time of the first union. He advises the man to indulge in them slowly as the woman is won over gradually by getting more and more excited. He points out the anatomical parts for the purpose of *Chumbana*, such as the forehead, locks of hair, cheeks, eyes, bosom, breasts, lips and the inside of the mouth. He has noted that the people of the Lata province indulge in *Chumbana* of the Urusandhi, Bahumula and Nabhimula also. But these are not in vogue in other provinces.

According to him there are three kinds of *Chumbana*s which, should be indulged in by maidens. These are *Nimitaka*, *Sphuritaka* and *Ghattitaka*. Some writers, according to him, mention four other kinds of *Chumbana*s for adult lovers, such as *Sama*, *Tiryag*, *Udbhranta* and *Avapiditaka*. There is also a subvariety of the *Avapiditaka*. He then enjoins that the female should resort to *Kapatadyuta* which should result in the pleasing *Chumbana-dyuta-Kalaha*. He then warns that this should be done only by those persons who are Chandavega. The *Chumbana* of the upper lip, though mentioned by him, is not generally liked for aesthetic reasons. *Samputaka Chumbana*, with a sound, is then mentioned by him for females and those males who have not grown a moustache. *Jihvayuddha* is then described which results in *Vadana* and *Radana-kalahas*. On other parts there should be *Sama*, *Pidita*, *Anchita* and *Mridu* types of *Chumbana*s.

All these kinds of *Chumbana*s are named differently according to Avastha, such as sleeping, discussing, returning home late and kissing the sleeping female. They are termed *Ragadipana*, *Chalitaka*, *Pratibodhika*, *Chhaya*, *Sankrantaka*, *Chumbana* of the fingers and of hands and feet. The *Abhiyogika* kind consists of two types of *Chumbana*s, *Uru* and *Padangushtha Chumbana*. They are indulged in by the woman while shampooing and when the lover falls asleep. Vatsyayana finally advises the lovers to pay each other in the same coin during *Abhiyoga* and *Samprayoga*, which would then result in increasing mutual pleasure.[17]

As against Vatsyayana and his commentator Yashodhara, Kokkoka[18] lays down that *Nimitaka*, *Sphuritaka* and *Ghattitaka* kinds of *Chumbana*s are to be given to maidens, and not by them to males. Kanchinatha, the commentator, has not fully grasped the meaning of *Jihvayuddha*, as given by Vatsyayana and explained by Yashodhara, and hence he has interpreted Kokkoka's *Jihvarana* differently (VII-6). Further, he has followed another reading, i.e., Abhyarthita in VII-7, and hence he has given a new variety: *Anvartha*, instead of four kinds as clearly stated by Vatsyayana and explained by Yashodhara (Kama Sutra II, 3-25).

Padmashri[19] does not give the list of anatomical parts but he classifies *Chumbana*s into *Sa-Shabda* and *Nih-Shabda*. Tripathi has remarked that Padmashri might have done so on the strength of a Sutra of Vatsyayana (Kama Sutra II, 7-18). In this, Vatsyayana clearly states that the female should return the *Chumbana* in the same way if the male has indulged in it with her, with a sound (*Sasitkritam*). These, *Stanita*, *Kujita*, *Shvasita*, *Sitkara*, *Putkara*, *Hikkrit* and *Dutkrit* are not given as *Chumbana*s by anyone else. However, it should be noted that Yashodhara does explain (Kamasutra, II, 3-32) that in *Samputa Chumbana* some particular sound must necessarily come out. Padmashri then gives seven kinds of *Nih-Shabda Chumbana*s. According to Tripathi, the commentator, these seven *Chumbana*s are to be indulged in by the male. Jayadeva[20] gives us a list of anatomical parts which includes Netra, Kantha Kapola, Hrid, Parshavadvaya, Griva, Nabhi, Mukha, Jangha (Kapola is given once more), Jaghana, Madanalaya and Stanayugma. He also gives *Mukhachumbana* with *Sitkara*.

Jyotirisha[21] in his list adds the nipples and gives six types of *Chumbana* but there is nothing striking in it. Praudhadevaraya[22] gives fourteen kinds of *Chumbana*s. In 3/30, he enumerates *Jihva* and *Yuddha* separately, while in 3/44 he does not distinctly describe *Rasanarana*. His list of anatomical parts is not exhaustive. Kalyanamalla,[23] like

Kokkoka and Jyotirisha, also says that *Chumbana* comes after Parirambha. Unlike Jyotirisha he gives nine kinds of *Chumbana* but like him, he also mentions that the female is in a joyous mood of dancing while indulging in *Samaushtha Chumbana*.

NAKHACHCHHEDYA – NAIL-MARKS

For a better understanding of this and the next component we will have to consider the essential phenomena of courtship in animals. It is well known that love inflicts and even seeks to inflict pain. Similarly love suffers and even seeks to suffer pain. This pain has a powerful stimulating effect and hence the partners in the love-combat willingly submit to temporary unpleasantness which would enable them to enjoy subsequent sexual excitement.

This pain becomes the servant of pleasure by supplying it with force. Everyone must have seen the display of force on the part of the male animal for winning over the female. The horse is found biting the mare before coitus; the male donkey seizes the neck of the female between his teeth; the he-buffalo is found pointing his horns at the she-buffalo; the he-goat is seen standing on his hind legs to pounce upon the she-goat with all his vitality. This is true even of birds. The love-combat of pigeons and sparrows is a common sight. Man, in his love-play, has not failed to imitate mammals and birds and perhaps improved upon the ways and means of the love-combat.

There are innumerable references to love-bites in the literatures of the world. Heine has described the marks of love-bites on the body of Harold whereby he was recognized by Edith. Shakespeare makes Cleopatra refer to amorous pinches. Indian writers have dealt with *Nakhachchhedya* and *Dantachchhedya* in detail. Not only writers on erotics but poets and dramatists of India have described these marks (nail- and teeth-) as adding to the beauty of the female, besides giving her extreme delight even in times of separation.

Kalidasa has described (Kumara, VIII, 18) how Parvati made the painful sensations of Shiva's teeth-bites on her red lips to cease by the cool rays of the crescent on Shiva's head. *Parvatirata* is further described in VIII-83. In IX-29 Kalidasa describes how Parvati experienced *Trapa* and *Romancha* simultaneously when she saw the reflections of the Sambhogachihnas in the mirror given to her by Shiva. Eharavi (Kirata, IX, 49, 59, 62) describes how embraces accompanied by deep nail-scratches, and kisses accompanied by sharp teeth-bites, were liked by ladies. They could see the beautiful reflections of teeth-bites in crystal glasses while drinking intoxicating drinks. Magha (Shishu, VI, 58-59) describes how the ladies experience more painful sensations on the lips due to teeth-bites, when the cold wind blows. Further (X, 86) he has described how marks of teeth-bites on the cheeks of ladies appeared red and beautiful. Kumaradasa (Janakiharana, VIII, 9, 15, 47, 52, 98, 101) describes how Sita's lip quivered at the thought of the love-bite; how she could utter a few indistinct words only; how, while drinking Madhu, the teeth-marks on the lips caused painful but pleasing sensations. Jayadeva (Gitagovinda, II, 6-6, XII, 23-2) describes the fingernail-scratches on the big bosoms of Radha and deep marks of teeth-bites on the lips of Krishna.

Both these marks are considered to be an ornament adding to the beauty of the female, besides being visible and tangible proofs of the deep affection of the lover for the beloved one. They also cause jealousy in the minds of co-wives and envy in the minds of other females for not being fortunate enough to receive such prize love-gifts. They not only give extreme pleasure to the female but also give a sort of warmth (ushma, Mallinatha on Megha, 101) and render all Shitopacharas ineffective. Fingernail-scratches made on the waist of the female give as much beauty to her form as a golden waistband would do. Magha (Shishu, X, 85, 90) thereby tries to convey to us that ornaments are redundant when these marks are made as the latter give enough beauty to the female form.

Now let us see how *Nakhachchhedya* is treated in works on erotics. Vatsyayana[24] says that nail-scratches are to be made after the lovers are sexually excited. The occasions on which they are to be done are:

first meeting, return from a journey, on being appeased after becoming angry and after being satiated by drinking intoxicating drinks. He clearly warns those that are Achandavega, against indulging in this way very often. He gives eight kind of nail-scratches and a list of anatomical parts on which they are to be made. They are the sides, breasts, neck, back, and Jaghana. Yashodhara quotes a verse which includes Katipristha also. This means that in Jaghana the waist is also included.

According to Suvarnanabha, there is no preferential anatomical part fit for nail-scratching as such, when once the battle of love has commenced. According to Vatsyayana, those who are Chandavega should have the nails of the left hand uni-pointed, bi-pointed and even tri-pointed and resembling the parrot's beak. Those that are Mandavega should have their nails very smooth and shaped like the inverted crescent. Vatsyayana has further given eight qualities of good nails and praised those of the people of Gauda province. According to him the nails of the people of Maharashtra are of a medium type and have fine qualities of both the long and the short ones.

The first nail-scratch is *Achchuritaka*, made very lightly with nails of all the fingers, giving out a sound when together and made on the chin, lower lip and breasts. This causes horripilation. When a grown-up female is shampooing or scratching the head, this type of nail-scratch may also be made by her. Or when she is to be teased or frightened, the male may do it. The *Arddhachandraka* nail-scratch should be made on the neck and breasts. Two such scratches facing each other are jointly called *Mandala* and should be made on Nabhi-mula, Kakundara and Vankshana. Each has its own beauty owing to the particular anatomical part.

Vatsyayana has warned that the scratches should not be long. A short one on any of the parts enumerated is termed *Rekha*. A crooked one, rising from the breast, is termed *Vyaghranakha*. Scratches with five nails and converging towards the nipples are called *Mayur-apadaka*. If these are very near each other, they are termed *Shashaplutaka*. *Utpalapatraka* is like the Utpala flower and made on the breasts and the waist. The *Smaraniyaka* scratch is made while separating and done for the sake of remembrance on the thighs and breasts. These scratches may be near each other and about three or four in number. Vatsyayana says that the sizes and shapes of scratches may be many. He enjoins that in case of other females, these scratches should be on parts that remain covered, and should be made for the sake of remembrance only.

Kokkoka[25] gives a list of anatomical parts and says that they should be made by those who are Chandavega. In case of others they should be done at the time of the first union, union after appeasement, after menstruation, after drinking intoxicating drinks, and prior to separation. He also gives six qualities of good nails and describes eight kinds of nail-scratches just like Vatsyayana. But, unlike him, he does not mention *Vyaghranakha* and *Smaraniyaka* and also does not praise *Nakhachchhedya*.

Padmashri[26] does not give the list of anatomical parts, occasions for making them and characteristics of good nails, but mentions eight kinds of scratches, omitting the *Smaraniyaka*. Jyotirisha[27] includes the forehead in the list of anatomical parts, giving eight kinds of scratches. He does not describe the *Vyaghranakha* but gives a new name, *Darduraka*, for *Smaraka*. Like Vatsyayana, he praises nail-scratches, but unlike him he does not give characteristics of good nails and occasions for making them. Praudhadevarayal[28] gives nine kinds of nail-scratches, a list of anatomical parts and describes one more: *Rekha*. Like Kokkoka he refrains from praising the *Nakhachchhedya*. Kalyanamalla[29] gives a list of anatomical parts and occasions for making scratches and characteristics of good nails. He gives eight kinds of nail-scratches, omitting *Vyaghranakha*. Like Kokkoka, he also does not praise them.

DANTACHCHHEDYA – TEETH-MARKS

Vatsyayana[30] mentions that except for the upper lip, the inner side of the mouth and eyes, all the anatomical parts included in the list while dealing with *Chumbana* are fit places for teeth-bites. He gives characteristics of good teeth and also mentions the defects of bad ones. He gives eight kinds of teeth-bites.

The teeth-bite called *Gudhaka* is mildly done with the Rajadanta (front teeth). This when done with force is called *Uchchhunaka*. These two and *Bindu* are done on the lower lip. The second and the fourth – *Pravalamani* – may be done on the cheeks also. Here, Vatsyayana lays down a very fine rule that *Karnapura*, *Chumbana*, *Nakha* and *Danta-kshatas* adorn the left cheek more. The fourth one is made on the left cheek with teeth and lower lip. When more marks are made (with other teeth also) it is termed *Manimala*. When done on the skin of a small portion of the body, with upper and lower teeth, it is *Bindumala*. Both *Manimala* and *Bindumala* should be done on the neck, sides and Vankshana as the skin is 'Shlatha' on these parts. *Bindumala* may also be made on the forehead and thighs. The round marks made by small, medium and big teeth on the breast is termed *Khandabhraka*. Yashodhara adds that it is easy to make on the breasts, and it adds to the charming appearance. The female may do *Kanthopagrahana* and then make such marks on the man's chest. If the lines made by these marks on the breasts are close together, many in number, long and appearing reddish in the middle, that mark is termed *Varahacharvitaka*. This should be made on the breasts only as there is much flesh there. *Khandabhraka* and *Varahacharvitaka* should be done only by persons having Chandavega.

Vatsyayana says that *Nakha* and *Dantachchhedyas*, if made when facial make-up and hairdo (such as Visheshaka, Karnapura, Pushpapida, Tamalapatra), are being done, increase the couple's inclinations for love, leading to further pleasant acts. He further lays down[31] that these should be done according to the general practices in vogue in the particular province and the nature of the female. If the male insists on doing these marks against the female's will, then she should retaliate by doubling those marks on his body. She must retaliate by doing *Mala* in case of *Bindu*, and by doing *Abhrakhandaka* if he has made *Mala*. She should resort to *Kachagraha* of the male and then kiss and bite him on the mouth. With one hand, she, lying on his chest, embraces his neck, and with the other hand, makes *Manimala* and any other desired marks. Unnoticed by others, she should feel amused during the day when the male tries to hide those marks on his body from the public gaze. In fact, she should show him the marks, made by him on her body, by making wry faces, and as if reproving him. Vatsyayana says that lovers living a pleasant life in this way do not find their love abating even after the lapse of a hundred years.

Kokkoka[32] mentions characteristics of good teeth and gives a list of anatomical parts fit for teeth-marks. He also cites eight kinds of teeth-marks like Vatsyayana. Kanchinatha, his commentator, has erred in explaining *Khandabhraka*. The correct technical and appropriate meaning is given by Yashodhara. Padmashri[33] does not give the characteristics and list of anatomical parts fit for teeth-marks but gives eight kinds of teeth-marks, like Vatsyayana. Jyotirisha[34] includes Shalatha in the list of characteristics, but apparently the printed text is incorrect here. He gives a list of anatomical parts fit for teeth-marks and adds that the female should give out *Sitkara*, *Hunkara* and do *Vicheshtita* also. He mentions only three kinds of teeth-marks, and says that *Kolacharva* should be made on certain specific occasions and for the sake of remembrance also.

Praudhadevaraya[35] mentions eight kinds of teeth-marks and a list of anatomical parts fit for the same. The last verse in the printed text (verse 75) should have 'Bahvyah' and the word 'Kroda' is meaningless. It should be 'Kola'. Kalyanamalla,[36] like Jyotirisha, says that sounds like *Sitkara* should be made by the female. He mentions a list of anatomical parts fit for teeth-marks and also gives a list of characteristics of good teeth and defects of bad ones. He gives seven kinds of teeth-marks, omitting *Manimala*. Another fact to be noted is that he specifically lays down that *Kolacharva* teeth-mark is to be done by the male on the body of the female, for the sake of remembrance when going out on a journey.

Nadikshobhana – the Clitoris

It is interesting to find that ancient Indian writers on erotics knew as well as Western writers all about the clitoris, parts in and around the female organ, and erotic stimulation resulting from friction by the male organ or fingers of the hand. These Indian authors found that in the human anterior mode of union, the clitoris generally does not come in close contact with the male organ and consequently it fails to receive powerful stimulation which is its due. Even a modern eminent sexologist like Adler states that this human method of union, even though it had added a new dignity and refinement, a fresh source of enjoyment to the embrace of the sexes, has failed to give unmixed advantage to the woman as she has, in this mode, to contend with an increased difficulty in attaining an adequate amount of pressure on that electric button which normally sets the whole mechanism in operation.[37] These writers, in order to overcome this natural defect, recommend *Nadikshobhana* and *Karikarakrida* which will be presently discussed.

All modern writers on the psychology of sex agree that the clitoris is the key to the genital apparatus in women, from the psychic point of view. To a certain extent it is the anatomical centre in their case. It is the rudimentary analogue of the male organ, but in its function it differs in as much as it only gets erotic stimulation under stress of sexual emotion, and transmits the stimulatory voluptuous sensations imparted to it by friction with the male organ. This was also known to the Arabs. There are definite names for clitoris in Greek and Latin. But in India its importance was long recognised and consequently *Nadikshobhana* formed an important ingredient of *Bahyarata*.

Vatsyayana does not mention *Nadikshobhana* as such, but it is Kokkoka[38] who says that the female organ is of four types. In the centre of the Bhaga there is a Nadika called Madanagamana-dola. If excited by rubbing with Tarjani and Madhyama fingers, profuse mucus comes out. Just above the Madanasadana there is Madana-chhatra full of sexual Madashiras. Inside the Madanasadana, there is a Nadi called Purnachandra. There are several other smaller Nadis also. But this triad is important. The male should cause the excitement thereof to rouse the female to the highest pitch of sexual emotion.

Padmashri[39] says that Madanachhatra is the source of twenty-four Nadikas which carry Mada (Sambhoghechchha). He names and describes six Madanadikas. It is in the centre of the female organ and it has to be excited with fingers and linga, and in that process, Kshobhana Mantra with three letters has to be recited by the male. He gives different ways in the case of Bala and others. The five Nadis – two for the eyes, two for the face, one for the mouth – are to be excited by Mukha. The sixth for the Angushtha is to be excited by the toe. The Mantras given by Padmashri are not given by others in such detail. Besides, he describes the characteristics of Madananadis and progeny resulting from successful excitement of these Nadis. Jyotirisha[40] mentions three Nadis – Samirana, Chandramasi and Gauri. The first is important. The last one, he says, if properly excited, helps a man in getting a son. Praudhadevaraya[41] describes these just like Kokkoka. He does not give anything new. Kalyanamalla[42] describes them but names Madanachhatra and Pumachandra. He describes the Nadi, in 'the centre of the yoni, as resembling Kaman-kusha'. He further states that the Nadi should be excited by the male organ. He does not add the fingers like Padmashri. It should be noted that all the other writers omit the linga and mention the rubbing by fingers only.

KARIKARAKRIDA – USE OF THE FINGERS

There appears to be some distinction between *Nadikshobhana* and *Karikarakrida*. In the first, certain Nadis are to be excited by fingers according to some; by fingers and linga according to one, and by linga only, according to yet another author. In the second, the *Mardana-kshobhana* is to be done in the Smaramandira by hand or fingers. Vatsyayana[43] says that this should be done before *Yantrayoga*.

This is explained by Yashodhara saying that the male should do it before he performs the union. There are two very technical terms used by Vatsyayana: 'Sambadha' and 'Gaja iva.' Yashodhara[44] quotes a verse which describes four kinds of female organs and says that, excepting the first, the remaining three kinds of organs give the female an excessive itching sensation, and that the hand should be rubbed against the same till the female gets orgasm. For the second technical term, Yashodhara quotes a verse which says that the three fingers Anamika, Pradeshini and Jyeshtha should be kept together like the trunk of an elephant. It is then called *Kritrima*.

Kokkoka gives various names for this, such as *Hastakshobhalila*, *Hastashakhavimarda*, *Karashakhayoga* and *Manmathagaramudrabhangakrida*. Jyotirisha and Kalyanamalla call it *Matangalilayita*. All the writers on erotics state that the male indulges in this to increase the sexual excitement of the female. Kokkoka adds that if she is not fully satisfied, then the male should indulge in *Angulirata*. Harihara, in his Smaradipika, states that a male with a delicate and short organ indulges in *Angulirata* and even in the use of artificial male organs. Thus it appears that there is some difference of opinion among these writers in as much as we find mention of various seasons and occasions for this love-play. Tripathi, in his commentary on Nagarasarvasva, adds that a male, in all forms of *Angulipravesha*, may rub the toe against Payu or Madanachhatra according to taste.

Kokkoka[45] has given four kinds of *Karashakhayoga* – *Karikara*, *Phanibhoga*, *Arddhendu* and *Kamankusha* – but he has not described any of them, which is strange. According to Kanchinatha, the commentator of Ratirahasya, *Bahyarata* is of two types – 1) Antar-bahya and 2) Bahir-bahya. The first consists of *Angulirata*, the second includes *Alingana*. The females of the Dravida province get sexually excited by inner and outer *Bahyarata* at the first union and get a profuse flow of mucus. He says that this *Angulirata* should be done before *Yantrayoga*, and expresses an opinion similar to that of Yashodhara for *Karikarakrida*.

Padmashri[46] has described six *Angulipraveshas*. *Karana* is that when

Tarjanika is inserted in the Varanga. *Kanaka* is that when Tarjanika is kept behind Madhyama while inserting. *Vikana* is that when the position of these two fingers is interchanged. *Pataka* is that when both, outstretched, are inserted. *Trishula* is that when these two along with Anamika are together inserted. *Shanibhoga* is that when the three fingers joined together are inserted. The learned editor and the commentator have not got any variant reading for *Shanibhoga*, but looking to the description, it should be Phanibhoga as the three fingers, when joined and bent, look like a serpent-hood. Tripathi in his commentary on this portion of the work of Padmashri quotes another verse defining *Karikarakrida* as joining of Tarjani and Anamika with Madhyama at the back. Jayadeva, the author of Ratimanjari [27], simply recommends *Mardana* of the Bhaga with the hand.

Jyotirisha does not deal with *Karikarakrida* separately, but Praudhadevaraya[47] mentions four varieties of *Karashakhabhirnardana* just like Kokkoka and describes the exciting of the Smaramandira by rubbing Tarjani and Madhyama against the same. Kalyanamalla, like Jyotirisha, does not describe this separately.

PRAHANANA – SADISTIC ACTS

Courtship is like a game and like any other game it is very likely to assume a serious form at one time or another. Cohn has therefore rightly described courting as a 'refined and delicate form of combat'. The female, equally like the male, delights in arousing to the highest degree the desire in him for certain favours and at the same time tries to withhold the same from him. Sanskrit literature abounds in exquisite descriptions of such acts on the part of females. Kalidasa, Bharavi Magha and Shriharsha, to name only a few, have beautifully described such acts in their works. As women are emotionally affected to a great extent by a show of strength and courage, certain components of tumescence in Kamashastra – *Prahanana* and *Sitkara* – have come to occupy an important place therein. Here it is necessary to point out at the outset that Havelock Ellis[48] has definitely misunderstood the terms '*Kila*' and '*Kartari*' through a French translation of Vatsyayana's *Kama Sutra*. These are very technical terms which have been explained in detail by Yashodhara and will be noted here in summary form.

In this connection it is interesting to compare remarks of Ovid (*Ars Amatoria*, lib. i) and those of Lucian (*Dialogues of Courtesans*) with those of Vatsyayana and others. Ovid says that force pleases a woman and that she feels grateful to the ravisher against whom she struggles. According to Lucian, a lover who does not heap blows on his beloved is no lover at all. Vatsyayana says that once the union has started, all thoughts of less or more pain are abandoned. *Prahanana* automatically is resorted to. The parties to the love-combat do not then think whether a particular matter is enjoined by the ancient texts or not. The ever increasing passion is the only important matter at that moment. Lovers then resort to Bhavas and Vibhramas which are undreamt of. Just as a galloping horse overlooks pitfalls in his way, the impassioned lovers indulge in the battle of love without being afraid of the results thereof. Vatsyayana says that a lover well-versed in this science of erotics should consider the 'Vega' and 'Bala' of the female and then indulge in it.[49] Males now definitely know that the manifestations of tears and cries in a female are quite normal ones and inwardly she desires the opposite of what she expresses by tears and cries and her withholding of favours from the male.

Now let us see how these two components of *Bahyarata* are treated in Sanskrit literature. According to Vatsyayana,[50] a pleasant coitus presupposes a combat – a struggle – between the two, the lover and the beloved, which even though apparently painful, is really pleasant in the end. *Prahanana* is thus an essential ingredient of the union. The anatomical parts of the female's body fit for doing it are shoulders, head, the space between the breasts, the back, Jaghana and the sides. It is of four kinds: *Apahastaka, Prahastaka, Mushti* and *Samatalaka. Apahastaka* is given with the palm, keeping the fingers apart, on the space between the breasts, when the female is lying on her back during the union. The force of *Apahastaka*, according to Vatsyayana, should gradually increase till she is sexually satisfied. *Prahastaka* is given on the head of the female, unsatisfied by the previous one, with fingers slightly bent like a hood and with a sound – Phutkara. This, like its predecessor, should also be given with force, gradually. *Mushti* is given while she is sitting on his lap. *Samatalaka*, the last one, is given with the palm, quite steadily. It is also given at the time of Ragavasana till the last moment as Priti resides in the region round about Linga and Jaghana

Besides these four kinds, Vatsyayana gives four others indulged in by males of the Southern province. These are explained in detail by Yashodhara[51] in his commentary. They are *Kila, Kartari, Vaddha* and *Sandamshika*. *Kila* is made by holding the palm in the form of a fist but keeping out the index and middle fingers. It is to be given on the bosom when the female has her head bent down. *Kartari* is of two types. When the fingers of one hand are straight and spread out, it is *Bhadrakartari*. When two hands are joined it is *Yamalakartari*. When the fingers are bent and the index finger is kept on the thumb, it is *Shabdakartari*, otherwise known as *Utpalapatrika*. *Kartari* is perhaps given on the head also. *Viddha* is made when fingers are bent so as to form a fist by keeping the thumb protruding from between the index and the middle fingers or from between middle and Anamika fingers. It is to be given on the cheeks. *Sandamshika* is made by pinching with the index finger and the thumb or the middle finger and thumb. It is done on the breast and the sides by pulling the fleshy part during the pinching. Vatsyayana, Kokkoka and even Yashodhara do not favour these four kinds of *Prahanana* in vogue in the South as harmful after-effects and even fatal injuries have happened in the past in certain well-known cases, by excessive indulgence in them.

Kokkoka[52] calls it *Tadana* and gives four types like Vatsyayana. According to him, they are to be given on the back, the sides, Jaghana, space between the breasts, and the head, as these are the Madanabhumis or erogenous zones. Padmashri[53] gives three kinds of *Prahanana* which he calls *Tadana*. *Shabdakartana* is done when all the fingers are bent and it is given on the head with a sound. *Mushti* is done when fingers are bent in the form of a fist and given on the buttocks and the back. *Viddhaka* is done when it is given on the neck with the thumb. Tripathi has explained that the first variety given by Padmashri is *Pataka*, given by Vatsyayana, but *Viddhaka* is quite new. I disagree with the last part of his remark and state that it is *Viddha* on the cheeks as mentioned by Vatsyayana. Jyotitisha does not mention it at all but on the contrary he describes *Santadita* which will be discussed later in its proper place.

Praudhadevaraya[54] describes the four *Prahananas* (*Apahasta*, etc.) and six others of the South, as given by Vatsyayana, omitting *Kila*. He mentions the anatomical parts fit for giving the same, but unlike Vatsyayana, Kokkoka and Yashodhara, he withholds any comment on their propriety. Kalyanamalla[55] calls it *Karatadana* and gives only the first four varieties (*Apahasta*, etc.) and also the list of anatomical parts for giving the same.

SITKRITA – SOUNDS OF JOY

This is a natural result of *Prahanana* which involves sound thrashing, thumping, fisting and even punching. According to Vatsyayana[56] it is of several kinds. He includes *Viruta* also in this class. Yashodhara explains that all *Virutas* are a form of sound and are a result of love. They are made by the female when undergoing *Prahanana* and they are pleasing to the ear. Vatsyayana says that the female should give out *Viruta* (accompanied by *Sitkrita*) resembling that of pigeon, cuckoo, parrot, bee or swan. The seven other sounds are *Hankara*, *Kujita*, etc. These may be made when *Apahasta Prahanana* is being given. There may not be any order. *Kujita* and *Phutkrita* are sounds made in the mouth of the female while she is being given *Prasrita Prahanana*. *Shavasita* and *Rudita* come out at the end of the union. *Dutkrita* resembles splitting up of a bamboo while *Phutkrita* resembles that made by a berry falling into water. *Stanita*, *Kujita* and *Rudita* are made by the female while being fisted by the male. Sounds like those of *Lavaka* and *Hansa*, are made by the female while *Samatalaka Prahanana* is being given. He further says that the female should cry out requesting him to desist if the male insists on indulging in *Prahanana*.[56a]

Kokkoka[57] also mentions *Sitkrita* and describes *Hinkrita*, and expressions or words with the Kantha and Nasika, requesting the male to stop the onslaught on her. He describes *Hinkrita* and *Stanita* which is not done by Vatsyayana. He also states when all these sounds are to be made. Padmashris[58] also mentions seven *Sashabda Chumbanas* perhaps because of a Sutra of Vatsyayana (II, 7-18) wherein he says that the female should retaliate by *Sitkrita* during *Chumbana*, etc. Padmashri's descriptions are also slightly different. In XVI, 12/13, he states that *Sitkara*, *Hakara* and *Shavasita*, made by a female, show her desire for the union. Jyotirisha[59] says that *Sitkrita* occurs when a male, finding the female not properly satisfied by a light-hearted union, bites her lip again and again and the female shrieks in pain. A female sexually excited during *Chitrasambhoga* makes sounds resembling those of a cuckoo with her mouth and teeth. This is called *Stanita*.

Praudhadevaraya[60] gives all the sounds like Vatsyayana and also the time when they should be made. He mentions four new ones – those for showing pain, helplessness, fondness and harshness. Besides these, he gives a sound quite new: *Kakaruta*. Kalyanamalla[61] gives five varieties. He describes *Sitkrita* as being like the hissing of a serpent, and *Phutkrita* as the sound very like the one produced by a drop of rain falling in water. He also says, like Jyotirisha, that during *Chitrarata*, the female gives out sounds like those of birds like *Lavaka*. He also states that *Sitkrita* is that sound made by a female when a male bites her lip again and again. These sounds are beautifully described by Kalidasa, Bharavi, Magha, Shriharsha and many others in their works while describing the love-play of important characters.

GRAHANA – HOLDING FAST

Now we come to those components of *Bahyarata* by which less pain is inflicted on the female. Padmashri[62] is the only author who describes *Grahana* of four kinds: *Baddhamushti*, etc. In *Baddhamushti* the various limbs are firmly and tightly grasped. *Veshtitalca* is when locks of hair are caught hold of by twisting hair round a finger. *Kritagranthika* is when fingers of the female are entwined. *Samakrishti* is when the thumb and index finger are joined so as to give a pinch on the neck and the breasts. This last one appears to be similar to Vatsyayana's *Sandamshika* as explained by Yashodhara. It is the same as modern *Chimta* or *Chunti*.

KACHAGRAHA-KESHAKARSHANA – LOVE-PLAY (HAIR)

Only two writers have described this love-play. Kokkoka[63] simply says that some persons pull the hair and kiss the eyes and the face. Padmashri[64] says that females of the Sindhu province are won over by the pulling of hair. Praudhadevaraya[65] says that some males pull the hair of the female for Ratipradipana on the Purnima.

According to Jyotirisha[66] it is of four kinds. He gives some characteristics of good hair – close and profuse, smooth, dark and long. He says that it is to be pulled when kissing in order to increase the female's sexual excitement. *Samahasta* is when the male pulls the hair with both hands and then kisses. In *Trangaranga* it is done with one hand. In *Kamavatansa* he pulls the hair near the ear and then kisses. In *Bhujangavalli* his fingers are entwined in the locks of hair. This last one is similar to *Veshtitaka Grahana* of Padmashri.

Kalyanamalla[67] adds that curly hair is also good. It should be pulled slowly while kissing. He also gives, like Jyotirisha, four kinds of *Keshagrahana*.[68] This appears to have been a very popular love-play in India in ancient times. Kalidasa refers to *Kachagraha* while mentioning the rape of Rambha by Ravana. According to Damodara[69] females consider themselves grateful if the male condescends to pull the hair while indulging in amorous dalliance. The author of Aryasapatashati[70] gives it the first place in love-play. Bana[71] refers to *Keshagraha* during the Rata and Magha[72] mentions *Kachagraha* of females for sexually exciting them. Amaruka has one fine verse wherein this is also mentioned.[72a] Instances can be multiplied but these are sufficient for our purpose.

MARDANA – LOVE-PLAY (HANDS)

We now come to another love-play in which the hand is used very prominently. There is a couplet in Sanskrit which says that if curds, betel leaf, breasts, cotton or sugar undergo *Mardana*, the result is that 'Guna' increases in each case. Here the root Mrid means a different thing in each case. If curds are *churned* again and again, we get tasty butter containing ghee. If betel leaf is *chewed* again and again it gives sweet taste. If cotton is *spun* again and again very thin thread can be had from it. The idea underlying it is that in this love-play both parties get pleasure.

Harihara in his Smaradipika gives a list of six anatomical parts that should undergo *Mardana*. They are the arms, the breasts, the female organ and the navel. Padmashri[73] is the only writer who decribes *Mardana* of four types. *Adipita* is done by fists. *Sprishtaka* is done by the palm touching all over. *Kampitaka* is done with a quivering hand. *Samakrama* is done, here and there, with pressure.

Even though Kokkoka and others do not describe *Mardana* separately they do refer to it, here and there, in their works. They particularly refer to *Kuchamardana*. All the poets of ancient India mentioned above refer also to *Kuchamardana*. Here it is necessary to refer to *Samvahana*, described by several poets. Kalidasa mentions the left thigh deserving shampooing (Meghaduta 101). Vatsyayana refers to *Urumula Samvahana* (Kamasutra, III, 2-33 to 35). He has also noted that some writers consider *Samvahana* as an *Alingana*, but says that it cannot be so, as Kalabheda, Phalabheda and Asadharanatva come in (Kamasutra, II, 28 to 29). Bharavi refers to *Samvahana* after the union, to relieve the female of the pain from love-play, and the union (Kiratarjuniya XI, 6). Several other poets have referred to *Samvahana* in the same way. No writer on erotics has treated it separately, but Kokkoka (XI, 17) and others make only a passing reference to it.

JIHVAPRAVESHA – LOVE-PLAY (TONGUE)

We now come to another love-play which is described in detail by Padmashri.[74] He states that this is of three kinds. *Suchi* is when the tongue is contracted and made pointed and then inserted into the mouth of the female. *Pratata* is when it is broadened while stretching inside the mouth. *Kari* is when it quivers inside the mouth of the female.

Vatsyayana, Kokkoka and Praudhadevaraya have not described *Jihvapravesha* separately, but in the *Chumbana* class Vatsyayana has one – *Jihvayuddha* – in which, according to Yashodhara, four *Chumbana*s with the *Jihva* (Antarmukha, Dashana, Jihva and Talu) are included. What Padmashri has described is slightly different from *Jihvayuddha* of Vatsyayana and others. It is simply a play of the tongue. The idea of *Yuddha* or *Rana* is absent here.

CHUSHANA – LOVE-PLAY (LIPS)

Padmashri[75] has treated *Chushana* separately, but in fact the varieties are included in the *Chumbana* class, as the lips have an important part to perform in this love-play. But as he has minutely described varieties of *Chushana* it deserves at least some notice. It is of four kinds. The *Oshtha-vimrishtha* kind is that when the tip of the tongue is sucked. *Chumbitaka* is that when the above one is done hurriedly. *Arddhachumbita* is that when the lip is bitten and then sucked. This is perhaps like *Avapidita Chumbana* mentioned by Vatsyayana. *Samputaka* is when both the partners suck the lips of each other. A look at the descriptions of *Chumbana*s, given by Vatsyayana, will convince us that some of the varieties of *Chumbana* of Padmashri are similar to certain *Chumbana*s as given by him. But as his descriptions differ in some details, his classification as a distinct love-play is accepted here.

RASAPANA – SUCKING

Harihara[76] is the only author who describes *Rasapana* in his *Smaradipika*. As a component of *Bahyarata*, it means that certain anatomical parts of the female are to be sucked by the male. There are five anatomical parts, such as breasts, lips,[76a] mouth, tongue and nipples. The *Rasapana* in the case of lips, mouth and tongue, is indirectly covered by some of the varieties of *Chumbana* given by Vatsyayana and others, but those of the breasts and nipples are quite new, not being mentioned by other writers on erotics or poets.

SANTADITA (STRIKARTRIKA)

We now have to deal with two other love-plays which form a class by themselves in as much as they are dealt by females only. According to Jyotirisha[77] this is done only by females, when they are in the reverse position, with the male on the ground lying on his back. *Santadita* is that when the female above gives blows with her fists on the male's chest. *Pataka* is that when the blows are given with the palm quite open. *Kundala* is that when it is given by her with the thumb and the middle finger. *Bindumala* is that when it is given by her with the thumb only.

Kalyanamalla[78] calls it *Tadana* and clearly says that the female inflicts these blows on the male when she is above him. There is one difference in the names of the first and third varieties of Jyotirisha. They are, according to him, called *Santanika* and *Kuntala* respectively. No other writer has dealt with this *Rata* by the female, as a separate and distinct one. Amaruka has a verse of Padatadana and says that the male who receives kicks from the red and delicate soles of a damsel is really favoured by the god of love.[78a]

KACHAGRAHA (STRIKARTRIKA)

Vatsyayana[79] says that the female should catch hold of the locks of hair on the male's head, raise his face and then impress a kiss and make teeth-marks. Yashodhara explains that this kiss is called *Adharapana*. The female holds the locks of hair by one hand, lifts up the chin by another, and kisses and embraces him lightly, simultaneously making teeth-marks on being fully sexually excited.

This *Kachagraha* is beautifully described by Kalidasa[80] who says that the pulls given by Parvati to the locks of hair on Siva's head were so hard that the moon suffered some pain. Again, he describes[81] how the queens caught hold of locks of hair on the head of the king and detained him to continue the love-play. He has also referred to Ganga[82] as catching the locks of hair on Siva's head and touching the moon thereon with her hands, in the form of surging waves, and laughing as it were with the foam at the frowns on the face of Parvati, her co-wife. Mallinatha, in his commentary, says that pulling of hair is done out of jealousy by co-wives, on the head of the husband.

NOTES

1   Ellis, H., *Studies in the Psychology of Sex,* I, pt. ii, p. 21 ff.

2   Kamasutra, II, 1-1.

3   Kamasutra, II, 2-1 to 5.

4   Kamasutra, II, 2-6.

5   Gitagovinda, II, 6-6, Rasamanjari of Shankara Mishra.

6   Kamasutra, II, 2-4, Jayamangala of Yashodhara, II, 8-30 to 35.

7   Kutanimata, 377-378.

8   Kamasutra, II, 2-31, 32; II, 3-13. Classical Sanskrit literature abounds
    in descriptions of such modifications, particularly: 1) Kalidasa,
    Kumarasambhava, VIII, IX, X; 2) Bharavi, Kiratarjuniya, IX; 3)
    Magha, Shishupalavadha, X; 4) Kumaradasa, Janakiharana, VIII; 5)
    Shriharsha, Naishadhacharita, XVIII, XX, etc.

9   Kamasutra, II, 3-2.

9a Amarushataka, 40.

10 Kamasutra, II, 2-7 to 23.

11 Kamasutra, II, 2-23 to 29. It is interesting to note that ancient writers
    have also noted sevenfold *Alingana* (Amoda, Mudita, Prema, Ananda,
    Ruchi, Madana and Vinoda) as quoted by Shabda Kalpadruma, from
    Kamashastra of Gaunisuta. Also *Alingana*s named after those
    practised by some birds and animals are known (Chakrahva, Hansa,
    Nakula, Paravata, etc.), see Kuttanimata, 581. For Nakula type, see
    Yogavasishta 6-109-13 and 14. The proper time for indulging in
    *Alingana*s is, 1) while appeasing, 2) when one is frightened, 3) when
    one is going out on a journey and therefore separating, 4) when
    returning from a journey and 5) at the time of coitus.

12 Ratirahsya, VI, 1-12.

13 Nagarasarvasva, XXIV, 1 to 9.

14 Panchasayaka, IV, 31 to 40.

15 Ratiratnapradipika, III, 4 to 27.

16 Anangaranga, IX, 1 to 10.

16a Amarushataka, 36.

17 Kamasutra, II, 3-4 to 34. Tripathi, commentary on Nagarasarvasva,
    XXV, 5, p. 82.

18 Ratirahasya, VII, 1 to 9.

19 Nagarasarvasva, XXI, 1 to 4. XXV, 1 to 5.

20 Ratimanjari, 19 to 22. 21

21 Panchasayaka, IV, 41 to 48.

22 Ratiratnapradipika, III, 28 to 48.

23 Anangaranga, IX, 11 to 21.

24 Kamasutra, II, 4-1 to 31.

25   Ratirahasya, VIII, 1 to 6.

26   Nagarasarvasva, XXII, 1 to 5.

27   Panchasayaka, IV, 49 to 58.

28   Ratiratnapradipika, III, 49 to 52.

29   Anangaranga, IX, 22 to 29.

30   Kamasutra, II, 5-1 to 18 and commentary.

31   Kamasutra, II, 5-34 to 43 and commentary.

32   Ratirahasya, IX, 1 to 4.

33   Nagarasarvasva, XXIII, 1 to 4.

34   Panchasayaka, IV, 59 to 63.

35   Ratiratnapradipika, III, 63 to 75,

36   Anangaranga, IX, 30 to 36.

37   Ellis, H., *Studies in the Psychology of Sex,* II, pt. 1, p. 132.

38   Ratirahasya, X, 5 to 9.

39   Nagarasarvasva, XVIII-XIX.

40   Panchasayaka, V, 1 to 4.

41   Ratiratnapradipika, IV, 35 to 39.

42   Anangaranga, IV, 32 to 35.

43   Kamasutra. II 7-10.

44   Kamasutra, II, 7-10, commentary. For other descriptions of female organs *see* Ratirahasya IV, Panchasayaka II; Ratiratnapradipika IV; Anangaranga IV; Ratimanjari 32–33, Naishadha, VII-90; XVI-96, XX-95 and Jivatu of Mallinasha.

45   Ratirahasya, X, 8.

46   Nagarasarvasva, XXXVI, 1 to 2 and Tripathi's commentary.

47   Ratiratnapradipika, IV, 39 to 40.

48   Ellis, *Studies in the Psychology of Sex,* I, pt. II, pp. 67-78.

49   Kamasutra, II, 7-30 to 35.

50   Kamasutra, II, 7-1 to 3, 9, 11-12, 14, 23 to 35.

51   Kamasutra, II, 7-23. commentary.

52   Ratiraliasya, X, 51 to 62.

53   Nagarasarvasva, XXXIII, 1 to 2 and commentary of Tripathi.

54   Ratiratnapradipika, VI, 55 to 58; VII, 1 to 18.

55   Anangaranga, X, 39 to 41.

56   Kamasutra, II, 7-4 to 20

56a   Amarushataka, 36, 40.

57   Ratirahasya, X, 54 to 63.

58   Nagarasarvasva, XX, 1 to 4.

59   Panchasayaka, V, 29 to 30.

60   Ratiratnapradipika, VII, 2 to 36.

61   Anangaranga X, 45 to 50.

62   Nagarasarvasva, XXXV, 1 to 2.

[63] Ratirahasya, II, 2.

[64] Nagarasarvasva, XX, 3.

[65] Ratiratnapradipika, I, 35.

[66] Panchasayaka, IV, 64 to 68.

[67] Anangaranga, IX, 37 to 41.

[68] Raghuvansha, X, 47. Kumarasambhava, VIII, 63, 83.

[69] Kuttanimata, 377.

[70] Aryasapatashati, 326.

[71] Kadanibari, Purvabhaga, para 2. Kane's edition.

[72] Shishupalavadha, X, 72.

[72a] Amarushataka, 98.

[73] Nagarasarvasva, XXXIV, 1 to 2.

[74] Nagarasarvasva, XX VI, I.

[75] Nagarasarvasva, XXVII, 1 to 2.

[76] Smaradipika quoted by Tripathi in his commentary on Nagarasarvasva, XXXVI, 2, p.105.

[76a] Amarushataka, 74.

[77] Panchasayaka, V, 26 to 28.

[78] Anangaranga, X, 42 to 44.

[78a] Amarushataka, 116, 128, 2.

[79] Kamasutra, II, 5-39. Sculptures beautifully portraying this love sport are at Khajuraho. This happens also when she is angry and while retorting, lifts up his chin a little and kicks him many times on the arms, head, chest or back. Kamasutra, II, 10-43.

[80] Kumarasambhava, VIII, 83.

[81] Raguvansha, XIX, 31.

[82] Meghaduta, 52 and commentary of Mallinatha.

CHAPTER III

DETUMESCENCE IN SANSKRIT LITERATURE

Rati or Kama or Shringara is the general denomination given to love and love-play and its culmination in Sanskrit literature. Rati is an emotional attitude of mind when one is attracted towards another person. This attraction may be towards a deity, king, teacher, parents, children, wife/husband or friend.[1] When one feels attraction towards a person of the opposite sex it is termed Shringara or Kama. Several writers on poetics and dramatics have minutely dealt with this subject, giving the various Bhavas, Anubhavas, Smaradashas and Sambhogavasthas.[2] Detumescence or *Surata* (Abhyantara Rata) is the climax of tumescence or Bahya Rata. It is an anatomico-physiological process intimately connected with the mind and yet quite independent of it.

According to Padmashri,[3] recitation of certain mantras excite the twenty-four Nadis, finally culminating in the sexual urge. Other writers mention only three Nadis and say that the origin of these Nadis is in the Madanatapatra or Chhatra. Kokkoka mentions besides this Chhatra, the Madanadola and Purnachandra Nadis. Jyotirisha mentions Samirana, Chandramasi and Gauri. Kalyanamalla mentions only Purnachandra. Both Kokkoka and Praudhadevaraya mention *Karikarakrida*, i.e. movements of fingers which result in exciting the woman.

Before we proceed further it will be interesting to know that Kokkoka and others who have followed him mention four types of female organs.[4] Jayadeva and Jyotirisha give additional descriptions thereof. Praudhadevaraya follows Kokkoka, but Kalyanamalla follows Jyotirisha. Maheshvara quoted by Padmashri favours only one type. Medical treatises like Nighantu Ratnakara and others have also classified them into different types. Jayadeva is the only writer who mentions two types of male organs. There are various names in Sanskrit works on erotics for the male and female organs and the clitoris.

It is said by some of these writers[5] that only particular females, avoiding relatives, those of low caste and others of higher social order, should be chosen for the sexual act. Even if we look into older works such as Smritis[6] we find that they also forbid sexual intercourse with near relatives and others of a higher social order. Certain purificatory ceremonies and observing of vows have been laid down without which the person committing the act cannot absolve himself of that sin.

These ancient writers[7] even say that certain places are to be avoided for intercourse. They give even the time when it should not be indulged in. It should be noted here that there is perhaps some difference of opinion among these writers and that these texts on erotics have certain corruptions in themselves.[8] This is evidently clear from the fact that these texts also give details of the waxing and waning of Chandrakala or Kamakala in women, in a month. Even the ways and means of stimulating this, for each type of women, are not altogether similar. In the Mahabharata we find accounts which do not follow standards laid down in these works.

Now if we turn to the positive side of this subject we find that these writers also give details of the place[9] where it should be performed. Vatsyayana and all others say that it should be large, lighted, white-washed, decorated with murals, fragrant with incense and resounding with music. Besides this neatness and cleanliness of the place, they insist on the woman being properly dressed, wearing ornaments, and the man similarly wearing garlands, fine garments, ornaments, and chewing betel leaf. They also say that he should anoint himself with fragrant oil.

Here it will be interesting to know how the ancient writers[10] have discussed the purpose and necessity of congress. In the Rig Veda we read about Lopamudra complaining to Agastya about the onslaught of old age. In the Mahabharata there is a dialogue between an old woman and Ashtavakra. The words of Vidura in this case are well known. The dialogue between Bhangasvan (in the form of a woman) and Shakra (in the form of a Brahmana), in the same epic, gives us an idea of the aim of the sexual union.

Now this leads us to the discussion about nature and quality of the partners. In Kuttanimata[11] we read details about an ideal lover as discussed by one person with another. He should be sweet in speech, amusing by his tales and anecdotes, endowed with sufficient means, and have a beautiful complexion. Further in the same text an elaborate list of physical characteristics and psychological traits of an ideal lover is given. This is corroborated and supplemented by the list in Bhava-prakasha where these and other qualities are mentioned. Just as we find mentioned the qualities of the male partner, there are in numerable instances in the Epics, Puranas and classical literature, where the qualities and characteristics of the female partners are given.

Now we may look at the way in which the ancient writers have treated this subject.[12] One poet has compared the act to a sacrifice.[12a] It is generally termed 'Battle of Love' or Ratisangara.[12b] Ancient writers have vividly described satisfactory sexual intercourse under ideal conditions.[12c] Damodara in particular has very beautifully described one such sexual act.[12d] Writers like Bharata, Amaruka, Rudrata, Damodara and several others have described the physical union, pointing out the perfect one under ideal conditions.[12e] Now we come to the act proper and find that Yashodhara[13] has fully explained what Vatsyayana has classified as Samanya and Vishesha Kama as follows:

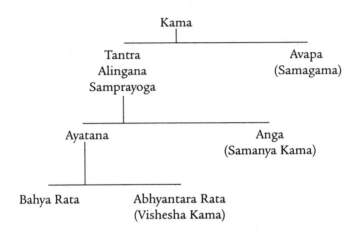

Vaysyayana[14] and others have classified the males and females according to the Ayama of the male organ and Parinaha of the female organ as follows:

Shasha	Harini
Vrisha	Vadava
Ashva	Hastini

They have then classified the union[15] (according to Pramana) into nine varieties of Sama, Uchcha, Nicha, Atyuchcha and Atinicha, as follows:

Shasha M	Harini F	
Vrisha M	Vadava F	These are Sama.
Ashva M	Hastini F	
Vrisha M	Mrigi F	These are Uchcha.
Ashva M	Vadava F	

Shasha M	Vadava F	
Vrisha M	Hastini F	These are Nicha.
Ashva M	Mrigi F	This is Atyuchcha.
Shasha M	Hastini F	This is Atinich.

It is accepted by all the writers on erotics that Sama types of Rata are the best.

Similarly there are nine more such Ratas[16] according to Kala. This Kala is Laghu or Shighra, Madhya and Chira. The classification then is as follows:

Laghu M	Laghu F	
Madhya M	Madhya F	These are Sama.
Chira M	Chira F	
Madhya M	Laghu F	
Chira M	Madhya F	These are Uchcha.
Laghu M	Madhya F	
Madhya M	Chira F	These are Nicha.
Chira M	Laghu F	This is Atyuchcha.
Laghu M	Chira F	This is Atinicha.

As regards duration,[17a] Indian writers have pointed out one 'yama' as the required time for the act. This is the reason why Kokkoka, Jyotirisha[17b] and others have assigned a particular 'yama' to Padmini, etc. Kalidasa in his Meghaduta mentions 'yama' which Mallinatha explains in his commentary.[17c] Shiva and Parvati and Devahuti and Kardama are described[17d] as immeasurably lengthening the duration of the sexual union. The epics and the Puranas and also in later literature, Kalidasa and others have beautifully described this.

Then there are nine such additional Ratas,[18] according to Vega or Bhava, which is Manda, Madhya and Chanda. The classification then is as follows:

Manda M	Manda F	
Madhya M	Madhya F	These are Sama.
Chanda M	Chanda F	
Madhya M	Manda F	
Chanda M	Madhya F	These are Uchcha.
Manda M	Madhya F	
Madhya M	Chanda F	These are Nicha.
Chanda F	Manda F	This is Atyuchcha.
Manda M	Chanda F	This is Atinicha.

Vatsyayana says that the total number of unions made by the various combinations is extremely large.[19] It is Yashodhara who gives in his commentary further classification of Surata into Shuddha and Samkirna. The latter is further subdivided into Sama and Vishama. With equal characteristics there are nine Sama Samkirna Ratas. With unequal partners there will be 72 Vishama Samkirna Ratas. So also in the case of Vadava, and the same is true in the case of Hastini. The total number of Ratas will thus be 243 x 3 =729.

Notes

1   Nagarasarvasva, Preface, ed. Tripathi.

2   Kamasutra, 5-1, Ratirahasya, 13-2 and 3, Panchasayaka, 6-19. Also commentaries of Mallinatha on Meghaduta 9, Raghuvasha 6-12, Kumarasambhava 4-17, and Kiratarjuniya.

3   Nagarasarvasva, XVIII, Ratirahasya, 10-6 to 9, Panchasayaka, 5-1 to 4, Ratiratnapradipika, 4-35 to 40, Anangaranga, 4-32 to 35. It must be noted that this is conspicuous by its absence in Kamasutra.

4   Ratirahasya, 10-5. Ratimanjari, 32-34. Panchasayaka, 2-33, 34. Ratiratnapradipika, 4-33, 34. Anangaranga, 4-30, 31. It must be noted that we do not find this discussion in Kamasutra. In the Mahabharata (4-14) Kichaka describes the Jaghana of Draupadi. In the same epic (3-46) private parts of Urvashi are described. In the Ramayana (7-26) Ravana describes such physical charms of Sita. Vishnudharmottara Purana (II, 8 & 9) also gives some hints about this matter. Bharata in his Natyashastra (XVI) gives a verse regarding physical beauty, Verses 77, 93, etc.

5   Panchasayaka, 4-25. Anangaranga, 8-15. Contrary statements in some respects are found in Ratirahasya, 4-28.

6   Amgira Smriti, 1. Yama, 26. Brihadyama, 2, 3, 4. Apastamba, 9, 10. Vasishtha, 21. Arti, 4, 7, 8. Manu, 4, 8, 11. Yagnavalkya, 24. Atri Samhita, 198-200.

7   Panchasayaka, 4-26, 27. Anangaranga, 8-25.

8   Ratirahasya, 2-4 to 28, 5-3. Panchasayaka, 1. Anangaranga, 2. Ratiratnapradipika, 26 to 68. Mahabharata, 1-121, 13-22, 13-93, 7-73. Baudhayana, 1-11. Manu, 3, 4. Vasishtha, 12. Yagnavalkya, 1. Vishnu, 69. These Smritikaras forbid intercourse on certain days of a month.

9   Kamasutra, 1-14. Ratirahasya, 10-1. Nagarasarvasva, 2-4 to 6. Panchasayaka, 5-3 1. Ratiratnapradipika, 4-26. Anangaranga, 8-26. Only one example from classical literature will be sufficient: Raghuvansha, 19-9.

10   Rigveda, 1-23-179. Mahabharata, 13-19, 5-39-79, 13-13-52.

11   Kuttanimata, 396, 1016, 966, 974. Bhavprakasha, 5. Skanda Purana, Kashikhanda. Bhavishya Purana. Varahamihira (Brihat Samhita, 7-7-13) says that women devoid of qualities are a source of anxiety, and trouble to males. Tripathi in his commentary on these verses in Kuttanimata has quoted from all these works.

12   (a) Nagarasarvasva, Tippani, p. 117.

     (b) Kuttanimata, 1051 and commentary.

     (c) Kuttanimata, 1053 and commentary.

     (d) Kuttanimata, 373 and commentary; Kira tarjuniya, 9-49 and commentary.

[e] Rasikapriya of King Kumbha on Gitagovinda, 2-3-6 and Kuttanimata, 387 and commentary; Amarushataka, 142.

13   Kamasutra, 1-1-86, 87 and commentary. Also 1-2-12 and commentary. Vatsyayana and others have classified males and females according to the Aya of the male organ and Parinaha of the female organ as follows:

14   Kamasutra, 2-1-1, 2. Ratirahasya, 3-1. Nagarasarvasva, 14-1. Panchasayaka, 2-1. Ratiratnapradipika 2-7 to 18, 23, 50. Anangaranga, 3-1.

15   All the above, chs 2, 3, 14, 2, 4, 3, respectively.

16   Kamasutra, 2-1-17. Ratirahasya, 3-11. Jyotirisha does not mention this category. Ratiratnapradipika, 4-7 to 11. Anangaranga, 3-12. Nagarasarvasva does not mention this category.

17   [a] Meghaduta, 102. Commentary of Mallinatha;
      [b] Ratirahasya, 1-22; Panchasayaka, 1-28, 29; Ratiratnapradipika, 1-10, 15, 19, 23; Anangaranga, 1-16, 17;
      [c] Meghaduta, 102;
      [d] Ramayana, 1-36; Mahabharata, 13-14; Vishnudharmottara. Purana, 1-228; Kumarasambhava, VIII and IX; Bhagvata, 3-23-46.

18   Kamasutra, 2-1-13 to 16. Ratirahasya 3-12. There is a mistake in the commentary of Kanchinatha, p.25. Panchasayaka, 2-7. Ratiratnapradipika, 4-11 to 15. Anangaranga, 3-13. Kamasutra, 2-1-66 and commentary of Yashodhara thereon. No other author or commentator gives this large number, viz., 243 x 3 = 729. Ratirahasya and other works give 9 + 9 + 9 = 27 only. They do not give further combinations as done by Yashodhara, shown above.

CHAPTER IV

POSTURES FOR CONGRESS

Most of the postures for congress described in the texts on erotics are found adopted by various peoples. They offer a vast range of variation. They are natural and not in the least vicious perversions.[1] Whatever may be the opinion of the ancient theologians and others, it is well recognised by modern physicians that variations from the ordinary method of congress are desirable in special cases. Kisch and Adler in their independent works recommend several variations of the position of congress and the advantages accruing from these positions and remark that such variations often call out the latent sexual feelings as by a charm.[2]

Readers are advised to refer to the excellent work[3] of Van de Velde, wherein he has given the scientific advantages of Normal, Extended, Flexed, Astride, Sedentary and Lateral attitudes in the case of Converse-Face to Face attitudes and those of Ventral, Posterior-Lateral, Flexed and Sedentary attitudes in the case of Averse-Front to Back attitudes. It is equally interesting to compare the reasons for certain variations in case of certain types of women given by Vatsyayana, Kokkoka and Padmashri, and minutely explained by their commentators, Yashodhara and Kanchinatha and Tripathi[4] respectively, with those given by Kisch, Adler, Havelock Ellis, and Van de Velde. This shows us the extent of the knowledge of the writers in India on erotics in the past. There is striking corroboration of their remarks with the scientific observations of eminent writers of the present day, mentioned above.

The main object[5] of the various postures for congress is to derive the maximum amount of pleasure from it even in cases of incompatibility due to differences in size/depth, protuberant belly, fleshy thighs or even inequality in stature[6] of the two parties. It will be observed that a slight change in any one position is termed a different posture, e.g., *Jrimbhitaka* and *Piditaka*. These different postures are made by mere change in the position of the legs.[7]

It is generally believed that there are 84 postures for congress.[8] But to our surprise we find that no printed text gives the complete list. Perhaps these extant printed texts are incomplete and corrupt at various places. Some of the cheaply printed books, which are not scientifically written, do give 84 names, but most of them are repetitions. The postures are generally termed A*sana Karana, Bandha, Laya, Samveshana, Samprayukta Vidhi*, etc. Now we find that Abhyantara Rata is classified as follows:

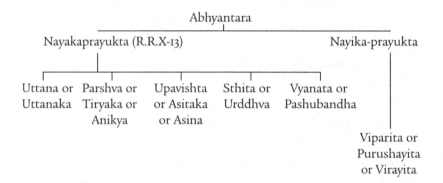

As regards the advantages, Tripathi, in his commentary on N.S., pp. 98-99, has observed as follows:

- ◆ *Uttana Rata* is pleasing to females as they experience 'Pidana' of 'Kamala' and 'Purvanga'.
- ◆ Females of Shankhini and Hastini types like *Parshva Ratas* because of the weight of the posteriors and 'Gadhatva' of the organ.

- *Upavishta Ratas* are liked because there is ample opportunity for indulging in tumescence.
- *Sthita Ratas* are not liked because they are difficult and even harmful.
- *Vyanata Ratas* are liked by those males who have a short phallus. Also it is easy to move the waist and there is 'Avaroha' of the 'Kamala'.

TABLE SHOWING POSTURES IN THE VARIOUS EXTANT TEXTS

Texts	Uttama	Parshva	Asina	Sthita	Vyanata	Purushayita
KS.	17a	3	*	1	10e	3
R.R.	26	2	3	4(chitra)	7	4f
N.S.	22b	7	2	6d	2	*
PS.	7	3	2	2	3	1
RRP	21c	4	3	6	7	2
AR.	12	3	10	3	5	3
RKK.	33	4	6	9	10	10

Note on the above

a – One more posture attributed to Vatsyayana by other writers is not found in the extant text.

b – In the colophon at the end of chapter XXVIII the author mentions 24 but there are only 22. Perhaps a stanza is missing in the extant text.

c – In the text there are 24 but three are out of place in that section.

d – One stanza is missing in the extant text.

e – Over and above this, Vatsyayana has 3, Kokkoka has 2 and Praudhadevaraya has 4 postures for congress in cases where in a union, members of one of the sexes are more than one. Vatsyayana has included Adhorata in Chitra Rata which is not done by any other writer.

f – Kanchinatha has added one in his commentary. One is quoted by Shankara Mishra from R.R.

NOTES

1   Ellis, *Studies in Psychology of Sex,* II, p. 149.
2   Ellis, ibid, II, p. 555.
3   Van de Velde, *Ideal Marriage,* Ch. XI and tables.
4   Compare the views of Tripathi given below with those of Van de Velde.
5   Shringaradipika, Prichchheda, 3.
6   Andromache was too tall to practise coitus with Hector and so Ovid recommended to little women, the male-superior position. (cf. *Ars Amatoria* III, 777-8). Also cf. Van de Velde, ibid, p. 195.
7   Tripathi, Nagarasarvasva, commentary, p. 98.
8   Tripathi, ibid, p. 99, mentions two works, Dinalapanika and Saugandhikaparinaya, wherein, according to him 84 coital postures are described. He has also mentioned (p. 98) several Chitra Ratas such as Stanatara, Kaksha, Janu, Padatalamadhya, Mushti, etc. Ellis also has mentioned inter-mammary coitus. Cf. ibid, iv, p. 272.

CHAPTER V

PURUSHAYITA, OR THE MAN SUPINE AND WOMAN ASTRIDE POSITION OF CONGRESS

This position appears to have been pretty old and popular all over the world. No wonder, the ancient authors of erotic works in India give minute details of its synonyms, psychological reasons for its appeal, various stages and variations. This position has very appropriate synonyms such as *Purushayita, Virayita, Viparita Rata, Upari and Rata.*

Vatsyayana says that this position is adopted in two ways: 1) the man during the congress is turned upside down so that he lies supine and the woman remains astride, or 2) the woman herself adopts this position from the commencement of the congress.[1] The psychological reasons[2] given for the woman preferring this position are:

- the husband being exhausted due to indulging in congress more than once
- dissatisfaction of the woman due to her passion not having subsided
- consent of the husband

- ◆ curiosity of the husband at the innovation, a pleasant departure from the usual mode

Yashodhara, in his commentary on K. S. 2-8-22 classifies this position into Bahya and Abhyantara. Describing the Bahya *Purushayita*, Vatsyayana says[3] that while the woman is astride:

- ◆ her hair gets dishevelled
- ◆ flowers drop down from her hair
- ◆ she breathes heavily and tries to laugh loudly
- ◆ she presses firmly with her bosom the man's chest to reach his mouth
- ◆ she repeatedly bends her head down
- ◆ she delivers blows on his body, asserting all the while to avenge his erstwhile aggression
- ◆ she points at him her index finger and with it she repeatedly pokes at him

The commentator while explaining Bahya *Purushayita*[4] says that it consists of loosening the Kaksha bandha of the man and similar other necessary things. As regards Abhyantara *Purushayita*[5] Vatsyayana says that the *Upasripta*, i.e., movements of the phallus are also included in this. He has enumerated the various movements, such as: 1) *Upasripta*, 2) *Manthana*, 3) *Hula*, 4) *Avamardana*, 5) *Piditaka*, 6) *Nirghata*, 7) *Varahaghata*, 8) *Vrishaghata*, 9) *Chataka vilasita* and 10) *Samputa*.

Vatsyayana mentions three particular variations of this position : 1) *Sandansha*, 2) *Bhramaraka* and 3) *Prenkholita*. Kokkoka follows Vatsyayana even though he does not specifically mention *Sandansha*. Kanchinatha, the commentator of Ratirahasya,[6] explains how it is implied in the description given by Kokkoka. Padmashri omits the subject altogether. Jyotirisha[7] describes only one position and designates it as *Viparita*. Praudhadevaraya[8] mentions *Bhramara* and *Prenkholita*. Kalyanamalla[9] gives three variations – *Viparita*, *Bhramara* and *Utkalita*. All these authors[10] strictly forbid any of these positions in any of the following cases due to the possibility of very bad after-effects.

- If the woman is in her periods
- If she has lately delivered
- If she is of the deer type
- If she is pregnant
- If she is extremely corpulent
- If she is a maiden
- If she is quite thin
- If she is deformed or bent down
- If she is recently married
- If she is down with fever

Now let us see how people of Western countries reacted to this position. It was familiar to the Romans. Ovid in his Ars Amatoria (III, 777-8) recommended it in case of women of small stature. The Greek writer Aristophanes referred to it in his works. The Greek language has some epigrams in which women boast of their skill.[11] The Roman poet Martial considered this so normal and obvious that he could not conceive of Hector and Andromache in any other attitude.[12]

Boccaccio described this method in his works. According to Ellis, the Christian and Mahomedan theologians did not approve of this position because of the superior position of the female herein, and they thought that it involved the subjection of the male as symbolic of moral subjection.[13] Ellis further says that many people are decidedly in favour of this inverse normal position since it enables the woman to obtain a better adjustment and greater control of the process and so frequently to secure sexual satisfaction which she may find difficult or impossible in the normal position.[14]

Van de Velde has explained in great detail how during the downward motion the woman increases the pelvic declination and stretches the vertebrae in the lumbar region. During her upward movement the pelvic angle decreases and the symphysis is raised and protruded upwards. The posterior rim of the vaginal orifice and the anterior portion of the perineum move in the same swing. He has further described the kind of stimulation and excitation resulting from this position.[15]

All Indian writers mentioned above refer to the excitement of the woman astride, but none of them has clearly referred to disadvantages resulting from the complete passivity of the man and the exclusive activity of the woman. The Western writers like Van de Velde are of the opinion that this is directly contrary to the natural relationship of the sexes and must bring unfavourable consequences if it becomes habitual. Thus psychologically and physiologically also this position in their opinion is not conducive to mutual happiness in the long run. However it is pleasing to note that all Western writers do agree with ancient Indian writers in forbidding this position in certain specific cases. This is a proof positive to show that the ancient Indian writers on erotics were very thorough in their scientific investigations and observations. Indian dramatists and poets of India have described Purushayita of the heroines in their works. Kalidasa[16] in his Kumarasambhava has minutely described the crumpled bed cover, with red spots of Alaktaka applied to the soles of the feet of Parvati. In another verse in the same work, he has described how Alaktaka powder fell in the eyes of Shankara supine, while Parvati astride was bending her head over him to kiss him. At another place he clearly describes Parvati astride. The commentator in all these cases explains the posture as *Purushayita*.

Jayadeva[17] in his Gitagovinda, while describing the amorous dalliance of Krishna with his lady love mentions the jingling of the anklets. At another place King Kumbha, the commentator, elaborates Jayadeva's reference to the lady bedecking herself with ornaments fit to be worn while in the astride position. Jayadeva has beautifully described the undulating earrings and jingling waist-band. King Kumbha at another place, explaining the beauty of the necklace and chest of Krishna, refers to *Purushayita* of his lady love. Krishna's request to his lady love to regale him by the jingling of her waist-band is explained by a commentator as indicating *Purushayita*. It is worth noting that Shankara Mishra, the commentator of Gitagovinda, refers to the posture as *Hamsalilaka* which is not found in any of the extant works on erotics.

One poet has very beautifully described the *Purushayita* of Lakshmi astride Murari, supine, thus: Lakshmi astride Murari lying supine, felt shy on seeing Brahma in the navel lotus and hence tried to close the right eye (the sun) of Murari thus indirectly making the lotus close its petals in the dark and consequently, avoiding the gazing of Brahma.[18]

Sculptors and painters have not lagged behind the poets and dramatists. In some panels at Bhubaneshwar, Konarak and Khajuraho there are representations of the astride posture. I have come across some very good paintings of the late Mughal, Rajput and Pahari schools, wherein the heroine is shown in the astride posture and the hero supine.

NOTES

1   Kamasutra, 2-8-2.
2   Kamasutra, 2-8-1.
3   Kamasutra, 2-8-3. Amarushataka, 3, 89, 147.
4   Kamasutra, 2-8-22, commentary.
5   Kamasutra, 2-8-11 to 21.
6   Ratirahasya, 10-47, 48.
7   Panchasayaka, 5-23.
8   Ratiratnapradipika, 5-39, 40.
9   Anangaranga, 10-32 to 34.
10   Number seven is mentioned by Kokkoka and others. Numbers eight to ten by Jyotirisha and Kalyanainalla. Praudhadevaraya does not mention the last three.
11   Ellis, *Studies in Psychology of Sex*, Vol. II, p. 147.
12   Van de Velde, *Ideal Marriage*, p. 195.
13   Ellis, ibid., II, p. 557.
14   Ellis, ibid., II, p. 556.
15   Van de Velde, ibid., pp. 195-196.

[16] Kumarasambhava, 8-19, 89 and commentary, 9-51 and commentary.

[17] Gitagovinda, 2-7–Prabandha 6; 6-4–Prabandha 12; 7-4–Prabandha 14;
      I1-2–Prabandha 22; 12-6–Prabandha 23; 12-3–Prabhandha 24.
      Commentaries of Kumbha and Shankara Mishra.

[18] Subhashita Ratnakara, Mishra Prakarana, Verse 17.

CHAPTER VI

CUNNILINGUS AND FELLATIO

According to Vatsyayana, the third Prakriti is of two types: the first having a female form and the second having a male form. The first has certain anatomical features of a female (such as breasts); the second has certain characteristics of a male (such as beard or moustache).

The female eunuch imitates a woman by her dress, voice, gait, laughter, delicacy, timidity, comeliness, impatience and shyness. The oral union with her is technically called *Auparishtaka*. She thereby gets pleasure and earns her livelihood also. The male eunuch does not do it openly. For oral union he desires the company of a male by taking up the job of a masseur. While massaging the Nayaka, the male eunuch gradually touches his thighs and by manual effects causes the Nayaka to be sexually excited and tries to laugh at his fickleness. There are eight types of oral unions. The outer ones are:

- *Nimita*
- *Parshvata*
- *Bahih Sandansha*
- *Antah Sandansha*
- *Chumbitaka*

- ◆ *Parimrishtaka*
- ◆ *Amrachushitaka*
- ◆ *Sangara*

According to Vatsyayana, the Nayaka should indulge in thumping or striking as other factors of tumescence are not practicable at this time. This act is also indulged in by those women who are devoid of morality, who are unfettered in their ways of life and by servants and masseurs. Vatsyayana follows the other ancient writers and says that one should not indulge in this act as it is against the tenets of the sacred law books and public morality. However, if one is involved in this act with a woman of low morals, he should repent and feel disgusted at having done it.

Because of an aversion for this act, the people of the East do not resort to the women who practise it. Vatsyayana says that courtesans indulge in this act with rogues, servants and mahouts. He clearly forbids learned Brahmins, ministers and those whom the public revere, from indulging in this act.[1] Smriti writers condemn this act. Vriddhaharita lays down some vidhis for atonement of this sin. Vasistha forbids it. Yagnavalkya lays down a fine for a person who indulges in oral union with his wife.[2] There are other Smritis which say that a woman's body is pure all over; a woman's mouth is pure at night; it is pure during union.[3]

Indian writers on erotics like Kokkoka[4] and others, even though aware of that practice, have not described it. This act is unhygienic and full of the danger of contamination. Yashodhara, commenting upon K.S. 2-9-39, mentions Lata and Sindhu provinces where oral coitus is not looked at with abhorrence. Kokkoka, while describing women of other provinces (R.R. 5-11), says that women living in the region of the Five Rivers cannot yield sexual satisfaction without oral union. However, there was a time when it was in vogue in some parts of India. Sculptural evidence from Bhuvaneshwar, Ellora and other places tells the same story.

Let us see how it existed in Western countries in the past. *Cunnilingus* is the apposition of the mouth to the female pudendum and *fellatio* is the apposition of the mouth to the male organ. *Cunnilingus* was adversely criticized by Greek and Roman writers. *Fellatio* has been equally well known from ages past. Both of them are practised by either sex. Scientifically speaking we know that close and prolonged contact of these regions under conditions favourable to tumescence sets up a powerful current of nervous stimulation.[5]

These practices derive a part of their attraction, more especially in some individuals, from a predilection for the odours of the sexual parts.[6] This is amply corroborated by Indian writers on erotics. Kokkoka[7] says that the mucous discharge of a Padmini smells like a blossoming lotus; that of a Chitrini smells like honey. Jyotirisha[8] describes the female pudendum. Kalyanamalla[9] also describes it like Kokkoka. Kalidasa[10] has indirectly described the Padmini-like characteristics of Shakuntala which is clearly explained by Raghavabhatta. The Mahabharata[11] describes Draupadi as having a lotus smell. According to Shrimad Bhagavata, Devahuti gave birth to beautiful daughters who had the fragrance of lotus flowers. Devahuti also saw one hundred maidens giving out a fragrant smell of lotus flowers in the Vimana in the sacred pond. Pururava spent several days in the company of Urvashi whose body smelt fragrant like lotus flowers and whose fragrant smell from the mouth had enchanted that king.[12] Shri Harsha[13] has described Damayanti as of Padmini type.

Instances can be multiplied which affirm that certain women do possess a peculiar type of attractive body odour which adds to their attractiveness, and which also acts as a powerful erotic stimulant to men who approach them. Among birds and other animals, smell plays an important part. A powerful musky odour is exhaled by the musk-drake. A peculiar and strong smell is also exhaled during the rutting or breeding seasons by crocodiles, deer, elephants, dogs and bats.

Notes

1   Vatsyayana, Kamasutra, 2-9-1 to 36.
2   Vriddhaharita, 9-3 13, 9-204; Vasistha smriti, 12-21; Yagnavalkya smriti, 24-293.
3   Vasistha, 28-9, 3-44/46; Shankha, 15-16; Atri smriti, 5-13 to 16; Atrisanhita, 141; Manu smriti, 5-130.
4   Kokkoka, Ratirahasya, 10-66.
5   Ellis, *Psychology of Sex*, II, 1-21.
6   Ellis, ibid., II, 1-75.
7   Ratirahasya, 1-11, 14, 3-21, etc.
8   Panchasayaka, 2-33/34.
9   Anangaranga, 1-8, 10, etc.
10   Shakuntala, Act I and commentary.
11   Mahabharata, 1-167-46, 1-184-10, 1-197-36.
12   Bhagavata Purana, 3-23-26, 48; 9-14-25, 10-47-60.
13   Shri Harsha, Naishadhiya, XVIII, 49.

CHAPTER VII

THE USE OF ARTIFICIAL DEVICES FOR CONGRESS AND AUTO-EROTICISM

Artificial aids to congress have been used a long time in India. Three charms in the Atharva Veda, in language not at all veiled, profess to promote virility.[1] Some people who perhaps did not believe in the efficiency of charms and prayers resorted to the use of aphrodisiacs and others made use of artificial aids. In the early centuries of the Christian era, these aids seem to have been much in vogue, as we find Vatsyayana enumerating Tarku Karma as a Kala wherein proficiency was essential for a successful and popular Nagaraka. The commentator explains it as Apadravya[2] saying that there should be a separate room for preparing artificial aids in the house of a Nagaraka.[3]

Vatsyayana has mentioned homosexual women who indulge in sexual practices with the help of artificial aids, which are of two types. They may be indulging in auto-eroticism by means of artificial aids. This practice of auto-eroticism, even though not clearly mentioned, can be inferred from some of the kinds of artificial aids.[4] Vatsyayana has clearly mentioned that males when they cannot have females for the sexual act, experience auto-eroticism with Viyoni, Vijati, figures of females and by Upamardana. As regards Viyoni, Vatsyayana has mentioned only two, but Tripathi has a larger number.[4a]

As regards females, they practise auto-eroticism by using 'kanda' – Aluka, Kadali, mula-root of Tala, Ketaki, 'fala' – Alabu and Karkati. Tripathi mentions brinjals and candles. The artificial phallus is called in Sanskrit Kritakadhvaja, Kritrima-linga or Apadravya generally. Vatsyayana mentions specific cases of Nicha Ratas, i.e., when a Hare-type male pairs with a Mare-type female and when a Bull-type male pairs with a Cow-elephant-type female.

According to Vatsyayana particular types of males have to make use of the artificial phallus. 'Nashta Raga' is 'Dhavasta' or 'Manda'. The 'Manda Raga' is either 'Pravartaka' or 'Apravartaka'. In the case of the first one, he recommends manual manipulation, karikara-krida, and for the second one, oral union. He recommends the use of Apadravyas in both cases. These may be used either in the natural way or when they are bored. The Apadravyas for the first (i.e., Aviddha) type of linga are made of gold, silver, copper, iron, ivory, horn, wood, etc. Those made of tin and lead are considered soft, cool and capable of withstanding forceful rubbings.

The Apadravya is of the size of the organ (stabdha, i.e., in its natural state). It has holes bored at the tip, and is rough on the outer side. It then fits properly like a valaya on the organ. This may have more than even two joints. That one which is of the size of the organ is called Chudaka. It is called Ekachudaka when a lead strip is wound round the organ and when covering it completely. The Apadravya has at the end, from where it is put on, two holes for inserting the string for tying it round the waist. It has also round rough balls resembling the testes. It is called Kanchuka when rough globules are on the sides. When it covers the whole organ it is called Jalaka. This is of two kinds. (It is Khara-kanchuka when its outer side is smooth. That one which covers the manibhaga is Arddha-kanchuka. This is called Maniraksha. It is called Utkirnajalaka when there are round globules on the sides. It is called Valaya when it has many holes. This is also Manijalaka.) When these materials are not available, Vatsyayana recommends stalks of Alabu and bamboo which are soaked and polished with oil and kashayas and tied with a string round the waist. This tube may have round wooden globules on its outer surface at certain points.

LINGA VYADHANA AND FITTING OF AFADRAVYA IN THE TRANSVERSE ORIFICE

Referring to the phallus with a hole bored at the tip, Vatsyayana mentions a custom prevalent among some races probably in South India. He compares it to that of boring holes in the earlobes. According to him the young man should remain in water till blood (due to the operation of boring the hole) stops coming out. The young man is then directed to indulge in sexual intercourse at night as many times as possible, to avoid the hole being closed up. Then, on alternate days, he should wash that part and continue to pierce the hole with small smooth pieces of bamboo to effect enlargement of the circumference of that hole. He has then to apply an ointment made of honey and 'Yashtimadhu'. He should cover the organ with 'Sisaka patra' and smear it with the oil of Bhallataka. In the hole thus made, the young man should insert Apadravyas of various sizes and shapes such as round, round on one side, one that is hollow like a mortar, one that is flower-shaped, one that is shaped as if thorny, one which is like the bone of Kanka, elephant's trunk, octagonal or square. These shapes are elaborately described by Yashodhara in his commentary.[5]

It will be interesting to know something about these devices from accounts and reports of journeys made by foreigners in India.[6] For example, we read in the Hakluyt Society Transactions on India in the fifteenth century that old prostitutes used to sell little bells of gold, silver and bronze which were sewn into the skin of the man's phallus. Consequently, it was swollen and thereby it gave great pleasure to the females in union. These bells were sewn to the phalli of boys when they attained maturity and were constantly changed for those of larger sizes as they grew up.

Similarly a passage in the account of the travels[7] of Nicolo de Conti contains the information that old women earned their livelihood by sale of bells of gold, silver and copper. Any young man without such bells sewn between skin and flesh of his phallus was repulsed. The metal varied according to the social status of the person. These old women also sewed these bells into the phalli of their youthful customers. Many young men used to have a dozen or more bells sewn into their phalli. Young men with bells were highly esteemed by women and if the jingling was heard while walking it was considered honourable. These appliances were common in Malaya, the Philippines, China and Russia and among the American Indians of the northern and southern continents. The existence of these appliances shows that painful stimulation is craved for by women to heighten the highly pleasurable state of tumescence.

In Borneo, the Kyans and Dyaks call it ampallang, palang, kambian, and it consists of a small rod of bone or metal, about two inches long, rounded at the ends. Before the union, it is inserted into a transverse orifice in the phallus, made by a painful and dangerous operation and kept open by a quill. Sometimes two or more such instruments are worn. Sometimes little beads are attached to each end of the instrument. The Bisayas perforate their phalli in the middle and put there a piece of lead sticking out on both the sides. On one side there is a star made of lead, and which can be turned round at the other end. There is a lynch pin to keep the instrument in place. Mantegazza describes another similar instrument saying that therein is placed a gold or leather cylinder as thick as a goose feather, having two ends, sometimes a kind of star with rays, or a disc-like head of a thick nail. This little cylinder still leaves the urethral canal open. In the Pintada Islands, males during infancy have a hole bored in their phalli in which they stick a piece of metal, in the form of a snakehead, in such a way that it cannot be dislodged. This is called Sagras, but now these are very rarely found. There is another instrument used by the Dyaks called palang anus, which is in the form of a ring or a collar of plaited palm-fibre, furnished with a pair of stiffish horns of the same wiry material. It is worn on the neck of the glans and fits tightly to the skin. In Borneo sometimes a tuft of horse hair is also worn. In Sumatra small stones are inserted by an incision under the skin of the phallus.

Paolo Mantegazza describes in detail his observations which are almost similar to those described by Vatsyayana. The perforation is executed with a silver needle, for affixing a silver or ivory needle perforated at both the ends. Two brushes are attached in the perforations forming a double-brush. Some phalli are perforated twice for the two instruments and for the changing of the position of the brushes. This operation is performed on adults only, by forcing back the string and placing the phallus between two small planks of bamboo. For about ten days it is covered with rags dipped in cold water. Then the glans is perforated, with a sharp bamboo needle. A feather dipped in oil is placed in the wound till it heals. Wet compresses are used during the healing period.[8]

In China, a wreath of soft, feathers with the quills solidly fastened by silver wire to a silver ring is slipped over the glans. Instruments similar to these are also known in Europe. In France, rings set with hard knobs were used by men. In Germany, condoms furnished with a frill are used. In Russia, elastic rings set with little teeth are used by fastening them around the base of the glans. In Argentina, the Araucanians use a little horse-hair brush fastened around the phallus. These instruments called gaskels are made by women and the workmanship is delicate.[9] In Borneo, a young lady who is in love with a young man keeps a cigarette at a particular place and thereby informs her lover the size of the ampallang that would be sufficient for heightening her sexual excitement. Brooke Low (who is quoted by Ellis), remarks that a woman once habituated to its use will never dream of permitting her bedfellow to discontinue the practice of wearing it.

The impulse to use such devices for sexual gratification is natural and has a zoological basis. Many rodents, ruminants and some of the carnivora group show development of the sex organ which resembles those artificially made and used by man. Guinea pig, cat, rhinoceros, sheep, giraffe, are cases in point. Butterflies are credited with having harpes which are beautiful and varied, taking the form of projecting claws, hooks, pikes, swords, knobs and strange combinations of these commonly brought to a keen edge and then cut into sharp teeth.[10] These devices serve to heighten sexual excitement which according to Vatsyayana is the primary aim of a union.

NOTES

[1]   Atharvaveda, 4-4, 6-72, 6-101; 2. S.B.E. XLII, pp. 3 1-32; Bloomfield, The *Atharvaveda,* p.62.

[2]   Kamasutra, 1-3-16. Kala No. 34 and commentary.

[3]   Kamasutra, 1-4-14 and commentary.

[4]   Kamasutra, 5-6-2 and commentary.

[4a]   Kamasutra, 5-6-5 and comm. As regards Viyoni, Nilakantha in his commentary gives different meanings: (i) low family; (ii) birds, etc. Cf. Mahabbarata, 13-104-33, 13-106-72, 12-228-15, 13-145-52/53.

[5]   (1) Kamasutra, 7-2, 15 to 24 and commentary. (2) Kandarpachudamani, 7-2-11 and 22.
Readers may refer to Mantegazza's book, pp. 71-78.

[6]   Mantegazza, *Sexual Relations of Mankind,* pp. 75-76.

[7]   Major, *India in the 15th Century. The Travels of Nicolo de Conti,* p. 11.

[8]   Ellis, ibid, I, 2, pp. 99-101. Mantegazza, ibid, pp. 76 to 79.

[9]   Ellis, ibid, I, 2, p. 99.

[10]   Ellis, ibid., I, 2, p. 100.

CHAPTER VIII

LITERARY SOURCES FOR A STUDY OF INDIAN EROTICS

TRADITION

Vatsyayana has preserved for posterity the tradition of this science in his Kama Sutra, saying that Prajapati, after creating the beings, prepared a treatise running into 100,000 Adhyayas. This treatise was meant to guide the beings in the pursuit of the Aims of Life. Svayabhuva Manu separated that part of this text which dealt with Dharma. Brihaspati did likewise to that part which dealt with Artha. It was Nandi, the attendant of Mahadeva, who separated the portion of the text which dealt with Kama into 1,000 Adhyayas. Auddalaki abridged this text of Nandi into 500 Adhyayas. Panchala Babhravya further abridged it into 150 Adhyayas covering the whole subject into 7 Adhikaranas. It was Dattaka who separately dealt with the 6th Adhikarana – Vaishika, at the instance of the prostitutes of Pataliputra. Charayana, Suvarnanabha, Ghotakamukha, Gonardiya, Gonikaputra and Kuchumara similarly dealt with the remaining six Adhikaranas – Sadharana, Samprayogika, Kanyasamprayuktaka, Bharya, Paradarika and Aupanishadika respectively.

As this science suffered several abridgements at the hands of writers in the hoary past, as each one of them dealt with a particular part, and as the work of Panchala Eabhravya was very difficult to be understood by ordinary persons, Vatsyayana himself wrote Kama Sutra.[1]

OTHER WRITERS ON EROTICS

Besides the names of these sages, Vatsyayana[2] quotes some previous writers, He mentions the names of some while indirectly referring to the others, such as Acharyah, Eke, Arthachintakah, Kalakaranikah, Gonardiya, Gonikaputra, Ghotakamukha, Charayana, Babhravya, Laukayatikah, Suvarnanabha. Kokkoka[3] mentions, besides Vatsyayana, Muladeva, Karnisuta, Muni, Munindra, Nandikeshvara. Damodara[4] mentions, besides Vatsyayana, Rajaputra, Madanodaya, Dattaka, Vitaputra. Jyotirisha[5] mentions, besides Vatsyayana, Rantideva, Kashyapa, Chandramauli, Mahesha, Munindra, Bhoja, Kavindra, Ishvara, Nandikeshvara. Padmashri[6] mentions, besides Vatsyayana, Masheshvara and Munindra. Kalyanamalla[7] refers, besides Vatsyayana, to Muni, Munindra, Budha, Vigna, Kavindra, Kavi, Praksuri, Munishvara. Devidatta Sharma quotes[8] from Katyayana. Pt. Mathura Prasada[9] mentions one Mallada.

Now if we look into these names we find some of them of interest to us for our study.

Auddaliki: He was the son of Uddalaka Aruni. This was his paternal name, the real name being Shvetaketu. Besides knowing him as a writer on erotics, from Vatsyayana's Kama Sutra and Kanchinatha's commentary,[10] we know from the Mahabharata[11] that he laid down certain rules of conduct.

Babhravya: That the text written by Babhravya Panchala was well-known, even up to the times of Jyotirisha and Yashodhara and perhaps Kanchinatha, is evident from quotations made by the last two in the commentaries Jayamangala[12] on Kama Sutra and Dipika on Ratirahasya.

Charayana: Charayana is referred to by Kautilya.[13]

Dattaka: As regards Dattaka we are now informed by Dr Raghavan[14] that a metrical résumé of Dattaka sutras exists in a fragmentary condition. Vatsyayana and Yashodhara refer to him.[15]

Ghotakamukha: He is also referred to (like Charayana) by Kautilya.

Gornardiya: He is referred to in the Mahabhashya.[16] That the text of Gonardiya was well known up to the time of Mallinatha,[17] is evident from quotations made by him in his commentaries.

Gonikaputra: Like Gonardiya, he is also referred to in the Mahabhahya.[18] His text also appears to have been well known even up to the time of Kanchinatha, since he has quoted from it.[19] Jyotirisha, before him, knew his work.

Ishvara: He is referred to by Jyotirisha,[20] but it is difficult to identify him. It is certain however from the references that he wrote a work on erotics.

Karnisuta: The editors of Kshemendra's Kalavilasa[21] say that Karnisutra, Kalankura and Mulabhadra are other names of Muladeva. It occurs in Subandhu's Vasavadatta, the commentary of which, quoting Haravali, gives Muladeva as his synonym thereof. The story of Karnisuta is referred to in Bana's Kadambari.

Kashyapa: He is referred to by Jyotirisha, but we do not know anything more about him as a writer on erotics.

Katyayana: He is referred to by Devi Prasada in his Tippani on Ratirahasya, but as in the case of Kashyapa, we do not know anything about him as a writer on erotics. Yashodhara refers to him in his commentary.[22]

Kavindra: In this case also it is not possible to identify him, though it is interesting to note that Jyotirisha once mentions Rantidava as Kavindra.[23]

Kuchimara: Besides references to him made by Vatsyayana we know of a work Kuchimaratantra dealing with special appliances and methods, the use of aphrodisiacs and mantras.

Madanodaya: We know that Raghava Bhatta[24] in his commentary on Shakuntala quotes from a work by this author. We do not know anything further. Here it is necessary to point out that Vishakhila as a writer on erotics, mentioned by Tripathi,[25] is a mistake since he is referred to by Damodara along with Bharata and Dattila as a writer on Kala. This is corroborated by Kavyalamkara Vrtti, 1-3-7.

Mahesha: He is referred to by Jyotirisha, but it is not possible to identify him. Chandramauli also is perhaps another name of this writer.

Maheshvara: He is referred to by Padmashri. Tripathi[26] says that he might be the same as Rudra, the author of Samara-Dipika. But in another place he mentions him as a writer on Kamatantra.

Mallada: He is mentioned by Pt. M. Prasada. Is it possible that this is but another synonym of Mallanaga Vatsyayana? This is merely a conjecture.

Muladeva: He is referred to both by Kokkoka and Jyotirisha. That the text of Muladeva was well known up to the time of Jyotirisha is evident from the reference made to him. Mulla is known to us from Kalavilasa[27] and Brihatkatha as an expert in the arts. He undertook to initiate one Chandra Gupta in the arts. He is known to be a writer on arts. The editors of Kalavilasa say that his other names are Mulabhadra and Karnisuta. Muladeva's karma, kala, karika, etc., are referred to by Yashodhara in his commentary.[28] While commenting upon Millechchhita, Yashocihara refers to Muladevi, a type of code difficult to be deciphered by others.[28a] The Mahabharata refers to Mulaprachara for removing the effects of poison given by an enemy.[28b]

Muni and Munindra: As regards Munindra, Kanchinatha[29] says that the reference is to Gonardiya, while he does not say anything when the name occurs further on. This may be correct in as much as Tripathi,[30] in his commentary says that he is different from Vatsyayana. As regards Muni, Kanchinatha[31] says that Vatsyayana is referred to by that name. But he does not say anything for 'Munayah' in 10-26, even though in 10-29 he explains 'Munibhih' as 'Gonikaputra and others'.

Nandi, Nandikeshvara: At least up to the time of Jyotirisha, his text must have been extant in as much as he says that he 'had seen' it, i.e., at least had gone through it, or was acquainted with it or knew it.

Rajputra: Tripathi[32] has quoted from Hastyayurveda (3-8-99) saying that he is referred to therein. Beyond this, we do not know anything more about him as a writer on erotics.

Rantideva: Jyotirisha calls him not only a king but also the best of poets. Nothing is known to us about him. Some Shishtas[32a] are referred to by Yashodhara. He also quotes[32b] Gautama and Bhrigu without naming their works.

Suvarnanabha: Nothing more is known about him than the references made to him by Vatsyayana.

Vitaputra: Nothing is known to us about him except that Damodara mentions him along with Vatsyayana, Dattaka and others. It is not also possible to identify the persons who are referred to generally by Kalyanamalla (mostly in plural), such as 'Buddha', 'Vigna', 'Kavi', 'Praksuri', 'Purvasuri'.

Let us now consider some of the old works wherein their authors have tried to depict erotic scenes, a perusal of which enables us to presume their knowledge of the science of erotics.

EPICS

In the Mahabharata[33] we come across excellent descriptions of the physical charms of Draupadi, Urvashi and Madhavi. In the Ramayana[34] we find Ravana describing the physical charms of Sita and Rambha, the heavenly nymph, Sita's own description of her bodily charms and a minute description of Ravana's harem.

PURANAS

We find equally good descriptions in the Puranas also. Agni Purana[35] and Garuda Purana[36] give descriptions of the physical charms of females. A portion of Harivamsha,[37] didactic in nature, deals with scientific eroticism, the Kama Shastra. It is in the form of a conversation between the wives of Krishna and Narada. The Devi Bhagavata[38] describes physical charms of Yashovati and Ekavali. Shrimad Bhagavata[39] describes physical charms of the Divine Body of Vishnu, King Kushapani, the lady (with her followers) who met King Puranjaya, Vishnu when he appeared before Virincha and Sarva, Vishnu when he adopted the female form, Krishna adored by Akrura.

CLASSICAL LITERATURE

Ashvaghosha[40] describes the musical parties in the royal palace, the hurried movements of the women of the city to see the prince, the amorous dalliance of beautiful young damsels with the prince, the sleeping beauties in the palace whose company the prince left to tread a higher and nobler path of life. Vimala Suri,[41] the author of Pauma-chariya (the oldest extant epic in Jaina Maharashtri Prakrit, written in about the 1st century AD), describes the physical beauty of Ravana, Anjanasundari and the wives of Ravana. Kalidasa[42] has described the physical charms of his heroes, heroines and even minor characters in his works. His description of the amorous dalliance of Shiva and Parvati in Kumarasambhava is quite well known. All these references cited above leave no doubt in our mind that the authors of these works must have known some text or texts on the art of love.

That Vatsyayana knew quite well some text or texts on erotics can be very easily inferred from the following discussion: Bharata in his Natyashastra (xxv) deals with Bahyopachara. There he refers to Vaishika and his qualities; Duti, her duties and qualifications, and behaviour of Veshyayas towards the lovers.[42a] Bharata[43] gives a classification of women on the basis of Shila, Svabhava, etc. This classification is followed to a certain extent by Kokkoka,[44] Jyotirisha[45] and Kalyanarnalla.[46] But it is not found in Vatsyayana's Kama Sutra. Kokkoka perhaps relied upon works like Gunapataka and authors like Muladeva alias Karnisuta. Jyotirisha gives one category which is neither given by Bharata nor Kokkoka and Kalyanamalla.

Similarly, the classification of women into Padmini, Chitrini, etc., though found in Kokkoka and other later writers, is not found in Vatsyayana's Kama Sutra. So also the fourfold classification of Nayakas into Bhadra, Datta, Kuchimara, and so on, found in Shrinagaradipika of Harihara[47] and Shringaramanjari of St. Ali Akbar Shah,[48] is not found in Vatsyayana's Kama Sutra. The author of Sringaramanjari speaks in unequivocal terms that this classification is in accordance with the opinion of Vatsyayana.

This raises another problem of the state of the present text of Kama Sutra; Ratiratnrathpika[49] (3-24 to 26) quotes verses as if they were those of Vatsyayana Maha Muni, but they are conspicuous by their absence in Kama Sutra while treating Udghrishta Aimgana. Shankara Mishra, in his Rasamanjari on Gita Govinda (8-4-17) quotes from Vatsyayana a Krodha bandha; but it is not found in the Kama Sutra. Moreover, Kalyanamalla gives (9-23) six qualities of nails, quoting Kama Shastra, but there are more in Kama Sutra, 2-4-8. At least one of them is quite the opposite of one given by Kalyanamalla.

KAMA SUTRA

Turning to the extant texts on erotics, we find Kama Sutra the first in the field. Vatsyayana wrote it in 7 Adhikaranas running into 36

Adhyayas, 74 (67) Prakaranas and 1,250 Slokas. In the first Adhikarana, Vatsyayana deals with general topics, such as pursuing the aims of life, the 64 Arts, the life of a Nagaraka, the various festivals, the Nayikas. In the Samprayogika Adhikarana he classifies men and women, the various types of union, embracing, kissing, scratching with nails, biting with teeth, postures for union, beating and screaming. In the Kanyasamprayuktaka Adhikarana he describes selection of the bride and marriage, taking her into one's confidence, ways and means of wooing a maiden without any extraneous help, employing agents in wooing the maiden. In the Bharya Adhikarana he deals with the life of a maiden who is married, her behaviour with the co-wives, the life of the wife indoors, and one's behaviour towards several wives.

In the Paradarika Adhikarana he deals with the character of men and women, women who can be won over easily, meeting and gradually winning them over, and guarding them indoors. In the Vaishika Adhikarana he deals with courtesans, and ways of those who resort to them for the gratification of their sexual desires. In the Aupanishadika Adhikarana he deals with special appliances and methods of use of aphrodisiacs, mantras, means of seduction, heightening of enjoyment, and so on.

Date of Kama Sutra: This is the first great treatise on erotics written in a style like that of Arthashastra. The style is dry and didactic and the morality of the work is that of Arthashastra. Its sociological and medical importance is so great that we find most of the later writers following him. To students of Sanskrit literature, it is well known how much later poets and dramatists such as Kalidasa, Magha, Bhavabhuti, Bharavi, Kumaradasa and a host of others depended upon Kama Sutra for depicting not only the physical charms of their heroes and heroines but also their amorous dalliance.

Shama Shastry[50] says that Vatsyayana flourished between AD 137 to 209. Some have been led to believe that Vatsyayana flourished after AD 225 from a reference to Abhiras, which is as inconclusive as is the reference to Kuntala Shatakarni Sata Vahana. Bhandarkar[51] puts his date about AD 100. According to Keith,[52] these references do not help us to arrive at a conclusive decision. His date may be before 4th century AD. H. C. Chakiadar has very ably discussed this problem,[53] and has concluded that Kama Sutra was written before AD 400 and after Mahabhashya and Arthashastra as Vatsyayana has quoted from these works.

His Name: Chitrava Shastri[54] says that Panchakarna Vatsyayana was the name of the author of Kama Sutra. Vatsyayana was his family name. There are some works such as Hemachandra's Abhidhana Chintamani and Yadava Prakasha's Vaijayanti, which say that Vatsyayana, Mallanaga, Kautilya, Dramila, Pakshiiaswami, etc., are names of one and the same person. Bhoja gives Katyayana instead of Vatsyayana, but we have the unfailing authority of Yashodhara[55] who says that Vatsyayana is the family name and Mallanaga is the name of the author of Kama Sutra.

ARTHASHASTRA

Here it will be worthwhile to know something about Kautilya's Arthashastra, even though it mainly discusses Artha. He devotes a chapter to courtesans, maidens and sexual offences. There is also a special chapter on Aupanishadika. In the preface to the second edition, Shama Sastry[56] has collected similar words and phrases found in Arthashastra and Kama Sutra and he has opined that Arthashastra was written 'before Kama Sutra'. According to Keith,[57] the work (Arthashastra) comes before Kama Sutra. That the work is a product of *c.* 300, written by an official attached to some court, is at least plausible if it cannot be proved. According to Winternitz,[58] Kautilya's Arthashastra is a work of the 3rd or 4th century AD.

RATIRAHASYA

After Kama Sutra, Ratirahasya,[59] stands second in popularity among the people. It is better known by its name after the author, Koka-Shastra. The author Kokkoka says in the first chapter that it was King Vainya (Vaishya v.1) Datta who commanded him to write it since he was curious about the science of love. Like the author of the Bhagavad Gita he also wrote this work after a study of previous works on the subject. In the colophon he says that his grandfather was Tejoka, his father was Paribhadra alias Gadya Vidyadhara Kavi. He calls his work Kama-Keli-Rahasya.[60]

This work is in 15 Parichchhedas. In the first, he gives fourfold classification of females and their characteristics; days which are congenial for each of these groups and ways and means of winning them over. In the second, he gives erogenous zones and gives days when each group gets sexually more excited. In the third, he gives classification of males and females according to the size of the organ and nine types of union as per size, nine as per duration and nine as per force. In the fourth, he gives classification and characteristics of females as per age, prakriti, satva, etc. In the fifth, he describes females of different provinces and their sexual characteristics. In the sixth, he deals with varieties of embraces; in the seventh, those of kisses; in the eighth, those of scratching with nails; in the ninth, those of biting with teeth; in the tenth, those of postures for union, end of union, union with the female above, beating, screaming, etc. In the eleventh, he deals with maidens, their selection and marriage, taking the maidens into confidence, etc. In the twelfth, he deals with the wife, behaviour with a co-wife, etc. In the thirteenth, he deals with stages of love, other females, those who can be won over, use of agents for enticing other women; in the fourteenth, ways and means of enticing women particularly with the help of mantras and other rites; in the last, with aphrodisiacs and special appliances for heightening enjoyment.

Date: It is not possible to fix the date of Kokkoka. We can, however, fix both the lower and upper limits in as much as a verse from his work (3-8) occurs in Jayamangala (2-1-26) a copy of which was stored in the library of Visaladeva who ruled at Patan from AD 1244 to 1264. Both King Kumbha[61] in his commentary (a) Rasikapriaya on Gita Govinda and Shankara Mishra in his commentary (b) Rasamanjari on the same work, have referred to Kokkoka and Ratirahasya. However, it is interesting to note that a verse 'Angesvedah' is quoted by Kumbha, as from Bharata, in his commentary on Gita Govinda 2-8-6, while Shankara Mishra in 3-6-14 quotes it as from Ratirahasya. Shankara Mishras three quotations in Gita Govinda 2-6, 7, 14, as from Ratirahasya, are not found in Kokkoka's work. Mallinatha,[62] in. his commentaries, quotes from Ratirahasya. Mallinatha has once wrongly referred to Kama Shastra.[63] This quotation is from Ratirahasya 11-8, while on Meghaduta 101, his quotations from Ratirahasya are not found in Kokkoka's work. Keith[64] is of the opinion that the date of Ratirahasya may be before AD 1200. It is not unlikely that he flourished even earlier as we find that Somadeva, the author of Nitivakyamrita, who flourished between the 10th and 11th centuries, has referred to Kokkoka.[64a] As regards the upper limit we have his reference to Haramekhala of Mahuka who flourished in the 9th century AD.[65]

KUTTANIMATA

Kuttanimata, known as Shambhalimata, is a poetical work by Damodara Gupta. It is a sort of cunning advice given by Vikarala, a procuress, to a dancing girl named Malati, who sought her help for enticing more lovers and leading them to their ruin – physical, moral and economic. This work is rich in information regarding the life, social customs, the state of society, religion and literature in the 8th century AD in Kashmir. The poet has tried to expose the evils of the society, the methods adopted by the deceitful procuresses and thus indirectly to warn the readers. The various cunning arts for decoying feeble-minded and innocent young men are described (88-174). The story of Samarabhata and Manjari contains descriptions of love sports by which the dancing girl ruins him (737-1056). The poet beautifully describes *Surata* (373, etc.) of Sundarasena and Haralata which can be compared with the description given by Bharavi in Kiratrajuniya 9-49. He describes *Bahya Rata* in 375-378, 402-403, 572-574, 581, etc. He also describes *Chaurya Surata* in 822. Embracing other women is beautifully described in 843; end of sexual union is described in 845.

Date: As regards the date, we know that Damodara was a minister of king Jayapida. According to Kaihana, Jayapida reigned in AD 751–782, but according to modern historical researches by Prof. Stein[66] the period should be from AD 779 to 813. The author refers to writers on erotics. His work was very widely known among later writers; but we know nothing beyond his name as regards his personal history and other literary work, even though stray verses are found attributed to him.

KALAVILASA AND OTHER WORKS OF KSHEMENDRA

Kshemendra, the prolific writer from Kashmir, wrote among others at least three very interesting works which have some relation to our present study. Samayamatrika or the Book of Conventions relates the story of a would-be prostitute who is introduced by a barber to Kalavati, an expert in her arts. The young maiden, by the instruction and advice of Kalavati, cheats a young man. In Kalavilasa, one Muladeva, an expert in the arts, initiates one Chandra Gupta in the line. Various follies of men are described. The author dilates upon cheats who practise hypocrisy and greediness. He describes love with the help of the story of Vasumati and Samudradatta. Thus the life of courtesans, Kayasthas, musicians, goldsmiths, different types of cheats and the various arts are described. Deshopadesha is also equally useful to us for knowing the state of society, the social customs and the daily life of the people in Kashmir.

Date: Kshemendra lived during the time of Anantaraja, AD 1028–1080.[67] In AD 1037 he wrote Bharatamanjari, in AD 1066 a Dashavatara charita. Jyotirisha refers to him along with the other writers in erotics. This is corroborated by the fact that Kshemendra is said to have written an epitome[68] of Vatsyayana's work.

NAGARASARVASVA OF PADMASHRI

In the 38th chapter the author says that one Vasudeva, by birth a Brahmin and a famous Pandita, was the person who made him write the work 'Flame of the Lamp of Love'. In the first chapter as well as in the thirty-eighth, he gives his name as Padmashri. He was a Buddhist by religion. He adores Arya Manjushri in the first chapter and worships Tara. The work runs into 38 parts of uneven size. In the third chapter, he describes beauties and faults of jewels which is not found in other works on erotics. In the fourth, he gives recipes for cosmetics, and in the fifth to eleventh, he gives bhasha, anga, vastra, pushpa, etc. The author says that a lover, even though endowed with proficiency in the 64 arts, is rejected by his lady love if he does not understand 'sanketa'. This subject like that of jewels mentioned above, is also not found in other works on erotics. In the twelfth, he gives applications of aphrodisiacs. He then describes hava and 16 cheshtas. In the fourteenth, he describes the classifications of males and females according to parinaha and aroha of their organs, and then deals with types of union. He then gives ways and means of enticing other women. In the sixteenth, he also gives classification of women according to age, and, the time of their suitability or otherwise for union and the process of fondling and caressing them. Further, he mentions erogenous zones and days when they are so affected; the various nadis and the manner of exciting them, and then he dilates upon madanadikas. In the twentieth, he gives charac-teristics of females of various parts of this country. Then he describes kissing (with sound), scratching, biting, embracing, kissing (without sound), licking and sucking. In the twenty-eighth, he describes

24 types of *Uttana*, 7 of *Parshva*, 2 of *Asina*, 2 of *Adhomukha*, 7 of *Utthita*, *Karanas* or postures for union. He then describes flagellation, massaging, pulling, fingering, etc. He then writes about tricks (Vamacharita) adopted by females. In the last chapter, 'Sutoday', he describes how to have children.

It is not easy to find out the exact date when Padmashri flourished, but we do find that he has quoted from Kuttanimata, and in one place he gives a verse which is simply another rendering of a verse (149) in Kuttanimata. Some quotations are found in Sharngadharapaddhati (particularly 3260, 3262, 3263). Hence we can say[69] that he flourished in about 1000 V.S.

RATIMANJARI BY JAYADEVA

This is a very short treatise running into sixty verses. In the very first verse, after adorning god Sadashiva, the author mentions his own name as Jayadeva, and that of his work as Ratimanjari. He further mentions that he has condensed the science of erotics in this treatise. He then proceeds to give characteristics of the four different types of women according to Jati – Padmini, etc., and those of the four different types of men corresponding to them who can satisfy them – Shasha, etc. Then he describes the four types of women according to their age and the means by which they can be won over.

Then comes the description of erogenous zones and the days on which they are affected. Next, we find the places fit for kissing in the female anatomy. The author goes on to describe how the male should perform the union; how and where he should scratch her body with nails; how and where he should bite her with his teeth; how he should squeeze her breasts; how he should catch hold of the locks of her hair. Then he describes the dalliance of the male in the case of each of the four types. He then gives characteristics of the female and male organs and their defects. Then we find descriptions of each of the four types of males. Next come the postures for union, only sixteen in number.

Scholars[70] are reluctant to ascribe this work to the author of Gita

Govinda and they are probably right. Poetical skill of the author of Gita Govinda is conspicuous by its absence here. Moreover, the dalliance of Krishna described and poetically immortalised in Gita Govinda is of such a high order that the descriptions of the ways and places of kissing, scratching, embracing, squeezing appear quite poor and mediocre in Ratimanjari. The argument put forth by Desai[71] regarding its authorship by Jayadeva, the author of Gita Govinda, is not at all convincing. However he appears to have come after Jyotirisha and before Kalyanamalla.

Panchasayaka of Jyotirisha alias Kavishekhara

The title of the work suggests that it is a treatise on erotics. It is divided into five Sayakas or Arrows of Cupid. After adoring Kama, the author gives out his name as Jyotirisha, the foremost of poets of his time. He condensed the science of erotics into this work after studying the works of Ishvara, Vatsyayana, Gonikaputra, Muladeva, Babharavya, Nandikeshvara, Rantideva and Kshemendra. He then proceeds to describe the characteristics of Nayakas and Pithamardas. Then he gives those of women classified according to Jati, their Tithis, erogenous zones and ways and means of exciting women for producing the orgasm.

In the second Sayaka, he describes males and females according to ayama and parinaha of their organs, their characteristics, types of union – *sama, attyuchcha, nicha* and *atinicha*. Then he describes women according to their age and provinces, different types of the female organs, etc. In the third Sayaka he gives ingredients of cosmetics, aphrodisiacs, collyrium, ointment, powder and sacred incantations and iconographic details of goddesses for attracting and enticing women. He then gives ingredients of medicines for lifting up sagging breasts, stiffening loose ones, contracting the vagina, menstruation, impregnation, sterility, depilation and even for growing hair.

In the fourth, he describes young maidens and youths; their outstanding characteristics and defects; eight different types of marriages; connections with other women; female messengers; women who can be easily won over; proper places and timings for a happy union. He then describes embraces, kisses, nail scratchings, biting with teeth and catching of locks of hair. In the fifth Sayaka, he describes nadi and then goes on to describe the postures for union and *Purushayita*. Then he deals with flagellation and ends with descriptions of eight types of Nayikas.

Date: It is possible for us to put down the upper and lower limits for the date of this work as he refers to Kshemendra in the first Sayaka, and Kshemendra, we know now, flourished in the first half of the IIth century AD. Jyotirisha flourished[72] in the first half of the 14th century. His patron was Arasinha who fought with Ghiyasuddin Taghlaq (1320-4). Shankara Mishra in his commentary Rasamanjari[73] on Jayadeva's Gita Govinda, has quoted several times from Panchasayaka. According to Manomohana Chakravarti (J.A.S.B., 1915, p. 414) he also wrote another work on erotics: Ragasekhara.

RATIRATNAPRADIPIKA OF DEVARAJA

This is a treatise on erotics running into seven Adhyayas. Some Adhyayas contain certain Adhikaras, e.g., in the third Adhyaya there are Adhikaras of *Alingana, Chumbana, Nakhakshata* and *Dantakshata*. Perhaps the author includes only these four in *Bahya Surata*. He[74] has referred to Nandisha, Gauniputra, Vatsyayana, Mailanaga, Kokkoka, Muni and Kovida. He also refers to Gunapataka. In fact, he has drafted his first Adhyya according to the views of Gauniputra and the sixth according to Nandikeshvara. The author calls himself Shri Praudha Devaraja Maharaja. Tripathi,[75] in his commentary on Kuttanimata, merely mentions him as Devaraja Maharaja. Devaraya II of Vijayanagara flourished from AD 1422 to 1466. Even Mallinatha wrote a work for this king.[75a] The author has perhaps closely followed Kokkoka. From him we know that the fourfold classification of females into Padmini, etc., is according to Nandisha and Gauniputra.

He has also given the threefold classification of females according to Vatsyayana into Mrigi, etc. There is also given the threefold classification of females according to Gunapataka into Shlatha, Madhya and Ghana. In his classification of females according to Prakriti he includes Gaja, Rakshasa and Danava which are not found elsewhere.

In the enumeration of 12 *Alingana*s he classifies them into *Jatarati* and *Ajatarati*. He gives 14 types of *Chumbana*, 9 *Nakhakshata*, 8 *Dantakshata*, 5 types of coitus, about 40 postures for union, 3 *Purushyita*, etc. He also gives eight types of *Surata* according to Adhikara. Then we are given 8 types of *Auparishtaka* done by females and another 8 types as performed by males. He also deals with *Prahanana* of 10 types and *Sitkrita* of 17 types.

SHARNGADHARAPADDHTI (C 1300)

This contains verses mentioning varieties of women in terms of God, demi-gods, etc. One Shridhara wrote these verses. He was probably a writer on Kamashastra, but unfortunately at the present moment we do not know anything about his works.

ANANGARANGA OF KALYANAMALLA

This is a work running into 10 Sthalas dealing with erotics. After adoring Kama the author says that he wrote this work for pleasing Ladakhan, son of King Ahmada of the Lodi dynasty. The author is none other than King Kalyanamalla. He studied the works of previous writers on erotics and then wrote this treatise. He then classifies women, their days and time most congenial for sexual excitement. Then he classifies men and women according to aroha and parinaha of their organs, different kinds of union, characteristics of three types of males and females, characteristics of women according to their age, humour, Sattva, etc., different variations of the female organ, characteristics of women of different provinces. Then, in the sixth Sthala, he describes ways and means of producing the orgasm, ingredients of aphrodisiacs for both the sexes, depilatory powders, hair-growing oils, stiffening loose and sagging breasts. In the seventh Sthala he describes marks, collyriums, powders, pills, incense, sacred incantations for captivating the hearts of women. He then gives ingredients of cosmetics, deodorant powders, etc. In the eighth, he describes characteristics and qualities of a maiden and a son-in-law; gives details of those with whom union is immoral; characteristics of female messengers; those of women who are difficult to be won over for union; places and times for union, etc. In the ninth, he describes various types of embraces, kisses, scratching with nails, biting with teeth, catching of locks of hair, etc. In the last, he describes different postures for union. Then he describes flagellation and its types, screams of various types, and lastly, the details of characteristics of the eight types of Nayikas.

Date: As regards Kalyanamalla[76] we can say that he flourished in the 16th century. Even though one Ahmad Khan flourished during the reign of Bahlul,[77] it is not known that the former had a son named Ladakhan interested in erotics. However, it is safe to say that Kalyanamalla wrote this work early in the 16 century AD.

KANDARPACHUDAMANI OF VIRABHADRA

This is a treatise on erotics modelled after Vatsyayana's Kama Sutra. It is divided into seven Adhikaranas. After adoring Bhairava, Krishna and Kamadeva, he traces the origin of the Vaghelas-Shalivahana, Birasinha, Virabhanu-Ramachandra and Virabhadra the author. He then traces the history of the works on erotics. In the course of time, these treatises either underwent great changes or went into oblivion, therefore Vatsyayana wrote Kama Sutra which is condensed into the present work.

In the first chapter, after describing the Trivarga and purpose of their study and practice, he deals with Nagaraka, Dutas, etc. Next he describes the various types of males and females, types of union, embraces, kisses, scratching, biting, postures for union, flagellation, *Purushayita, Auparishta*, method of beginning and ending the union, etc. From the third to the fifth Adhikarana he deals with maidens, marriage, consummation of marriage, choice of the male partner, ways and means of captivating her heart, different types of marriages, daily life of certain types of women, intercourse with other women and types of such men and women, employment of messengers and their duties and life in harems. In the sixth, he deals with courtesans. In the seventh, he gives ingredients of aphrodisiacs and those of improving defects in the anatomy for a better enjoyment of union. As regards the date, we know from the colophon that he wrote in 1633 V.S.

SHRINGARAMANJARI OF ST. ALI AKBAR SHAH

Bhanudatta compiled Rasaparijata. Therein we find mentioned the four classes of women, Padmini, etc. Shringaramanjari is closely related to Rasamanjari of Bhanudatta[78] and its commentary Arnoda. Akbar Shah alias Bade Saheb was the son of Shah Raja. The author has explained that his name Akbar (A-Ka-vara) denotes that even Vishnu and Brahma are not superior to him.

This Akbar wrote a book in Telugu named Shringaramanjari, and the present work is its Sanskrit version. Shah Raja was the teacher or the guru of Sultan Adul Hasan Qutb Shah of Golconda, known as Tana Shah, who was the last Qutbshahi king and who died in 1704. Dr Raghavan, after discussing the problem of the date, concludes: 'It is quite natural to suppose that some Telugh and Sanskrit poets associated with both the king (Thana Shah) and his spiritual preceptor and were connected with the production of this Shringaramanjan in Telugu and Sanskrit.' This work mainly deals with Nayakas and Nayikas. We are concerned only with his reference to the fourfold classification of Nayakas and Nayikas, to which a reference has already been made.

RATIKELIKUTUHALA

This is written by Pandita Mathura Prasada[79] in 1949. In fifteen Tarangas, he discusses masturbation and its effects, use of aphrodisiacs, classification of males and females, coital postures, prescriptions for overcoming sterility, increasing fecundity, prostitution, venereal diseases and medicines for their cure, ways and means of enticing the other party, and lastly, planned parenthood. This is a very good work, even though it appears quite modern. It is encyclopaedic in nature and has been written after a thorough study of previous works on erotics and the author's personal experience.

OTHER WORKS

Besides these, there are two other works, Ratishastra and Shringaradipika of Harihara. The latter is profusely quoted by Tripathi in his commentaries on Kuttanimata and Nagarasarvasva. It should be noted that Harihara gives the classification of Nayakas – Panchala, Kuchimara, Datta and Bhadra. Thus he differs from Vatsyayana and Kokkoka and those that followed them. There are other works which are perhaps unpublished as yet, such as Dinalapanika, Kamasamuha,[80] Kamapradipa, Ratikallolini, Samaradipika of Minanatha, Saugandhikaparinaya, Smaradipika of Maheshvara alias Rudra, Rativilasa, Kamasarvasva, Rasikasarvasva,[81] etc. Dr Gode has mentioned three more works.[82] I possess a printed copy of the Ratishastra which is in the form of a dialogue between Shiva and Parvati. It gives the fourfold classifications of males and females, their characteristics, qualifications of marriageable girls, fruits of their union at a particular time of the night, types of beds of the four kinds of females and methods of pleasing them. This appears to be an extract from some Purana.

Dinalapanika, besides treating other aspects of this science of erotics also gives the *Karanas* (postures for union). Similarly, Saugandhikaparinaya of Krishnaraja also gives these *Karanas* and also brings out the provincial variations. Smaradipika of Minanatha and that of Rudra are several times quoted by Tripathi. The Rativilasa is utilized by Raghava Bhatta in his commentary on Shakuntala (Act ii) and Kamasarvasva is quoted by Kumbha in his commentary on Gita Govinda and by the Tippanikara also. Ratisarvasva is quoted by Mallinatha in his Sanjivini on Meghadutta 102. Perhaps this work is the same as Kamasarvasva often quoted by Kumbha. Gunapataka referred to by Kokkoka is perhaps referred to by Mallinatha in his Sanjivini on Meghduta 108 as simply Pataka, while in his Sanjivini on Raghuvamsha 8-92, he does not mention the name, although he quotes the same verse. Shri Devidatta Sharma, in his introduction to the Tippani on Ratirahasya, adds the names of Pururawa, Bharata, Dandi, Daivagna-Surya, Shamaraja, Viranaradhya and Badarayana. But at present we know nothing about works on erotics by any of these writers.

COMMENTARIES

Here it is necessary to mention the commentaries of Arjunadeva (Amaruka Shataka), Kumbha (Gita Govinda), Shankara Mishra (Gita Govinda), Tripathi (Kuttanimata and Nagarasarvasva), all of which are extremely useful for a study of Indian erotics.

NOTES

1 (i) Vatsyayana, Kamasutra, 1-1-6 to 1-1-86; (ii) Schmidt, *Das Kama Sutram des Vatsyayana. Die Indische Ars Amatoria,* pp. 6-10. Yashodhara refers to the legend that when Mahadeva was engrossed in amorous alliance with Utha, lasting for one divine year, Nandi guarded that place and during that period wrote Kama Sutra.

2 Vatsyayana, ibid: (a) 1-2-21, 1-3-4, 2-1-70, 2-2-2, 2-4-24, 2-9-22, etc.; (b) 1-5-27, 2-2-4; (c) 1-2-45; (d) 1-2-37; (e) 1-5-25, 4-1-4, 4-1-21, 4-2-42 (f) 1-1-5, 1-5-34; (g) 1-5-24, 3-1-3, 3-1-10, 3-2-17; (h) 1-4-20, 1-5-22; (i) 1-5-33, 2-2-22, 2-6-21, 3-2-3, 4-2-40; (j) 1-2-30; (k) 1-5-23, 2-6-32.

3 Kokkoka, Ratirahasya: (a) 5-22; (b) 4-21; (c) 10-13, 26, 29; (d) 6-8, 11, 8-4; (e) 2-5.

4 Damodara, Kuttanimata, 77 and 123.

5 Jyotirisha, Panchasayaka: (a) 1-3, 3-36, 3-42; (b) 4-20; (c) 5-2; (d) 4-56; (e) 4-44, 47, 50, 53, 5-18, 39; (f) 3-6; (g) 2-7, 3-42; (h) 1-3; (i) 1-2-3.

6 Padmashri, Nagarasarvasva, 1, 16, 17, 24, 38.

7 Kalyanamalla, Anangaranga: (a) 1-4; (b) 9-3, 10-9; (c) 3-23, 25, 8-24, 9-10, 23, 25, 32; (d) 9-36; (e) 4-13, 10-11-20; (f) 3-5, 9-15; (g) 3-1, 4-35; (h) 7-41.

8 Ratirahasya, 10-18. Tippani.

9 Pt. M. Prasada, Ratikelikutuhala, 1-2, 7-33.

10 Ratirahasya, 13-91, comm. Kamasutra 1-19 comm. and 6-6-34 comm.

11 Mahabharata, 1-122-16 to 20.

12 Kamasutra, 2-1-67; Ratirahasya, 13-91 comm.

13 Kautilya, Arthashastra, 5-5-93.

14 Madras Triennial Catalogues, R. No. 3220(b) referred to by Dr Raghavan in his introduction to Shringaramanjari of St. Ali Akbar shah, p. 35, n.4.

15 Kamasutra, 6-3-44, 1-1-11 and comm., 6-3-19 and comm.

16 Mahabhashya, I, III, and VII.

17 (i) Kumarasambhava, 7-95, comm.; (ii) Raghuvamsha, 19-16, 29, 31, comm.

18 Mahabhashya, 1-4-51.

19 Ratirahasya, 13-91, comm. Nagoji Bhatta has identified him with Bhashyakara.

20 Jyotirisha, Panchasayaka, 1-3.

21 Kshemendra, Kalavilasa, 1, Note 1, pp. 36, 37.

22 Kamasutra, 6-3-45, 2-6-16, comm.

23 Jyotirisha, Panchasayaka, 3-42.

24 Shakuntala, 1-26.

25 Damodara, Kuttanimata; Tripathi's commentary on verses 504

(p. 145) and 124 (p. 28).

26 Padmashri, Nagarasarvasva, 16-2, comm., p. 52 an4 p. 120.

27 Kshemendra, (1) Kalavilasa, 1-9 and note. (2) Brihatkatha, 9th and 10 lambakas.

28 Kamasutra, comm. Mulakarma in 4-1-26, 6-1-16, 6-2-36; Mula Kala in 1-3-15; Mulakarika in 4-1-20, 4-1-9; Muladeva in 6-1-17, 2-4-25.

28a Kamasutra, 1-3-16, comm. on Art. No. 45.

28b Mahabharata, 3-233-14.

29 Ratirahasya, 6-8, 11; 8-4, comm.

30 Nagarasarvasva, p. 121.

31 Ratirahasya, 10-13; 10-26; 10-29, comm.

32 Damodara, Kuttanimata, 77, comm. p. 18; 123 comm. p. 28.

32a Kamasutra, 2-6-17, comm.

32b Kamasutra, 2-6-33, comm.

33 Mahabharata, (a) 2-65, 4-14; (b) 3-46; (c) 5-116.

34 Ramayana, (a) 3-46; 6-12; (b) 7-26; (c) 6-48; (d) 5-9, 10.

35 Agni Purana, 244.

36 Garuda Purana, 65.

37 Harivamsha, Punyaka Vidhi, 136, 140-7722-7956.   -

38 Devi Bhagavata, 6-21.

39 Shrimad Bhagavata, 2-2, 3-15, 4-21, 4-25, 8-6, 8-8, 9 and 9, 10-39.

40 Ashvaghosha, Buddhacharita, 2, 3, 4, 5.

41 Vimalasuri, Paumachariya, 11, 14, 26, 70.

42 (i) Raghuvamsha, 3, 7, 19; (ii) Kumarasambhava, 1, 7, 8, 9, etc. Keith has remarked that Kumara 3-68, 7-77, and Raghu 6-81 violate Kama Sutra, cf. *History of Sanskrit Literature*, p. 469, n.1.

43a Bharata, Natyashastra (Kashi ed. 25). This whole chapter deserves to be studied comparatively with Kamasutra V-4 and VI.

43 Bharata, Natyashastra, 22 (Kashi ed. 24).

44 Kokkoka, Ratirahasya, 4.

45 Jyotirisha, Panchasayaka, 1.

46 Kalyanamalla Anangaranga, 4.

47 Harihara, Shringaradipika, quoted by Tripathi in Kuttanima4, 652, comm.

48 St. Ali Akbar Shah, Shringaramanjari, p. 54. Raghavan. Introduction to Shringaramanjari pp. 16-18.

49 Devaraya, Ratiratnapradipika, 14-74-75, quoted by Tripathi in his commentary on Kuttanimata, 823.

50 Kautiliya, Arthashastra, ed. Shama Shastry, Intro., p. II.

51 Bhandarkar, Proc. Oriental Congress, Poona, I, p. 251.

52 Keith, *History of Sanskrit Literature*, pp. 51, 461, 467-469.

53 *Social Lfe in Ancint India*, pp. 11-35. Prof. S. K. De while evaluating the

merits of the Kamasutra has not at all discussed this problem. Cf.
De, *Ancient Indian Erotics & Erotic Literature,* pp. 85-104.

54   Shastri, Prachina Charitra Kosha, pp. 307, 520. Taittiriya Aranyaka,
      I-7-2.
55   Kamasutra, I-2-33, comm., Schmidt, *Das Kamasutra,* p. 24.
56   Kautiliya, Arthashastra, ed. Shama Shastry, Intro., p. 14.
57   Keith, ibid, p. 461.
58   Winterniz, *History of Indian Literature,* p. 519, n. 3.
59   Mahika, Haramekhala, Pts. I & 2. Mabuka the son of Madhava
      finished his Haramekhala in V. S. 887. It deals with various kinds of
      incenses, treatment of some diseases, secret recipes for extra virility,
      etc. Kokkoka has actually referred to him and acknowledged his
      indebtedness to this author, in his Ratirahasya (Ch. XIV). A number
      of verses in Ratirahasya, chapters XIV & XV, bear very close resem-
      blance to some verses in Haramekhala Parichchedas, 2, 3, 4, etc.
60   Ravana, Uddisha Tantra with Hindi commentary. Uddisha Tantra by
      Ravana is in verse. It contains Kavachas and Mantras and Chapters
      on Vashikarana, Akarshana, etc. Kokkoka in his Ratiraliasya, admits
      having studied and availed of the material in Uddisha Tantra. The
      present work therefore may be before the 10th century AD.
61   Gita Govinda: (*a*) Rasikapriya, I-12, 2-3-5, 2-3-7, 8, 8-4, II-I-3, etc.
      (*b*) Rasamanjari. 2-3-5, 2-3-7, 8.
62   Kumarasambhava, 8-6, 9; (*b*) Raghuvamsha, 19-25, 32; (*c*) Meghaduta,
      29, 83.
63   Kumarasambhava, 7-94.
64   Keith, ibid, p. 461.
64a   Pandita N. Prerni, Jaina Sahitya and Itihasa, pp. 61-92.
65   Mahuka, Haramekhala Introduction, T.S.S., CXXIV, Pt. I.
66   Keith, ibid, p. 236.
67   (*i*) Kavyamala 10, Samayamatrika; (*ii*)Kavyamala Ist Guchchha,
      Kalavilasa; (*iii*) Deshopadeshamala; (*iv*) Keith, ibid, 136, etc; (*v*) *The
      Sanskrit Drama,* pp. 236, 240, etc.
68   Kavyamala Ist Guchchha, pp. 34-35.
69   Nagarasarvasva, Tippani, pp. 15, 116.
70   Keith, ibid, pp. 467-470.
71   Desai, *Shri Forbes Sabha Mahotsava Grantha,* p. 258.
72   Jyotirisha, Varnaratnakara, ed. by Chatterji, p. 13, etc.
73   Gita Govinda, Rasamanjari, 2-5-6, etc.
74   Ratiratnapradipika: (*a*) I-4; (*b*) I-4, 40, 68; (*c*) 2-34, 76, 3-26, 44, 69,
      5-27; (*d*) 5-16; (*e*) 4-16; (*f*) 4-24, 5-47; (*g*) 5-47, 7-27; (*h*) 2-36.
75   Kuttanimata, 403, comm.
75a   Gode, *Studies in Indian Literary History,* Vol. I, p. 281, n.l.

[76] Keith, ibid, p. 470.

[77] *Cambridge History of India,* Vol. III, Ch. IX, pp. 229-230.

[78] Raghavan, ibid, pp. 5-9.

[79] Pt. M. Prasada, Ratikelikutuhala, 1, 2, 3.

[80] Gode, *Studies in Indian Literary History,* Vol. I, pp. 494-500 and Vol. II, pp. 176-181. Ananta the son of Mandana wrote Kamasamuha in V.S. 1514. He was a Nagara Brahmin and hailed from Ahmedabad. His guru was Anandapurna. His work Kamasamuha is an anthology bearing on Kamashastra and its several topics.

[81] Jagaddhara composed one Rasikasarvasva which is perhaps the same as the one quoted by Kumbha.

[82] Shringarakallola is a love poem by Rayabhatta who flourished before AD 1550. Shringaralapa by Rama is a big anthology of Shringara verses written before AD 1556. Shringarasanjivini of Harideva is a poem of about 100 verses on Shrhigara, written between AD 1650 and 1700. Gode, ibid, Vol. II, pp. 62-64; 97-106; 211-215.

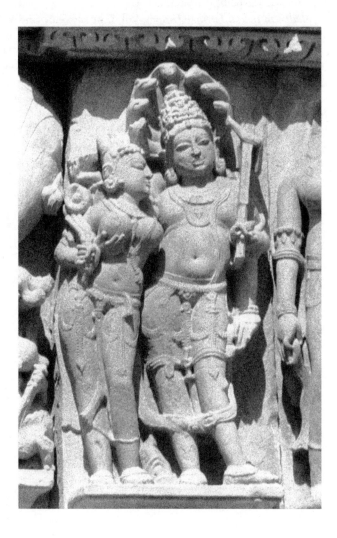

PART I

GENERAL

CHAPTER I

INTRODUCTION TO THE SUTRAS

SUTRAS 1-4

Salutation to Dharma,[1] Artha,[2] and Kama.[3] The three Aims of Life that are dealt with in this Shastra (scientific treatise). Salutation also to those masters who have made a deep study of these subjects, and to those sages who have disseminated their teaching. Indeed, the work of both has great bearing on our present subject.

SUTRAS 5-10

In the beginning, the Lord created men and women, and having regard for their well being, He revealed in 10,000 chapters, the ways of securing the threefold Aims of Dharma, Artha and Kama. Of these, some chapters dealing with Dharma were gleaned by the self-born Manu; others dealing with Artha were propounded by Brihaspati, and the remaining chapters that dealt with Kama were collected by Nandi, the follower of Mahadeva, into 1,000 chapters.

Later, Shvetaketu, son of Uddalaka, condensed Nandi's work into 500 chapters, while these in turn were further abridged by Babhravya, a native of the Panchala province, into 150 chapters under the following seven sections:

- ◆ General observations.
- ◆ Union of man and woman.
- ◆ Selection of the bride, marriage, etc.
- ◆ Position and conduct of one's wife.
- ◆ Extra-marital relations with wives of other men.
- ◆ Courtesans and their ways.
- ◆ Secret formulas, tonic medicines, and so forth.

SUTRAS 11-17

The sixth section dealing with courtesans was separately elaborated by Dattaka at the request of the courtesans of Pataliputra, and following Dattaka's example, Charayana detailed the first section. Other writers similarly treated the remaining sections thus:

- ◆ Suvarnanabha   the second part
- ◆ Ghotakamukha the third part
- ◆ Gonardiya   the fourth part
- ◆ Gonikaputra   the fifth part
- ◆ Kuchumara   the seventh part

In this way, the work became so mutilated in the course of time as to be almost lost. Furthermore, since the work of Babhravya was too long and intricate, and since the works of Dattaka and the other authors mentioned above treated only the isolated aspects of the whole subject, Vatsyayana condensed their individual contributions as concisely as possible, and composed the present work.

NOTES

1   Dharma is the practice of religion.
2   Artha indicates material prosperity.
3   Kama includes sensual pleasures.

CHAPTER II

THE PURSUIT OF THE THREE AIMS OF LIFE

SUTRA 1. Man is said to be granted a life span of a hundred years. He should pursue the three Aims of Dharma, Artha and Kama at different periods in his life, either one or more at a time but in such a way as to harmonize with each other and not clash in any way.

SUTRAS 2-4. In childhood, he should devote himself to acquiring knowledge; in youth, he should engage in worldly pleasures, and in his old age, he should aspire to salvation through the practice of Dharma.

SUTRAS 5-6. Since life is riddled with uncertainties, a man may pursue these in any manner he chooses, provided he observes celibacy during his term of study. (Otherwise, instead of imbibing knowledge, he will become impious and harm his own interest. There is, however, no restriction on owning land or property during the period of study.)

SUTRAS 7-8. Dharma implies acting according to the injunctions of the sacred texts, such as performing sacrifices, which are supernatural, and whose effects are not humanly visible;. Dharma also forbids certain things like eating meat, which have visible effects on human beings. Dharma should be learnt from these sacred texts and from those conversant with them.

SUTRAS 9-10. Artha is the acquisition of knowledge and wealth in the shape of land, gold, cattle, food-grains, utensils, friends, and so forth. One should learn about Artha from merchants who are well-versed in the ways of trade and commerce.

SUTRAS 11-13. Kama is the enjoyment of objects with the help of the five senses – of hearing, of speech, of sight, of taste and of smell, according to the dictates of his mind in consonance with his soul. Actually, Kama is that special pleasure experienced when the sense of touch operates, and when it is in contact with the object that generates pleasure. Kama is to be learnt from the Kama Sutra and also from the worldly-wise citizen.

SUTRAS 14-17. As the three Aims stand, Dharma, Artha and Kama, the former is better than the latter, i.e., Dharma is better than Artha and Artha is better than Kama. But this order of procedure is not applicable in all cases. With a king, Artha is of prime importance, since the very livelihood of his subjects depends on it. Similarly Kama comes first with courtesans.

OBJECTION I

SUTRAS 18-21. Some learned men say that it is proper that Dharma should be treated of in a learned text, since the effects of the precepts are elusive and supernatural: they maintain similarly that Artha can also be learnt only through books, since it is practised by special methods. But they argue that since Kama is instinctively practised even by the animal world, a learned text on the subject becomes redundant.

ANSWER

SUTRAS 22-24. This is not true. The ways of men and women differ from those of the lower animals, and there are other important considerations relating to their intermingling. A clear enunciation of these therefore becomes essential and this can be seen in the Kama Sutra of Vatsyayana. Among the lower animals, however, the females are free to do what they like: moreover, they have congress purely by instinct and only during certain periods, hence instructions for them, it is true, are rendered rather superfluous.

OBJECTION 2

SUTRAS. 25-30. The Lokayatikas[1] contend that since the fruits of religious rites may only be tasted in afterlife, and since those benefits are usually a matter of doubt anyway, religious rites need not be performed. Indeed, which sane person forfeits his own possessions to another? As the old adage goes, a pigeon in hand today is better than a peacock tomorrow; and a coin we are certain of obtaining, though it be of copper, is preferable to a gold one which may or may not be ours.

ANSWER

SUTRA 31. Vatsyayana's reply to that is that religious precepts must be obeyed for the following reasons:

- The sacred texts which ordain the practice of Dharma, do not admit of a doubt.
- Sacrifices for exorcising evil spirits certainly have visible results.
- The constellations the sun, the moon, the stars, the planets, exert their influence as if intentionally for the good of creation.
- The affairs of this world are wholly dependent on the conduct of men throughout their four classes[2] and their four stages of life.[3]
- A seed is sown in anticipation of its further blossoming.

OBJECTION 3

SUTRAS 32-37. Believers in the force of destiny maintain that it is useless to pursue Artha, since at times it eludes one in spite of great effort. At other times, Artha comes to a man unasked, and as if by sheer chance or accident. All this is the doing of destiny. It is destiny alone which brings wealth to a man, hurls him into poverty, crowns him with victory, brings defeat to him, showers happiness on him, and heaps misery on him. It was destiny that raised Bali[4] to the throne of Indra: it was also destiny that wrought his subsequent downfall, and only destiny could have reinstated him.

ANSWER

SUTRAS 38-39. To this Vatsyayana replies that every object that is gained or enjoyed by man presupposes at least some effort on his part. Even if a thing is destined to happen, it can only happen after some effort in that direction has been made. Good things never come to the inactive.

OBJECTION 4

SUTRAS 40-45. The champions of Artha argue that the pursuit of Kama, or life's pleasures, is detrimental to the other two Aims of Life – Dharma and Artha. It leads him into the company of wicked persons, undesirable occupations, unclean habits and impure deeds; it also deprives him of future prospects. It engenders rashness and undue haste, and makes him unacceptable and untrustworthy in the eyes of all.

Many are the devotees of Kama one hears of in history, who have been vanquished en masse. For instance,[5] take King Dandakya of the Bhoja dynasty, who became enamoured of the Brahmin maiden and perished with his kinsmen and kingdom. (The story goes that when King Dandakya set out on a hunt, he came upon this Brahmin maiden, the daughter of Bhrigu, and was smitten by her. He kidnapped her in his chariot. Bhrigu, returning to his hermitage after gathering fuel for his daily sacrifices, missed her, and discovered what had happened. He cursed the king and his kingdom and both perished in an incessant shower of dust. That place is still known as Dandakaranya.) Similarly, Indra, the most powerful of gods, was enamoured of Ahalya the mighty. Kichaka lusted for Draupadi; Ravana overpowered and abducted Sita – these and many others were disgraced through their subjection to Kama.

ANSWER

SUTRAS 46-48. To this Vatsyayana's reply is that the pleasures of Kama are as essential for the proper maintenance of the human body as is food. Moreover, they take their very roots in Dharma and Artha. Granted, one must, however, acknowledge and beware of the dangers. Do people refrain from cooking food simply because there are beggars? Do they not sow the seeds of barley in spite of the deer eating their sprouts?

SUTRAS 49-51. In this way, a man who pursues Dharma, Artha and Kama, experiences untrammelled happiness both in this world and in the world to come, unimpeded. Wise men direct their actions without undue regard to what will result from them in afterlife, but with due regard to their own welfare. That action which is conducive to the Aims of Dharma, Artha and Kama together, or to any two of the three, or even to one of them is to be desired, but certainly not such an action that will further one at the expense of the other two Aims of Life.

NOTES

1. The followers of the Lokayata system, who were essentially materialists.
2. Hindu society was in those days divided into four classes: The Brahmin, or the priestly class; the Kshatriya, or the warrior class; the Vaishya or the merchant or peasant class; the Shudra, or the menial class.
3. The four stages in a man's life are: that of a student; that of a householder; that of a hermit, and that of an ascetic.
4. Bali in Hindu mythology was a demon who desired to dethrone Indra, but was subsequently banished by Vishnu to Patala.
5. Kautilya, Arthashastra, 1-6-3.

CHAPTER III

THE STUDY OF THE VARIOUS ARTS

SUTRAS 1-4. Man should study the Kama Sutra and its subsidiary arts alongside the arts and the sciences contained in Dharma and Artha. A maiden should study the Kama Sutra and the subsidiary arts before marriage, and in the event of her marriage, should study the same with her husband's consent. (The husband's consent is necessary, otherwise she is likely to be branded as coquettish and wayward.) Here some learned men object with the argument that since women are barred from studying the sacred texts, their initiation into this science is meaningless.

SUTRAS 5-11. Against this Vatsyayana contends that women are already familiar with the practice of this science, and this text is merely the summing up of the science into a set of principles; therefore, it is not in any way out of place or meaningless.

This argument holds not merely in the case of the Kama Sutra: everywhere in this world one finds that while the practice of a particular science is known to all, only a few are acquainted with the rules and the laws on which the science is based. Indeed, the Shastra of the text is the fountainhead, however remote, of the practice of every science. For instance, take the priests presiding over sacrificial rites: even though they themselves are not grammarians, they freely use the 'Uha' in the rites, fully recognising the fact that there is a standard grammar. ('Uha' is thoughtfully guessing the meaning of a word and then using it. The priests, though no scholars of grammar, are able to do it through habitual practice and traditional knowledge.) A similar instance is of people who perform good deeds and pious actions on auspicious days, who are themselves no astrologers, but who simply believe that they are acting according to the dictates of the science of astrology. Again, horsemen and mahouts are found training horses and elephants, even though they have not studied the science of horse-training and elephant-training. In the same way, people in the most far-flung districts of a kingdom obey the laws, knowing that, there is a king in authority. The study of the Kama Sutra on the part of women is exactly analogous to these instances.

SUTRA 12. There are, however, some courtesans, princesses and daughters of ministers whose minds are literally befogged through excessive effort at learning the texts.

SUTRA 13. It is advisable therefore that a woman should study this text or part of it and also the practical application of its principles privately with the help of a person worthy of her confidence.

SUTRA 14. A maiden should study in private the sixty-four practices detailed in the text of the Kama Sutra.

SUTRA 15. Her instructor should be one of the following persons:
- The daughter of a nurse brought up with her and already married.
- A woman companion, sweet-spoken, who can be trusted in everything and who is also married.
- The daughter of her mother's sister and her equal in age.
- A trusty old woman servant, who is to the maiden like her own mother's sister.
- A woman who is experienced, but who is now a mendicant.

◆ Her own elder sister who can always be trusted.

(Among these, the mendicant woman is recommended because of her varied experiences gathered during her wanderings, while the elder sister is mentioned as a suitable instructor because she would be free from malice or envy.)

SUTRA 16. The sixty-four arts which are auxiliary to the Kama Sutra are enumerated below:

1. Vocal music.
2. Instrumental music.
3. Dancing.
4. Painting.
5. Cutting of different designs on the Bhurja leaf for adorning the forehead.
6. Making various designs with rice-grains and flowers (in temples of Sarasvati, Kamadeva, etc., or on floors set with jewels).
7. Arrangements of flowers (in temples and homes).
8. Colouring teeth, garments, hair, nails, body and other toiletries.
9. Fixing coloured tiles on the floor.
10. Arrangement of the bed, the settee, the divan (according to bedtime mood and food partaken).
11. Creating musical sounds with water. (Jalataranga.)
12. Splashing and squirting with water. (Jalakrida.)
13. The various secret formulas and mantras and their application (other than those mentioned by Kuchumara).
14. Making various garlands (for worshipping deities and adorning one's self with).
15. Making head decorations known as Shekharaka and Apida. (The Shekharaka garland hangs down from the top of the head. The Apida is worn round the head and supported by a wooden frame.)
16. Dressing and decorating the body (according to time and place).

17. Making designs called Karnapatra (with ivory and conch materials for additional decoration to costumes).
18. The preparation and proper use of perfumes.
19. Making ornaments (joined or stringed ones such as necklaces with jewels and pearls; whole ones such as bracelets, round earrings, etc.).
20. Magic and creating illusions.
21. Preparation of ointments (for additional physical charm and virility. These recipes are expounded by Kuchumara).
22. Deftness in manual work (for instance, in games where throwing and snatching money and other things are included).
23. Cooking and similar culinary arts. [It is interesting to note that food and drink were divided into four sections, viz., Bhakshya (eating), Bhojya (chewing), Lahya (licking) and Peya (drinking).]
24. Preparing sherbats and drinks.
25. Needlework (including making new garments and mending of old ones, darning, making mats, etc.).
26. Creating patterns from yarns or threads (such as the parrot motif, flower motif, tassels and so forth).
27. Playing on the Veena and the drum called Damaruka.
28. Composing and solving riddles and rhymes (for play and discussion).
29. A game in which one party recites a verse and the opposite party recites another which begins with the same letter as that on which the last verse ended.
30. Reciting verses difficult to repeat, tongue twisters and so on.
31. Recitation from books (generally from the Epics).
32. Knowledge of dramas and stories.
33. Composing other lines when one is given. (This takes the form of a game in which one person is given the last out of four lines and is challenged to compose the first three on the spot.)
34. Caning of wood-frames of cots, chairs and so forth.
35. Making of mechanical aids. (This refers particularly to those

recommended for use during congress, and which are usually made of silver, gold, steel, bone, or ivory.)

36. Carpentry (making wooden furniture for sitting, reclining and sleeping).

37. Knowledge of architecture and house construction.

38. Knowledge of precious metals and precious stones (especially the ability to distinguish between genuine and fake gems).

39. Knowledge of metals (extracting, refining, alloying, etc.).

40. Knowledge of jewels, colours and mines. (Crystals are coloured for sale, while knowledge of mines is considered important for purposes of income.)

41. Horticulture and gardening. (This includes sowing and growing plants in a nursery.)

42. Art of cockfighting, ram-fighting and quail-fighting. (This is one of the games of wagering where animate things are made use of.)

43. Training parrots and mynas to speak and sing. (If trained properly, these birds can memorise messages and carry them where their owner wishes.)

44. Proficiency in pressing, shampooing and dressing hair.

45. The art of understanding writing in cipher, and the writing of words in a peculiar way.

46. Talking in a language with deliberate transposing of words or letters. (This takes various forms: for instance, when the beginning and the end of words are interchanged, or when unnecessary letters are added in between syllables of a word and so on.)

47. Knowledge of languages of other provinces and of various dialects.

48. Art of making flower-carriages; Dolis, Palakhis, etc.

49. Art of addressing spells, charms, auspicious and bad omens, etc.

50. Constructing mechanical aids (such as those for riding, drawing water from well and for use in warfare, etc.).

51. Memory training.

52. Recitation of verse. (This game is played in company with

others. While one recites from a book, another recites it alongside him purely by hearing.)

53. Deciphering by code (when a message or verse is left incomplete but with designs of flowers, etc.).

54. Knowledge of etymology (of Sanskrit, Prakrit and Apabhramsha).

55. Knowledge of lexicography.

56. Prosody and rhetoric.

57. Art of impersonation. (Deceiving others by impersonating and assumed personality: Shurpanakha and Bhima did this successfully.)

58. Wearing garments artfully (in a way that will conceal torn or ill-fitting garments).

59. Various games to be played with the dice.

60. The game of dice called Akarsha. (Nala and Yudhisthira, history tells us, lost in this game because they did not know the niceties and intricacies of the game. It is to be played on a board.)

61. Making dolls and playthings for children.

62. Knowledge of proper behaviour. (In other words, knowledge of etiquette in public and in private gatherings. In another sense, 'Vainayiki' also implies the training of elephants and other domestic animals.)

63. Knowledge of the science of victory. (Knowledge of 'Aparajita Vidya' is essential for divine purposes, while knowledge of the science of warfare is essential for the purposes of this world.)

64. Physical culture.

PHYSICAL CULTURE.

These sixty-four arts are an essential part of the science of Kama Sutra.

A list of 64 Mulakalas (the knowledge of which is essential) is given. There are 24 arts which are technically called Karmashraya, i.e., which require some use of technical skill and physical exertion.

They are:

1. Vocal music.
2. Dancing.
3. Instrumental music.
4. Script of other provinces.
5. Graceful speech.
6. Painting.
7. Doll making.
8. Cutting Bhurja leaves according to designs.
9. Making garlands and bouquets.
10. Cookery with special knowledge of mixing of tasty ingredients.
11. Distinguishing genuine gems from fake ones.
12. Needlework.
13. Preparing colours and dyeing garments.
14. Keeping ready required quantity of flour, etc., before cooking.
15. Weights and measures.
16. Source of daily and future livelihood.
17. Veterinary science.
18. Magic, jugglery and tricks.
19. Proficiency in games.
20. Knowledge of other people.
21. Cleverness.
22. Shampooing.
23. Toilet.
24. Hairstyles and adorning the forehead.

There are 20 arts based on wagering. Out of these, 15 are Nirjiva and 5 Sajiva. They are:

25. The game of three dice.
26. The art of jingling them and playing by scattering them advantageously on the floor.
27. Holding out the closed fist full of dice and questioning

regarding the quantity concealed therein.

28. Knowledge of the places of their movements.
29. Extracting money from the husband when the reply is correct.
30. Giving correct and indisputable decision.
31. Snatching the amount placed as wager.
32. Different wagering games.
33. Keeping the amount in the fist and questioning about its quantity and then showing it.
34. Settling of accounts – loss and gain.
35. Taking away the money won, without loss of time.
36. Account of the amount won.
37. Carefully proceeding further at each turn in the game.
38. Misguiding the other party.
39. Giving away the amount (which is wrongfully taken).

These fifteen (25-39) are Nirjiva as the things played with are inanimate.

Now there are 5 Sajiva dealing with animate things, such as:
40. Keeping ready the birds or animals for games.
41. Encouraging their mutual fight.
42. Calling them by particular sounds and cries.
43. Releasing them for the actual action, e.g., flying or fighting, etc.
44. Making them dance.

There are 16 bedroom arts. They are:
45. Knowing the mood of the other person.
46. Expressing one's sentiments.
47. Offering oneself physically.
48. Teeth- and nail-marks.
49. Unloosening of the waistband.
50. Physical contact.
51. Dexterity in love-sport.

52. Giving extreme pleasure to the other person.
53. Obtaining complete satisfaction and reciprocating it.
54. Encouraging the other person in love-sport.
55. Showing slight anger and continuing the love-sport.
56. Controlling anger properly at the right time.
57. Propitiating the angry person.
58. Leaving the sleeping partner.
59. The way of sleeping last (or the last sleep).
60. Sleeping with the body properly covered.

There are four Uttarakalas, i.e., those which are to be done last. They are:
61. Exchanging words with tears.
62. Putting one's name before the husband, as a means to let him refrain from undertaking a journey.
63. Following him if not refraining from separating.
64. Looking in his direction if going away without hearing her appeals.

There are 518 Antarakalas in these 64 Mulakalas. In the Kama Sutra (Sutra 16 above), 64 Aupayiki Kalas are enumerated by manipulation of the first 44 Mulakalas. The remaining 20 Mulakalas are described in Part II dealing with sexual union.

SUTRAS 17-19. The sixty-four Panchalika arts, however, are different from these sixty-four mentioned above. We shall speak about them at the proper time, when dealing with the congress of sexes in Part II. They are actually of the very essence of Kama.

SUTRA 20 (verse). A courtesan, endowed with character, beauty, and virtues attains an honoured place among the public and acquires the rank of Ganika if she is an expert in these sixty-four arts.

SUTRA 21 (verse). Such a woman is ever honoured by the king and lauded even by the virtuous, and since she is sought after, and courted by one and all, she becomes the cynosure among her class and enjoys universal regard.

SUTRA 22 (verse). A princess or a daughter of a highborn official, as long as she cultivates these sixty-four arts, will certainly enjoy her husband's favour in spite of his having a thousand wives in his harem.

SUTRA 23 (verse). A cultivated woman like that can happily survive with the help of these talents in the face of great calamity of separation from her husband or even in foreign lands.

SUTRA 24 (verse). Similarly, a man who is an expert in these arts, who is well spoken and well mannered, instantly wins over women's hearts, though he be a total stranger to them.

SUTRA 25 (verse). A person's good fortune arises from the proper cultivation of the arts. However, he must always bear in mind the fitness of time and place before he puts them into practice. (He may exercise his talents, for instance, in the presence of citizens who like fairs and excursions and theatrical performances. On the other hand, he may desist if he feels that he is among citizens who cannot appreciate them and his talents, or if he finds that there is famine or drought and if the citizens are in no mood to be entertained.)

CHAPTER IV

THE DAILY LIFE OF A CITZEN

SUTRA 1. After a man has acquired learning, it behoves him to start his life as a householder with whatever money he is fit to earn: either through the acceptance of alms and gifts (as a Brahmin may do), or through conquests (as a Kshatriya may do), or through the sale of merchandise (as a Vaishya may do) or through serving these three classes of men (which it is the lot of a Shudra to perform); and having done so, he should assume the duties of an educated and cultivated gentleman. (A poor man cannot adopt the role of a refined and educated gentleman.)

SUTRAS 2-3. He should take up his abode in a capital city (of 800 villages), or in a provincial capital, or even in a smaller town dominating either 400 or 200 villages. Wherever his residence, it must at least be in the vicinity of cultivated and refined people, and must be within easy access of his workplace.

SUTRA 4. There he should construct his house with two blocks (one of them must be for sleeping, and the other for cooking and so forth), amidst sylvan surroundings and where water is available in plenty. It must have separate rooms for different domestic requirements.

SUTRA 5. The outer block should house the bedroom where a cot should be placed supporting a soft bed with two pillows on either side and covered with clean bed linen. There should be another cot nearby. (Since the sacred texts forbid the pious man to sleep in the same bed after congress with a woman, the other bed becomes essential for that purpose. The second bed is usually lower than the main bed.)

SUTRAS 6-8. A mat must be placed adjoining the head of the main bed (for the purpose of worshipping the family deity). Near it should be a platform (an arm-length by another arm-length square and as high as the bed, with a tiled surface) for putting the remains, left at night, of sandal-paste, flowers and garlands, pots of collyrium and perfumes, betel leaves and the bark of the citron tree. (The box of perfumes contains leaves of the Tamala used as a deodorant, and the bark of the Matulunga for removing bad breath; the betel leaves, which are kept ready with proper ingredients, are eaten at night.)

SUTRA 9. On the floor should stand a spittoon.

SUTRA 10. While along the wall, on separate ivory pegs, should be hung the Vina, materials for painting and sketching, a book (which the citizen is currently reading), and garlands of the amaranth flowers. (The Vina must be kept covered, while the flowers lend charm to the pleasures of love, specially since they do not crush and wither easily. The amaranth flowers are considered to be auspicious for love. These various objects hanging on the wall reflect the good taste of the citizen.)

SUTRA 11. Not too distant along the ground, a circular mat with a cushion must be arranged.

SUTRA 12. Also handy must be one board for the dice game and another for other games. (These must stand against the wall.)

SUTRA 13. Birds domesticated for sport should be in cages hanging outside the bedroom. (These should be hung on pegs outside, since otherwise the room will be filled with a foul smell.)

SUTRA 14. A separate place must be allotted for the making of artificial aids for congress. (Usually a separate room is set aside for women to indulge in indoor games, out of sight of other people.)

SUTRA 15. Beyond this in the garden a whirling swing should be situated under a canopy of flowering creepers, in such a way that the seat of the swing is perennially covered with flowers (dropping from above).

So much regarding the construction of the citizen's abode.

SUTRA 16. The citizen, having awakened early in the morning, and after performing the necessary duties imposed by nature, cleaning his teeth, applying cool sandalwood paste while performing the morning worship, burning incense, decorating himself with flowers and garlands, applying wax and red Alaktaka, (liquid made from lac), admiring his own mien in the looking glass and chewing betel leaf and other sweet-smelling ingredients, should then attend to his daily work. (Such is a citizen's daily toilet. The sandal-paste is used sparingly. The Alaktaka stick should be moistened slightly before it is applied to both lips evenly, and the betel leaf is then chewed to heighten the red colour. Wax is then applied to the lips to preserve the colour for a long time, while betel leaves, already prepared with the proper ingredients, are carried in a small box for ready use.)

SUTRA 17. Bathing should be a daily affair; limbs must be massaged on alternate days; every third day, Phenaka, a foam-producing and cleansing substance must be applied to the thighs, every fourth day, the face must be shaved while every fifth or every tenth day, other parts of the body must be shaved. These chores must be performed without fail. (Bath is necessary for cleanliness and lustre. Massage is required for keeping the limbs sturdy. Phenaka is to be applied on the day affixed, as otherwise soft parts will be rough. The Shastras lay down that shaving of beard and moustaches should be done thrice in a fortnight, i.e., Ayushya type of shaving should be done on the fourth day; the Pratyayushya type of shaving should be done on the tenth day.)

SUTRA 18. Now and again, perspiration should be wiped off from the armpits in case they are covered. (Normally armpits are kept uncovered, but this is not always possible and when it is not, the citizen must keep a handkerchief handy for the purpose, otherwise the stale smell will brand him as unrefined.)

SUTRA 19. Meals should be taken in the forenoon and in the afternoon. (The day is divided into eight equal parts. The first three are devoted to work; the fourth, to bathing and meals; and the late afternoon, to the evening meal.)

SUTRA 20. Even Charayana is of the same opinion in this matter. (*But* the afternoon meal is not so conducive to health and strength as is the evening meal).

SUTRA 21. After the forenoon meal, the citizen should indulge in teaching and listening to domesticated birds such as parrots, mynas and so forth; watch fights between quails, cocks and rams, and generally indulge in other artistic pastimes; then in the company of the Pithamarda, the Vita and the Vidushaka,[1] he should entertain himself with repartees and witticisms; and finally, he should enjoy a siesta. (The Shastras forbid the afternoon nap except in the summer or during convalescence.)

SUTRA 22. Later during the afternoon, the citizen having donned his proper garments, should go out to converse with his friends.

SUTRA 23. In the evening, there should be music.

SUTRA 24. And afterwards, he and his friends should await the arrival of the ladies in the bedroom, in his own house, decorated and filled with the fragrance of burning incense. Either he should send lady-messengers to fetch the ladies or he should go to fetch them himself.

SUTRA 25 After their arrival at his house, he and his friends should welcome them and entertain them with pleasant and agreeable anecdotes. Should the ladies be travelling from a distant place, and should their make-up be smudged by rain, the citizen should himself attend to it again.

So much regarding the duties for the day. (The post-reception part of his duties at night is dealt with in Part II of this text.)

SUTRA 26. He should occasionally undertake such diversions as are mentioned below:

- ◆ Going out to festivals and worship in an organized group.
- ◆ Gatherings of cultured citizens for discussions on topics of art.
- ◆ Social parties.
- ◆ Excursions to public parks, picnics.
- ◆ Sports and parlour games.

FESTIVALS

SUTRAS 27-33. Every fortnight or every month, an assembly of Niyuktas (appointed for religious duties) must be convened on a certain auspicious day in the temple of the goddess Saraswati. Also present must be the accredited temple actors from near and far, who should give a performance on the first day for the benefit of the citizens. On the second day of the festival, the actors should be rewarded by the temple authorities. (There are usually two types of actors: those whose fees are fixed earlier and those whose fees are not fixed. The latter usually received gifts from the citizens spontaneously, during or after the show.) The actors should repeat their performance if there is a strong demand, or else return gracefully. It is the duty of the citizens. to cooperate with the temple authorities in every way – in difficulties or in celebrations. (The show must proceed without hindrance from the audience. Again, in case of emergency, the temple authorities may require the help of a guest artist, from a member of the audience, to which request he must comply.) The duties of the host require him to attend to the needs of those actors, Nagarakas, etc., who have travelled to the festival from afar.

In this way, other festivals should be celebrated in honour of the various deities on the time and place auspicious to each one of them.

Cultural Gatherings

SUTRAS 34-36. The term 'Goshthi' refers to a conclave of citizens of similar age and wealth, learning, intelligence and character, who meet either in the house of a courtesan, or of another citizen or in a pandal, and engage in agreeable discussions. Topics dealing with poetry, drama and the other arts are here discussed. (At the end of these discussions, usually the most brilliant and the most popular speaker is honoured with rewards. Quite often these happened to be courtesans who in those days were fluent debaters.)

Social Parties

SUTRAS 37-38. Social parties should be organized in the house of every citizen by turn. At these parties, courtesans should ply the citizens with the fare provided, and they should themselves share the various delicacies of salts, fruits, green vegetables, pungent, bitter and acid-flavoured dishes.

Picnics

SUTRAS 39-40. The preceding Sutra also explains how excursions should be arranged. The citizens, having dressed with care and mounted their horses, should embark on the excursion in the forenoon, followed by their lady-companions and attendants. Then, having performed the day's duties and having watched and wagered heavily on fights between cocks, quails and rams and thus having passed the time, they should return, preserving some mementos (of flowered wreaths and so forth) of their pleasant excursions. (These picnics should be fortnightly or monthly; the mementos of blossoms should be worn on the head, ears and the neck).

Sports and Parlour Games

SUTRA 41. The preceding Sutra also explains how aquatic sports are to be arranged during the summer months in spacious wells and reservoirs, specially constructed so that there is no danger of crocodiles. (Reservoirs should be cared for like holy places, so that there is no lurking danger from marine creatures. Water sports are considered uncongenial in any other season except in the summer.)

Other Social Diversions

SUTRA 42.

- Spending the night playing with dice.
- Celebrating the full-moon night in the month of Ashvin. (The games include swinging, etc.)
- Spring festivities (of singing and dancing, dedicated to the god of love).

Other special games are:

- The game in which the mango fruits have to be plucked.
- The game in which grams are to be roasted on the fire and then eaten.
- The game in which lotus stalks are to be eaten.
- The game in which sprouting leaves are to be eaten.
- The game in which water is to be squirted at others. (This is popular in the Madhyadesha.)
- The game of the people of the Panchala country where various stories are enacted. (This is popular in Mithila.)
- The game to be played on the Shalmali tree laden with blossoms. (This is popular with the people of Vidarbha country.)
- The game wherein scented powder of barley is to be sprinkled. (This is on the fourth day of the bright half of the month of Vaishakha. This is popular in the Western countries.)

- The game of the swing. (This is on the third day of the bright half of the month of Shravana.)
- The festival of the god of love. (Here the image of the god of love is to be worshipped.)
- The game in which one has to adorn the ear of the other with Damanaka flower.
- The Holika festival. (This is on the fifteenth of the bright half of the month of Falguna when water, coloured with Kinshuka flowers, is to be squirted on others, with syringes shaped like horns and coloured and scented powder is to be thrown in handfuls at others.)
- The game in which Ashoka flowers are to be used for wearing on the head.
- The game of plucking and collecting flowers.
- The game in which tiny mango-tree twigs are to be used (for head and ear ornaments).
- The game of cutting sugar cane (and making beautiful designs with those pieces).
- The game in which Kadamba flowers are to be thrown at each other. (The party is to be divided into two groups as if in an army and then one group should strike the other group with these wild flowers.)

Both these groups of games should be played by the citizens collectively and in a competitive spirit. (Petting each other with sticks and hurling brick-bats, although the Paundras indulge in it and though it is popular in some parts, is however crude, and not to be recommended. The group of the first three games is fairly universal in its appeal, while the following seventeen are somewhat provincial. The cultured citizen should be able to discriminate between the refined and the crude diversions, and abstain from the latter.)

SUTRA 43. The amusements listed above may be indulged in either by a lone citizen in the company of a courtesan, according as his income allows, or by a courtesan in the company of her maidservants or in the company of other citizens.

SUTRAS 44-47. The Pithamarda is a poor man whose sole possession is his own body, but who always carries with him the Mallika² seat and Phenaka.³ Hailing from a civilized part of the country, and being well versed in the arts, he ekes out a living by practising them for the benefit of citizens and courtesans. (The Pithamarda usually carries his seat on his back, and supports himself on it when he goes about exhorting his pupils.)

The Vita is one who has tasted the pleasures of life and enjoyed good fortune and is endowed with good qualities. He lives with his wife, and is honoured everywhere by citizens and courtesans, and depends on them for his daily bread.

The Vidushaka or the Vaihasika (i.e., one who provokes laughter) is acquainted with only a few of the arts, is chiefly a jester and one who enjoys everybody's confidence. (The Vidushaka is either poor or otherwise: he has a wife, he may choose to be a member of the household or not, as he wishes. He often has the right to reprimand an erring citizen or courtesan.)

These are the counsellors of courtesans and citizens alike, appointed to mediate between their quarrels and reconciliations.

SUTRA 48. These descriptions also apply to mendicant women, widows with shaven heads, slave women and aged courtesans.

SUTRA 49. Rural Nagarakas should encourage intelligent and inquisitive villagers of similar age and caste to discuss the urban Nagaraka's way of living and to emulate it. They should organize gatherings for this purpose and themselves grace the occasion; and by rendering assistance to them, they should set an example for them to oblige each other.

SUTRA 50 (verse). While conversing with them, they should use neither very pure Sanskrit nor completely the local dialect. In this way they will achieve popularity.

SUTRA 51 (verse). A wise man should avoid gatherings disliked by the public, which are not governed by any rules, and which malign others.

SUTRA 52 (verse). A wise man attains success only by cooperating in gatherings approved by the public, and where only innocent amusement is provided.

NOTES

1 These three are stock characters in the ancient dramas and Bhanas who generally perform duties of jester, messenger of love and pander to the hero of the play; more is heard about them in Sutras 44-47 in this chapter.

2 The Mallika seat is made from a staff, with a seating platform, and is portable.

3 Phenaka is a soapy, lathering substance.

CHAPTER V

THE DIFFERENT TYPES OF WOMEN, FIT AND UNFIT TO CONSORT WITH, AND ABOUT MESSENGERS OF LOVE

SUTRAS 1-3. The practice of Kama by the men in the four castes with women of similar castes who are virgins in accordance with the rules of ancient texts is conducive to progeny, besides bringing them a good name and being accepted as legal and binding. However, marital relationship with a woman of higher caste, who has already been married once, is absolutely forbidden. Union with women who are of lower caste, or who are excommunicated, or with those once married and later deserted or widowed, or with courtesans, is neither commended nor condemned, since this relationship is entered into for mere pleasure (i.e., there is no desire for progeny).

SUTRA 4. Therefore Nayikas[1] are of three kinds: the maiden, the woman once married and later deserted or widowed, and the courtesan.

SUTRA 5. According to Gonikaputra, however, there is yet a fourth type of Nayika, Pakshiki: one who is already married to another, but who is resorted to for some special reason (i.e., other than the reasons of procreation or pleasure).

SUTRAS 6-7 When a man considers a woman to be of a free will and knows her to be morally depraved and thinks it would not be impious to approach her like a courtesan, then he should accept her as a Nayika, even though she be of higher caste. There is no doubt that such a woman qualifies as a Punarbhu (referring to the second type of Nayikas enumerated in Sutra 4), since she has belonged to another man before.

SUTRA 8. When a man wishes to possess the wife of another, he thinks thus 'This woman is capable of influencing her husband who is very powerful and who is friendly with my enemy. If, therefore, she is united with me, she can make him abandon my enemy altogether.' Or, he thinks:

SUTRA 9. 'This woman, whose influential husband is prejudiced against me is capable of reinstating me in his favour.' Or, he thinks:

SUTRA 10. 'With the friendly assistance of this woman I can oblige some friend or frustrate my enemy, and perhaps accomplish some onerous task.' Or he thinks:

SUTRA 11. 'If I can do away with this woman's husband, I shall inherit all his wealth which I covet.' Or he thinks:

SUTRA 12. 'My attachment with this woman is not dangerous, and since I am poor and destitute, and in great need of subsistence, I can acquire her vast wealth with no great difficulty.' Or he thinks:

SUTRAS 13-15. 'This woman is utterly devoted to me, and if I do not respond to her, she may expose all my weaknesses. She will accuse me of the unlikeliest deeds, which outsiders will believe and which I will never be able to refute, and will bring about my downfall. She will break my friendship with her influential husband, and unite him to my enemy; or she will herself join the enemy.' Or he thinks:

SUTRA 16. 'This woman's husband has taken liberties with my wives: I shall therefore pay him back in his own coin, and consort with his wife or wives.' Or he thinks:

SUTRA 17 'With the help of this woman, I shall gain access to the king's enemy who is sheltering with her, and slay him, as the king has commended me to do.' Or he thinks:

SUTRA 18. 'The woman I love is under the control of this woman: I can therefore approach the former only through the latter.' Or he thinks:

SUTRA 19. 'This woman can help me to have the maiden who is otherwise beyond my reach, but who is endowed with beauty and wealth and under her control.' Or he thinks:

SUTRAS 20-21. 'My enemy is hand in glove with this woman's husband. I shall therefore bring my enemy and this woman together and thus create enmity between the husband and my enemy.'

For these and other similar motives, a man may resort to other men's wives. But it must be clearly understood that such actions are undertaken not for mere pleasure, but rather as desperate measures.

SUTRA 22. Charayana contends that there is a fifth class of Nayikas, consisting of widows. They may be attached either to a minister or to a king or to any member of their respective families, or a widow who helps a man in his work and to whom she is attached.

SUTRA 23. Suvarnanabha enumerates yet a sixth class of Nayikas comprising widows who have renounced the world.

SUTRA 24. Ghotakamukha adds that there is a seventh class, composed of unmarried or unattached daughters of courtesans, or unmarried maidservants.

SUTRA 25. The eighth type of Nayika, according to Gonardiya, is the (young) maiden born of good family, after she comes of age.

SUTRA 26. Vatsyayana maintains, however, that the first four classes of Nayikas automatically include the remaining ones, since the motives for resorting to them are much the same in both cases. (The widow and the recluse belong to the Parakiya class; the daughter of a courtesan and the maidservant, to the Veshya class; and the high-born maiden is included in the Kanya class. Other classes need not be separately mentioned, the author argues, since they are not generic, and differ from province to province, and from decade to decade.)

SUTRA 27. According to some people, the eunuch constitutes the fifth class of Nayika, because of a very marked difference (with the first four classes mentioned above).

SUTRAS 28-31. There is one type of Nayaka for all types of Nayikas (Kanya, Punarbhu and Veshya). Actions of the second type are not known to the public: he accomplishes his specific object in complete secrecy. This class of Nayakas is divided into three groups – the best, the better and the lowest type, according to his qualifications. These qualifications of the Nayaka and the Nayika will be described later in Part VI of this book when dealing with courtesans.

SUTRA 32. Physical union with the following is strictly forbidden:

- One who suffers from leprosy or a similar contagious disease.
- One who is mentally deranged.
- One who is morally depraved.
- One who divulges secrets.
- One who flirts with the Nayaka openly.
- One whose charms of youth have faded altogether.
- One who is very white.
- One who is very dark.
- One who emits a foul smell.
- One who is a near relative (friend of one's brother, son or sister).
- One who is a friend (of one's wife).
- One who is a recluse.

- One who is related (wife of the teacher, pupil or brother).
- One who is the wife of a friend.
- One who is the wife of a Brahmin, well versed in the sacred texts and religious rituals.
- One who is the wife of a ruler. (Physical union with a queen is totally forbidden because she is considered equal to the wife of the guru of all the four classes of Hindu society. This is the opinion of all the masters of the science of love.)

SUTRA 33. The followers of Babhravya opine that a woman who has had intimate relations with five men, becomes fit to resort to.

SUTRA 34. But Gonikaputra dissents from this view and urges that even if this is the case, that woman should not be resorted to if she happens to be the wife of a relative, of a friend, of a learned Brahmin, or of a king.

SUTRA 35. Friendship develops in nine different ways:

- With one who has been a playmate in childhood.
- That engendered by mutual obligation.
- From similarity of temperament and habit.
- From being co-students.
- With one who knows the other's lapses.
- With one who knows the other's secrets.
- From mutual acknowledgement of each other's lapses and secrets.
- With the child of the nurse.
- With one who is brought up together.

SUTRA 36. The friends should possess the qualities of:

- Hereditary friendship.
- A congenial temperament.
- Unwavering respect for truth.
- Being obedient.

- ◆ Constancy.
- ◆ Being free from covetousness.
- ◆ Being firm in friendship.
- ◆ Faithfully guarding secrets.

SUTRA 37. Friends of the citizen may include a washerman, a barber, a florist, a perfumer, a wine merchant, a mendicant, a cowherd, a betel-leaf dealer, a goldsmith, a Pithamarda, a Vita, a Vidushaka, and so on.

SUTRA 38. Vatsyayana maintains that citizens should be on friendly terms with the wives of these men also.

SUTRA 39. Any person who is a common friend of the citizen and the Nayika, loving them equally, but who is trusted more by the Nayika, can adequately perform the functions of a love-messenger.

SUTRA 40. Desirable qualities in a messenger are: Eloquence, pushing and courageous nature, insight into men's behaviour and motives, cool-headedness, knowledge of other people's inner thoughts, reliability, ability to give, evasive answers, knowledge of the neighbourhood, awareness of the propriety of time, capacity to decide quickly in case of doubt, resourcefulness shown by using trivial means for solving difficult problems, quick and ready application of remedies.

SUTRA 41. Thus a prudent man who has a large circle of friends, who performs his duties conscientiously and who is aware of the propriety of time and place, can win over a woman effortlessly, even though she be unapproachable.

NOTES

1. The term 'Nayika' refers to any woman fit to be enjoyed without sin, for either of the two purposes – procreation or pleasure.

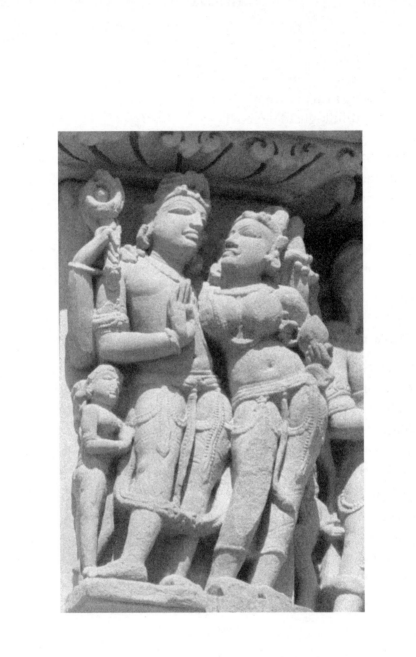

Part II

ON THE UNION BETWEEN MAN AND WOMAN

CHAPTER I

KINDS OF UNION, COMMENSURATE WITH DIMENSION, INTENSITY AND DURATION

SUTRA 1. There are three types of men according to the size of their phallus[1]: the rabbit type (small), the bull type (medium), and the horse type (large).

SUTRA 2. Similarly, there are three types of women depending on the depth of their respective pudendas[2]: the deer type (small); the mare type (medium) and the elephant type (large).

SUTRAS 3-4. Thus there are three equal unions between persons of corresponding dimensions, and six unequal unions in which the dimensions do not correspond (making a total of nine).

EQUAL

No.	Men	Women	Opinion
1	Rabbit	Deer	Excellent
2	Bull	Mare	Excellent
3	Horse	Elephant	Excellent

UNEQUAL

No.	Men	Women	Opinion
4	Rabbit	Mare	low
5	Rabbit	Elephant	lowest
6	Bull	Deer	high
7	Bull	Elephant	low
8	Horse	Deer	highest
9	Horse	Mare	high

SUTRAS 5-6. In these unequal unions, when the man exceeds the woman in dimension, his union with a woman immediately next to him in size is called a high union, and is of two kinds, while his union with a woman most remote from him in size is declared the highest union, and is of one kind only.

SUTRAS 7-8. On the other hand, when the female exceeds the male in point of size, her union with a man immediately next to her in size is called a low union, and is of two kinds, while her union with a man most disparate to her in size is called the lowest union and is of one kind only.

SUTRAS 9-12. However, amongst all these unions, the equal ones are the best, while those between extremes in size, viz., highest and lowest, are the worst. The rest are normal, but even among these the high ones are better than the low ones.

Similarly, there are nine kinds of unions based on the intensity of desire:

No.	Men	Women	No.	Men	Women
1	Small	Small	4	Small	Middling
2	Middling	Middling	5	Small	Intense
3	Intense	Intense	6	Middling	Small
			7	Middling	Intense
			8	Intense	Small
			9	Intense	Middling

SUTRAS 13-14. A man is considered to have small passion when he has little desire for union with a woman, who does not exert himself much at the time, and whose flow is scanty. He also evades the woman's teeth-marks. When a man has some force of passion, he belongs to the second class (Madhyama) and if his passion is very strong, he qualifies for the third, namely, intense class (Chanda).

SUTRAS 15-16. Similarly, women are reckoned to have the three varying degrees of passion, and nine different combinations, exactly like those based on dimensions.

SUTRA 17. Again, there are three types of men and women according to the duration of their individual passions – the short-timed, the medium-timed and the long-timed (and similarly, they give nine different combinations).

SUTRA 18. But on this subject of duration, there is a difference of opinion regarding the woman.

SUTRAS 19-22. Auddalaki says: 'The woman does not discharge in the same way as the man. While the man, by merely uniting with the woman, is able to fulfil his passion, the woman takes pleasure in the consciousness of desire and this gives her the kind of pleasure that is totally different from the man's.'

SUTRAS 23-24. The contention is that the pleasure experienced by the man is intangible: it is impossible for the man and the woman to describe to the other how each feels his or her own peculiar pleasure.

SUTRA 25. To the question as to how this is concluded, Auddalaki replies: 'After the culmination of the union, the man ceases automatically, while woman does not.'

SUTRA 26. This opinion, however, is disputed, since it is an established fact that women are better pleased with men who can perform protracted unions: they detest men who perform unions for a very short duration, and this would seem to prove that the woman emits also.

SUTRAS 27-31. Against this it is argued that the last statement is not correct. It takes a long while to allay a woman's passion, and during the whole time, she experiences intense pleasure and it is therefore quite natural that she should want it to be protracted. Auddalaki's verse corroborates this: 'Women realise great enjoyment during their union with men: their real pleasure, however, springs from the consciousness of it being realised.'

SUTRAS 32-34. Babhravya and his followers opine that the woman's fluid continues to fall from the very beginning of protracted union, while the man's pleasure comes at the very end. (The woman's pleasure permeates like water spreading everywhere when a water-pot is broken, while the man experiences it when the fluid is discharged. Since there is no consistency between the timings of the two sorts of pleasure, it is obvious that classification of unions into nine groups according to duration is not possible. The nine groups can only be based on the intensity of urge.) Conception would never take place if women did not have the flow of this fluid.

SUTRAS 35-36. Here too there is room for objection and counter-objection. It is argued that if the women takes pleasure in protracted union, why is it that at first she is so indifferent and shows so little endurance, and only at the very end comes to the culmination of her desire and, disregarding all physical pain, is at last inclined to stop?

SUTRAS 37-40. The answer to this is that just as the potter's wheel or the spinning top at first starts rotating slowly and only gradually gathers speed, so the woman's passion has perforce to start slowly before it culminates in the final intensity of pleasure. (Hence the protraction of early period of preparation is absolutely essential.) Therefore the objection is invalidated.

SUTRA 41 (verse). Corroborating this is the verse by Babhravya: 'While the man experiences pleasure towards the end of the union, the woman's pleasure, however, continues throughout, and when they have both shed their fluid, they desire its discontinuation.'

SUTRAS 42-43. The final objection is: Since it is clear that the pleasure experienced by the woman is much the same as that experienced by the man, and since both are engaged in bringing about the same result, why should they have different work to do?

SUTRA 44. The answer is: The difference may arise from the difference between their respective attitudes and feelings.

SUTRA 45. How is this?

SUTRAS 46-48. Again the answer is: The difference between their respective attitudes is purely nature's work. The man takes the active part whereas the woman's is the passive role. In the result therefore, the man's pleasure differs from the woman's. Thus, due to the difference in approach, not only the feelings but the resultant pleasure is different in each case.

SUTRA 49. Vatsyayana concludes therefore that the man takes pleasure in the belief that he is active, while the woman feels it in the knowledge that she is united with the man.

SUTRA 50. Again, it may be alleged that since their respective approaches are different, it is reasonable to suppose that the feelings engendered are also divergent.

SUTRAS 51-55. Well, this objection is groundless; there is a reason behind the difference in approach, arising from the basic difference between the role of the man (which is active) and that of the woman (which is passive). However, there is no reason for the difference in pleasure they feel, because they both derive pleasure naturally from the same act that they both perform.

SUTRA 56. Here one may ask that since several factors combine to produce one result (as in cooking food) and since the man and the woman have their own divergent objects in mind, how can there be the identical feeling in the result?

SUTRAS 57-62. This is not really inconsistent for we find that sometimes two things are affected equally by the same action: for instance, in ram-fights, where both rams receive the shock on their heads at the same time, or in throwing one wood-apple against another, and also in a fight or struggle of wrestlers. If, at this point, it is contended that in these cases the protagonists are of the same kind, it can be answered that even in the case of men and women, there is no real dissimilarity of nature, except the one imposed by sex – nature's creation! It follows then that men and women experience the same pleasure.

SUTRA 63 (verse). There is a verse on this subject: 'Since men and women are similar as far as feelings are concerned, and since equal pleasure for both is the ideal, it behoves the man to arouse the woman earlier, before the final union is attained.'

SUTRA 64. Having established that men feel the same pleasure as women, it follows that in regard to duration, there are nine different unions, similar to the nine classified earlier, each according to dimension and intensity of pleasure.

SUTRA 65. The synonyms of Rati or the union between men and women are as follows:

- ◆ Rasa: pleasure experienced physically.
- ◆ Rati: that experienced mentally.
- ◆ Priti :   pleasure due to contact of minds.
- ◆ Ehava: when love is generated through physical union (kamita bhava).
- ◆ Raga: when love fills the soul.
- ◆ Vega: when the fluid drips during physical union.
- ◆ Samapti: the culminating point for both parties.

The synonyms for the act of physical union are:

- ◆ Samprayoga: the pleasurable physical union of man and woman.
- ◆ Rata: the union of body and spirit alike.
- ◆ Rahah: mutual love of man and woman where other men and women are totally excluded.
- ◆ Shayana: when, according to injunctions, the citizen moves himself from the usual to the smaller bed nearby.
- ◆ Mehana: when pleasure from union removes entirely the other occupations of the mind.

SUTRA 66. It will be seen therefore that since there are nine types of unions belonging to each of the three categories based on dimension, intensity of pleasure, and duration, their total is very large indeed. (In actual fact, the total number is 243 x 3 = 729.)

SUTRA 67. Vatsyayana says that from all these types of unions, therefore, a man should choose intelligently the type most suited for the occasion.

SUTRAS 68-69. The opinion of the learned men on this subject is that while the man's passion at the outset is short-timed but intense, and the woman's is long-timed and gradual, until the fluid flows, subsequently the position becomes reversed.

SUTRA 70. According to the firm belief of the masters of this science, those women who have naturally delicate limbs experience pleasure in a short time with men.

SUTRA 71. Educated and cultured persons will find these details regarding the union of men and women sufficient for their culture and education; further exposition of the subject is undertaken after this.

ON THE DIFFERENT KINDS OF LOVE

Verses 1-7. Experts learned in this science have detailed four kinds of love:

1. Love born of continual habit.
2. Love arising from the imagination.
3. Love resulting from self-belief and belief of others.
4. Love resulting from perception of external objects.

1. This kind of love results from the constant engagement of the senses in actions such as hunting, riding, and so forth.
2. This is the sort of love which results not from any direct action dictated by the senses, but from the anticipation of doing so.
3. Love in this category is mutually recognised by the man and the woman and so convincing that others recognise it too.
4. The perception and enjoyment of external objects results in the kind of loving pleasure which is well recognised in the world. Actually this kind of love is generic and embraces the other three varieties mentioned earlier.

A person has to be able to distinguish between these varieties of love according to the texts, and decide for himself which one he should adopt after determining the inclination of the other person at the proper time.

NOTES

[1] 'Lingam' or 'Phallus' are terms used throughout to describe a man's reproductive organ.
[2] 'Yoni' connotes the woman's vagina.

CHAPTER II

ON EMBRACING

SUTRAS 1-4. According to the ancient writers, the union of the sexes is an integral part of the sixty-four arts, collectively named Chatuhshashthi. Each of these arts is connected in one way or the other with the subject of the union of the sexes, and hence the name 'sixty-four' is in vogue. Some others, however, opine that one passage containing sixty-four *Riks* appearing in the Rig Veda was composed by a Rishi named Panchala; and since the chapter on the union of the sexes was also written by a person named Babhravya Panchala, the name Chatuhshashthi (meaning sixty-four) came to be applied to this part of the work.

SUTRAS 5. The followers of the Babhravya school of thought enumerate eight stages during the union:

- ◆ Embracing
- ◆ Kissing
- ◆ Marking with nails
- ◆ Marking with teeth
- ◆ Uniting in congress
- ◆ Shrieking and crying
- ◆ The woman assuming the role of a man
- ◆ Oral congress

Each of these is supposed to have eight subdivisions, making a total of sixty-four.

SUTRA 6. However, in the opinion of Vatsyayana, the total is only approximate. Acts such as *Prahanana*, *Viruta*, etc., are also dealt with additionally, and the name 'sixty-four' is applied loosely, in the same way as we apply the words 'the tree of seven leaves' and 'the oblation of five colours,' etc., to things which are not in fact, so.

SUTRAS 7-8. A man and a woman who have not met before can display their mutual love through four kinds of embrace, in each of which the name signifies the action involved:

SUTRA 9. *Sprishtaka:* In this embrace the man confronted by the woman during the play of love, pretends to pass by with some other purpose, but moves in a manner as will make the bodies of both of them touch each other.

SUTRA 10. *Viddhaka:* In this embrace, the woman discovers the man sitting or standing quite alone, dashes against him with her bosom (pretending to snatch away something from his hands). The man, on his part, pressing her holds her tightly in his embrace. (While *Viddhaka* can be practised either by the man or the woman, the Apaviddhaka can only be done by the woman.)

SUTRA 11. Both these (*Sprishtaka* and *Viddhaka*) happen in the case of those Nayaka and Nayika between whom much talking has not taken place.

SUTRA 12. *Udghrishtaka:* When in the dark or in a crowd, or in a lonely place, or while walking together, the bodies of both the man and the woman are rubbed against each other frequently, it results in this sort of embrace. (The word Ghrishtaka applies when only one of the two indulges in this embrace, while the word *Udghrishtaka* applies when both indulge in it together.)

SUTRA 13. *Piditaka:* This covers the above-mentioned *Udghrishtaka* embrace, in as much as the woman here is heavily pressed against a wall or a pillar while standing. (This embrace can either be practised by one or by both.)

SUTRA 14. The last two embraces are practised particularly by the man and the woman who understand each other's sexual inclinations.

SUTRA 15. There are four varieties of the embrace to choose from at the time of the actual union:

◆ *Lataveshtitaka*	practised by the woman alone
◆ *Vrikshadhirudhaka:*	
◆ *Tilatandulaka*	practised by both
◆ *Kshiranira*	

SUTRA 16. *Lataveshtitaka:* A woman, entwining herself round the man like a creeper to a Shala tree should pull his face down to her own, and holding it up should then utter a slow shriek; or, supporting herself against his body, should pretend to see something wonderful in his face (*Lataveshtitaka*). (This can be done in three ways: with the man standing face to face with the woman, or with the woman embracing one of his sides, or with the woman embracing his neck.)

SUTRA 17. *Vrikshadhirudhaka:* When the woman, keeping one of her feet on that of the man, presses against his thigh and entwines it with the other, and keeps one hand firmly on his back, and with the other hand, presses down his shoulder a little, shrieking and cooing, attempting to climb him for kissing, it results in this embrace (*Vrikshadhirudhaka*).

SUTRA 18. Both these embraces require both the participants to be standing.

SUTRA 19. *Tilatandulaka:* In this embrace, both the man and the woman, lying down on their sides on the bed, press their thighs and arms against each other's with great pressure, embracing mutually (*Tilatandulaka*).

SUTRA 20. *Kshiranira:* Almost blinded by passion and impervious to any damage to their limbs, the man and the woman in this embrace merge into each other (Kshirajala). The woman may be either in the man's lap or may be facing him or be lying in bed. (This embrace is like the mixing of two lumps of clay, or like the mixing of milk and water. It also includes the earlier-mentioned *Tilatandulaka.*)

SUTRA 21. The last two embraces are practised when both participants feel the urge for the union strongly. It must be timed just before the woman's pleasure culminates into the actual union.

SUTRA 22. These embraces have been recounted by Babhravya.

SUTRA 23. Suvarnanabha, however, details four varieties of the embrace at the time of the union: it is in fact Ekangopaguhana, as one limb of each participant is mutually pressed.

SUTRA 24. *Uruvaguhana:* When one or both thighs are pressed against each other mutually. (Both participants may practise this embrace. The pressure on the muscular part results in much pleasure, and the stronger thighs usually play the active part.)

SUTRA 25. *Jaghanopaguhana:* In this embrace, the woman covers up the man with her hair dishevelled, and her Jaghana (i.e., the part of the body from the navel downwards to the thighs) pressed with her lifted thigh, inviting the man for the union. (The woman appears very beautiful in this embrace, displaying as she does the large and pleasing shape of the Jaghana.)

SUTRA 26. *Stanalingana:* When a woman with her bosom brings pressure to bear upon the man's chest, it results in this embrace. (The participants may either sit or lie on their sides.)

SUTRA 27. *Lalatika:* When both participants press each other's mouth, eyes and forehead intensely, the result is this embrace. (Again, either the standing or the lying down position can be chosen. The forehead should be pressed over and over again. Actually the woman is the active agent in this case.)

SUTRA 28. According to some, even *Samvahana* (massaging or shampooing) is a kind of embrace, as it involves mutual physical contact. The three varieties of this embrace are determined by the three elements involved – the skin, the muscular part and the bones.

SUTRA 29. But Vatsyayana dissents from this opinion, since he maintains that shampooing belongs to a different time and a different purpose. Moreover, shampooing is not always pleasant for both participants.

SUTRA 30 (verse). It has been declared in this connection: even those who merely question and hear and those who narrate the details of the embrace, feel the urge for enjoyment gathering within them.

SUTRA 31 (verse). If there are other kinds of embraces not described in, this text on Kama, they should certainly be made use of for greater enjoyment – with due regard to their utility.

SUTRA 32 (verse). Texts on the science of Kama are of help only till passion is not excited: but once the wheel of passion starts to roll, there is then no Shastra and no order.

CHAPTER III

ON KISSING

SUTRA 1. When once a man's passion is aroused, there is no order of precedence among the various steps such as kissing, marking with teeth and nails, etc.

SUTRA 2. As a rule, these are indulged in before congress, while shrieking and striking and other sadistic acts accompany the actual union.

SUTRA 3. But Vatsyayana is of the opinion that all these (five) can be indulged in at any time, since passion is unpredictable (i.e., there is no telling when passion is aroused sufficiently to shun any rules).

SUTRA 4. These five modes of arousing passion should not be used all at once at the time of the first union. While the woman's confidence is still growing, and her passion increasing gradually, one or the other of the modes may be used.

SUTRA 5. After that, all the five modes (with their twenty variations) may be used rapidly for arousing and sustaining the flame of passion. (Otherwise, the union is likely to be devoid of pleasure. Once the participants have gained mutual confidence, no set order need be followed.)

SUTRA 6. The proper places for kissing are: the forehead, hair, the eyes, the man's chest, the woman's bosom, the upper lip, and the inside of the mouth (the palate).

SUTRAS 7-8. The people of the Lata province, however, indulge in kissing also the joints of the thighs, the armpits and the Nabhimula, but according to Vatsyayana, these practices are not to be followed by all, since they are in vogue in one particular province and are peculiar only to their state of passion.

SUTRA 9. There are three sorts of kisses for a young maiden:
- *Nimitaka* or the nominal kiss.
- *Sfuritaka* or the throbbing kiss.
- *Ghattitaka* or the touching kiss.

(Even though ,she has come forward for the embrace, the maiden is still inexperienced and bashful).

SUTRA 10. *The nominal kiss* is said to be done when the maiden is forcibly pulled towards the man and his mouth is pressed against hers, but she does not herself do anything.

SUTRA 11. *The throbbing kiss* is said to be performed when the maiden, setting aside her bashfulness a little, responds to the man's kiss by pressing his lower lip quiveringly, without moving her upper lip.

SUTRA 12. *The touching kiss* is effected when the maiden, holding the lip of the man between her own lips, closes her own eyes and covers his eyes with her hands, and then with the tip of her tongue, presses against his lip.

(These three modes of kissing follow one another.)

SUTRA 13. Other authors describe four other varieties of kisses:

- The straight kiss
- The slanting kiss
- The turned kiss
- The pressing kiss

The straight kiss results when simply the lips are in contact, facing each other. The slanting kiss requires one of the participants to slant the kissing lips diagonally against the other's. The turned kiss is effected when one of the two lovers turns up the face of the other by holding the head and the chin, and then kisses. The pressed kiss takes place when any of the three varieties mentioned above is done with some force. It can again be subdivided into:

(a) the pure kiss where only the lips are pressed.
(b) the tongue kiss where the tips of tongues come into play.

SUTRA 14. There is also a fifth kind of kiss, which is actually another variation of the pressed kiss. This is effected by holding the lower lip between the thumb and the index finger, and shaping it to an 'O', and then kissing it with the lips only, without using the teeth.

SUTRA 15. While, these kisses are indulged in, mock contests should be held. (This may tend to increase mutual passion.)

SUTRA 16. The person who grasps the other's lower lip first is declared winner. This contest can be carried out either in a frank or a shy manner.

SUTRA 17. If the woman loses, she sobbingly shakes her hand, pushes the man, bites him, turns away, disputes the result of the contest if drawn, and keeps forcibly asking for a fresh contest. If she loses a second time, she repeats these acts with redoubled force.

SUTRA 18. Continuing the quarrel arising from this mock contest, the woman should suddenly hold the lower lip of the unsuspecting and unwary man between her teeth, laugh (in triumph), proclaim her victory, threaten him with biting his lip, strain her limbs and invite her lover to another contest, with eyebrows dancing and eyes sportively rolling, laughing derisively and saying many things at once. (The man, whether victorious or defeated, should pay back in the same coin.)

SUTRA 19. Similarly, contests and quarrels can be staged between the lovers in marking each other with nail and teeth marks and such other sadistic acts. (Contests in these cases consist of inflicting the marks on the other person without his or her knowledge.)

SUTRA 20. However, these contests are found congenial only by those people who are intensely passionate. (Those with small passion avoid them as they cannot suffer to go through the scuffle.)

SUTRA 21. *Uttarachumbita,* or 'the kiss of the upper lip' takes place when the man, seeing the woman kissing him, holds her upper lip and kisses it.

SUTRA 22. *Samputaka,* or 'the clasping kiss' results when a man with both his lips, grasps those of the woman and kisses them. (This kiss may be varied as 'the straight,' 'the oblique,' 'the turned' and 'the pressed kiss'. The fifth variant is not to be indulged in here.) The woman should not employ this kiss with a man who has a moustache.

SUTRA 23. When one of the lovers who has been kissed with 'the clasping kiss' rubs the tongue against the teeth of the other and then stretches it to explore the palate, and again straightens it to rub against the other's tongue, it becomes 'the fighting of the tongue'.

SUTRA 24. The same description applies to kisses involving forcible grasping or offering of the mouth and the teeth.

SUTRA 25. There are four other kinds of kisses bestowed on other parts of the body besides the lips:

- *Sama* which is given on the joints of the thighs, the sides and the chest.
- *Pidita* which is given on the bosom, the cheeks and the navel (Nabhimula).
- *Anchita* which is given on the bosom and the sides.
- *Mridu* which is given on the forehead and the eyes.

(The names of these kisses are given according to the intensity of the kiss: *Sama* – balanced; *Pidita* – forcible; *Anchita* – lightly touching; *Mridu* – gentle or affectionate.)

SUTRA 26. When a woman, acting from her own urge, gazes at the sleeping man and then kisses him,[1] it increases the intensity of her passion (*Ragadipana*). (It also accelerates the man's passion when he wakes up and realizes this. The same mode can be employed when both are awake, but only during the actual union.)

SUTRA 27. When a woman kisses the man when he is absorbed (either in music or painting, etc.) or engaged in quarrelsome discussion, or when his attention is diverted to some other object, or when he is inclined to sleep, and she kisses him to ward off his sleep, it is named the *Chalitaka* kiss. (This kiss is proper for women only.)

SUTRA 28. When a man, returning home late at night, kisses the sleeping woman to convey his rising passion, it is called the *Pratibodhaka* kiss.

SUTRA 29. She, on her part, desiring to find out his state of passion, awakes from a pretended sleep, while actually awaiting the moment of his arrival. (These three kisses are indulged in by those who have already met several times, or by those who have been intimate for a long time.)

SUTRA 30. When a man, in order to indicate his rising passion, attempts to kiss the woman's reflection in a looking glass, or in the water or on the wall, it is called *Chhaya-Chumbana*.

SUTRA 31. When a man kisses either a child or a painting or an image in the woman's presence, it is named *Sankranta*. The same name also applies to that type of embrace. (Both the *Chhaya-Chumbana* and the *Sankranta* kiss are to be used on particular occasions only. They are indulged in by men and women who are not able to have any physical contact or meetings or private trysts.)

SUTRA 32. Kissing the fingers of the hand is usually done at night or in a public place or at a gathering of relatives. The woman may kiss the feet of the man who is sleeping near her. (But it is considered undignified for a man to kiss the woman's feet.)

SUTRA 33. When a woman, while shampooing or massaging her lover's supine body, rests her head on his thighs, indicating her feelings towards him, it is named the 'demonstrative kiss' (*Uruchumbana*). Such a kiss on the thighs and the toes has the effect of arousing great passion. (This kiss belongs to the *Abhiyogika* or the 'demonstrative' type, while *Chhaya-Chumbana* and the others belong to the *Prayoganta* or 'instrumental' type.)

SUTRA 34. Every lover must reciprocate the beloved's gesture with equal intensity, kiss by kiss and embrace by embrace. (If there is no reciprocity, the beloved will feel dejected and consider the lover cold as a stone pillar. It will result in a highly unsatisfactory union. To keep the passion alive and inflamed, reciprocity is absolutely essential.)

NOTES

[1]   Cf. Amarushataka, 37.

CHAPTER IV

ON NAIL-MARKS

SUTRA 1. When love becomes intense, scratching the body of one's lover with one's nails is practised.

SUTRAS 2-3. It is done only on certain occasions: at the time of the first union, or on returning from a journey, or on embarking on a journey, or when the woman is placated after a quarrel, or when she is intoxicated after a party. This amorous sport is not agreeable to people with small or middling passion, nor is the sport involving marking with the teeth.

SUTRA 4. Nail-marks are of eight kinds:

- ◆ Of limited pressure
- ◆ Crescent-shaped
- ◆ Circular
- ◆ Lineal
- ◆ Tiger's claw-like
- ◆ Peacock's foot-like
- ◆ Leaping hare-like
- ◆ Like the petal of a lotus

SUTRA 5. The proper places for nail-marks are the armpits, the bosom, the neck, the back, the waist and the posterior, and the thighs.

SUTRA 6. Suvarnanabha, however, maintains that at the actual time of the union, nail-marks can be imprinted anywhere on the body. (Some nail-marks of particular design are good to look at – 'Rupavat' – while others are ugly – 'Arupavat'.)

SUTRA 7. Those whose passion is intense and who are going to indulge in this play should have their left-hand fingernails freshly manicured into two or three points (like a saw blade). Persons with medium passion should have their nails slightly polished at the pointed ends like the beak of a parrot, while those with small passion should have their nails pointed to a crescent.

SUTRA 8. Nails should possess the following qualities:

- A faint line down the middle
- A flat even surface
- Brightness
- Cleanliness
- Absence of cracks
- Healthy growth
- Softness
- Smoothness

SUTRA 9. The Gaudas possess long and beautiful nails which enhance the beauty of their hands, and which women find very attractive. (The Gaudas, however, do not indulge in this game of marking with nails, being content with merely the pleasure by touching.)

SUTRA 10. The people of the South, though they possess small nails, still use them for making designs without the nails breaking.

SUTRA 11. The Maharashtrians possess medium-sized nails, and have the advantages of both the long and the short nails.

SUTRA 12. Now, the eight varieties of nail-marks mentioned earlier are made in the following manner:

(1) **Of limited pressure**: This is done by keeping all the fingers close together and exerting just enough pressure to arouse a hair-raising feeling but without leaving any scratches. The thumbnail is gradually rubbed against the others, producing a slightly audible sound (Achchhuritaka).

These marks should only be done with fingernails of the medium type, and only on the chin, the bosom and the lower lip.

SUTRA 13. They are made on the woman's body by the man when he wants to unite with her, or while he shampoos her limbs, or while he scratches her head, or when he opens small eruptions on the skin, or when he wishes to agitate the unresponsive woman, or when he wishes to frighten her. (They may also be made by the man when he wishes to induce confidence in the maiden.)

SUTRA 14. **Crescent-shaped**: This mark is usually made on the neck and the bosom. (On the neck, the mark faces outwards; on the bosom it faces upwards. It is made with the help of the nail-tip of the middle finger).

SUTRAS 15-16. **Circular**: When two such marks are made facing each other, it is called 'Mandala' and is usually bestowed on the navel, the sides of the hips and the joints of the thighs.

SUTRA 17. **Lineal**: This can be made on any part of the body, provided it is small.

SUTRA 18. **Tiger's claw-like**: The same line when it is curved is so named, and usually adorns the breast and neck.

SUTRA 19. **Peacock's foot-like**: Again the same line, when it is made with all the five nails in the shape of a peacock's foot, comes to be known as that, and is usually made around the nipples.

SUTRA 20. **Leaping hare-like**: When marks of the peacock's foot are made close to one another near the nipples of the breasts, it becomes like the leaping of a hare and, is usually much admired by a passionate woman.

SUTRA 21. **Like the petal of a lotus:** This mark in the form of a lotus petal, is made on the bosom and the waist. (It is like jewels presented by the man to the woman.)

SUTRA 22. When the man, about to embark on a journey, imprints three or four line-marks all at once on the woman's thighs and bosom, it is named the 'remembrance mark'. (The woman may also indulge in this according to the dictates of the time and the custom of her people).

SUTRA 23. Many other shapes and forms (such as birds, flowers, pots leaves, creepers) may be thought of and made.

SUTRA 24. As the learned men of this science have said, there are far too many shapes and forms, in addition to the eight mentioned above, to be enumerated individually. They all require expertise in execution and constant practice. Again, since some marks are thought of on the spur of the moment, under the influence of intense passion, it is difficult to detail them.

SUTRA 25. In the opinion of Vatsyayana, however, just as variety is necessary in love, it is equally true that love is to be mutually aroused through variety. Hence, those courtesans who are clever and who are acquainted with the varieties of love-sport are generally more in demand; if in the science of warfare and archery, variety is considered necessary, how much more important it is for this science of love! (Here lies one of the differences between an untutored rustic and a cultivated citizen.)

SUTRA 26. Nail-marks should never be made on the body of another man's wife, but certain other kinds of marks may be made on her hidden parts, like the thigh joints, etc., for the sake of remembrance. Such marks become a constant reminder for the woman of her trysts with her lover.

SUTRA 27 (verse). When a woman looks at the nail-marks on her body, hidden from other's view, she finds her love resuscitated and renewed even after a long lapse of time.

SUTRA 28 (verse). Without them, she could never revive her memories of her own beauty, youth, charm and other qualities.

SUTRA 29 (verse). Even a stranger who notices nail-marks on the bosom of a young maiden from a distance, begins to feel esteem and love for her.

SUTRA 30 (verse). In the same way, a woman feels attracted to a man who carries nail-marks on his body, even though she be of a cool and firm temperament.

SUTRA 31 (verse). Actually, there is nothing more effective for arousing passion in a man or a woman than the effects of marks made by fingernails.

CHAPTER V

ON TEETH-MARKS. WOMEN OF DIFFERENT PROVINCES: THEIR LIKES AND DISLIKES, AND THEIR WAYS OF LOVE

SUTRA 1. The places proper for biting or for teeth-marks are the same as those fit for kissing, with the exceptions of the upper lip, the tongue and the eyes. (In other words, the forehead, the lower lip, the neck, the cheeks, the bosom, and the places favoured by the Latas, viz., the thigh-joints, the armpits and the navel – all these places are suitable for teeth-marks.)

SUTRA 2. Good teeth should have the qualities of being even, shiny, of an attractive colouring, proportionate, close-set and pointed.

SUTRA 3. Teeth are considered rather defective when they are blunt, protruding from the gums, hard, uneven, sticky, broad, and loosely set. (These are considered to be defects either because they are unsightly or because they are ineffectual for making teeth-marks.)

SUTRAS 4-18. Teeth-marks are of eight varieties:

- *Gudhaka* or the 'hidden' teeth-mark is that which leaves no red mark afterwards, and is only done from passion. (The Rajadanta only is used here.)
- *Uchchhunaka* or the 'swollen bite' is done when pressure is used during the 'hidden bite'.
- *Bindu* or 'spot bite' is effected by making teeth-marks with two teeth on a small area of the skin (on the neck, it is the size of a Mudga grain; on the lower lip, it is of the size of a sesame seed).
- *Pravalamani* or the 'line of corals' results when the 'swollen bite' is made on the cheeks with the help of the upper teeth and the lower lip. (The mark is red, but leaves no permanent scar.)
- When *Pravalamani* or the 'line of corals' is made one after the other, it is called *Manimala*, or the 'jewel chain'.
- *Bindumala* or the 'line of points' is effected when teeth-marks are made in a row by all the teeth. Both the 'jewel-chain', and the 'coral chain' should be imprinted only on the neck, and sides and the thigh joints. (The skin at these places is usually quite tender and soft.) However, the 'coral chain' may also be imprinted on the forehead and the thighs. (On the thighs, it should be like a row of sesame seeds.)
- *Khandabhraka* or the 'broken cloud' is made when broad, medium and small teeth are used all together to make a circle on the breast. (This is an easy process, and considered to lend great beauty to that part of the body. The woman may use this method on the man's armpits during the *Kanthopagraha* embrace.)
- When the teeth-marks are close to one another, sustained and continuous and slightly reddish in between, it is called *Varahacharvitaka*, because it appears like the 'biting of a boar'. This is done on the breasts only. The last two modes of

imprinting teeth-marks should be practised only by those whose passion is intense.

So much regarding teeth-marks.

SUTRA 19. When these shapes made by the nails and the teeth are implanted on either the Bhurja leaves or the blue lotus petals used as ear-ornaments or the flowers used as a crown or the betel leaf or the fragrant Tamala leaf, and sent to the beloved person, they indicate one's passion and act as code-messages. (Sometimes actual messages are also written.)

Now, we describe women of different provinces, their likes and dislikes and their ways of love.

SUTRA 20. When dealing with his relationship with a woman, a man must consider well the prevailing customs and practices of that particular province. (The same applies to the woman.)

SUTRA 21. The people of the Madhyadesha are of the pure stock, clean in their habits in love, detesting as they do the second, third and the fourth modes of nail- and teeth-marks (mentioned earlier). They favour embracing, but are not very keen on thrashing as a love-sport.

SUTRAS 22-23. The women of Bahlika and Avanti also have similar tastes, detesting kissing, but favour *Chitrarata* – (unions with unusual postures).

SUTRA 24. The women of Maiwa and the Abhira country are aroused and won over by the use of the first four modes of love-sport (mentioned earlier in this chapter) and also by oral congress, but they dislike marks or scars to be left on their bodies. They are also excited by thrashing and similar sadistic love-sports.

SUTRA 25. The women of the country around the Indus and the five rivers (viz., Vipat, Shatadru, Iravati, Chandrabhaga, Vitasta), being exceedingly passionate, are easily excited by oral congress.

SUTRA 26. The women of Aparanta and Lata are also very passionate, and enjoy shrieking and cooing softly. (They also enjoy the third and the fourth love-sports mentioned earlier, and also thrashing, if done slowly or lightly.)

SUTRA 27. Also very passionate are the women of Strirajya and Koshala. They favour thrashing and similar sadistic actions, and are keen on using mechanical aids during the union.

SUTRA 28. The women of the Andhra province are by nature quite delicate yet they do have a taste for impure things, and do not observe rules for a good and healthy life. (They do not tolerate thrashing and yet they enjoy strong movements after intromission.)

SUTRA 29. The women of Maharashtra are fond of all the sixty-four arts and all the modes for arousing passion. They use strong and harsh words, and prefer a speedy, forceful and sudden union.

SUTRA 30. The Nagariki women (of Pataliputra) are in many ways like the women of Maharashtra, except that they prefer their union to be in complete privacy.

SUTRA 31. The women of the Dravida province like to indulge in excessive love-play, but reach their culmination rather slowly.

SUTRA 32. The women of Vanavasa are moderately passionate, and while they endure all forms of love-sport, they conceal physical defects, laugh at those of others and refuse to unite with a man who is, in any way, vulgar.

SUTRA 33. The women of the Gauda province are soft-spoken and delicately built.

SUTRA 34. According to Suvarnanabha, in matters of love natural inclinations should take precedence over provincial customs. (In other words, one should indulge in the various modes of love which are in vogue in that province only when they are favoured by the other partner. In case of doubt, these should be avoided and actions confined only to those favoured by the other partner. However, there are others in whose opinion, contrary to Suvarnanabha's, local customs should be practised in any case, whether favoured by the other partner or not, but Vatsyayana agrees with Suvarnanabha in as much as he does not refute his opinion.)

SUTRA 35. One should also bear in mind that in the course of time, certain customs and habits of dress infiltrate from one province into another (and hence one has to be careful as to which of these are authentic and which are borrowed, and choose from them judiciously).

SUTRA 36. The six modes of arousing passion which are mentioned earlier in this chapter are stated in their order of precedence: each succeeding one is more effective than the previous one, but quite different in the result.

SUTRA 37 (verse). If a man persists in making nail- and teeth-marks in spite of the woman's resistance and beyond her endurance, she should retaliate by making similar marks on the man, with double the force. (When the woman can endure them, she should respond in a similar way – not with greater force, since there is no quarrel.)

Sutra 38 (verse). In retaliating, the women should pretend to be angry in a quarrel and make the following marks:

- ◆ A 'coral chain' in answer to the 'spot bite'.
- ◆ A 'broken cloud' in return for the 'coral chain'.
- ◆ A 'biting of the boar' in return for the 'broken cloud'.
- ◆ A 'swollen bite' in return for the 'hidden bite'.
- ◆ A 'spot bite' in answer to the 'swollen bite'.
- ◆ A 'line of points' for the 'swollen bite'.

(The 'broken cloud' and the 'biting of the boar' get deep into the skin, while the rest are superficial marks.)

SUTRA 39 (verse). When a woman's passion is so aroused that she is beside herself, she should employ the *Adharapana* kiss by grasping her lover's locks of hair and raising his face, and then closely embracing him and making teeth-marks on the same places that he had used. (With one hand, she clutches his locks; with the other she upholds his chin.)

SUTRA 40 (verse). A woman, clasping the man and raising his face with one hand, and resting her other hand on his chest, should make the 'jewel chain' and other beautifying marks on the neck. (Vatsyayana opines that there should be a variety of teeth-marks on the neck.)

SUTRA 41 (verse). When a man displays the marks made on his body by a woman and then points in her direction, she should simply smile to herself, unobserved by others. (She should not be seen smiling even by the man, otherwise both will be considered rustic in manners.)

SUTRA 42 (verse). The woman in return should show chagrin, and point out the marks made by him on her body, making a wry face and pretending to rebuke him (conveying to him that he only got what he deserved).

SUTRA 43 (verse). When a man and a woman enjoy their life in this way, with due shyness and modesty and mutual consent, their love does not fade even after a lapse of a hundred years (which is considered the normal life span of a man). Just as food, even when it is excellent, if repeatedly eaten day after day loses its charm, so it is with love.

CHAPTER VI

ON POSTURES FOR CONGRESS

SUTRA 1. When passion is roused to a pitch, the woman of the Deer-type uniting with a man in *Uchharata* or 'high congress' should lie down on her back with her legs wide apart. (However, when the man is of the Bull-type, she should lie naturally, and if he is of the Horse-type she should engage in 'high congress'.)

SUTRA 2. A woman of the Elephant class, uniting with a man in *Nicharata* or 'low congress', should lie down with her legs as close to each other as possible. (However, when the man is of the Bull-type, she should lie down naturally; and if he is of the Rabbit-type, she should contract her thighs, as indicated earlier.)

SUTRA 3. When both lovers are equal, and they engage in *Samarata* or 'equal union', the woman should lie down quite naturally (that is, without deliberately contracting or widening her thighs).

SUTRA 4. The woman of the Mare class should adopt the same postures as those adopted by the Deer and the Elephant class, as already indicated (that is, when uniting with a man of the Horse-type in 'high congress', she should widen her legs, but when the man is of the Rabbit-type, she should engage in 'low congress', and keep her legs contracted).

SUTRA 5. When the woman has decided to which of the three classes she belongs and which posture she is going to adopt according to her lover's dimensions, she should prepare for the congress.

SUTRA 6. Artificial aids for congress are needed only when the woman resorts to *Nicharata* or 'low congress'. (In other words, only when the Mare-type of woman unites with the Rabbit-type of man, or when the Elephant-type of woman unites with the Bull-type of man. In cases of *Samarata* or 'equal union', aids are not necessary. When artificial aids, however, are used in cases of 'low congress', the woman should not contract but widen her thighs. In cases of *Uchharata* or 'high unions' these aids again become redundant.)

SUTRA 7. There are three postures suitable for the Deer-type of woman:

SUTRA 8. *Utfullaka*: or 'the widely open position', when she lies on her back, presses down her upper half of the body and raises her hips as high as possible. (It is so named because the abdomen appears to be fuller and rounder because of the assumed position.)

SUTRA 9. In doing this, (both) should recede a little after congress, since sudden intromission is painful to both, and it results in the injury known as 'Avapatika' to Indian medical men.

SUTRA 10. *Vijrimbhitaka*: or 'the yawning position', when the woman lies on her back and raises her thighs keeping them well apart, and then allows intromission.

SUTRA 11. *Indrani*: or 'the position of the consort of Indra', when the woman holding her bent knees and thighs together and keeping them well apart, holds them pressed to her sides. This requires some practice. (It was adopted and popularized by Indrani, consort of the god Indra. Here, too, both have to recede a little after congress to avoid pain.)

SUTRA 12. This posture can also be adopted in 'higher-congress'. (The Deer-type woman can unite in this posture not only with the Bull-type man, but also with the Horse-type man. With the Bull-type man, she can unite also in 'the widely open position' and 'the yawning position'. Similarly, the Mare-type woman can unite with the Horse-type man in both these postures.)

SUTRA 13. In the case of 'the low congress', the *Samputa* or 'the clasping position' should also be used (for instance, when the Elephant-type of woman unites with the Bull-type man).

SUTRA 14. In the case of 'the lower congress', the Elephant-type of woman should also adopt this posture. For her there are four suitable postures:

- *Samputaka* or 'the clasping position'
- *Piditaka* or 'the pressing position'
- *Veshtitaka* or 'the twining position'
- *Vadavaka* or 'the mare's position'

(In these postures, she can unite with the Rabbit-type man also, just as the Mare-type woman can.)

SUTRA 15. When, during actual congress, the legs of both the lovers are straightened and stretched, it is called *Samputaka*. (It is also so named because the union of both is perfect, like *Samputa*.)

SUTRA 16. *Samputaka* can be of two varieties:
  (a) *Parshva,* or 'sidewards' when both lovers lie on their sides facing each other.
  (b) *Uttana,* or 'supine', when the woman lies on her back; however, when the man changes his position, the posture comes to belong to another sub-variety.

(*Samputaka* is differently described by Katyayana. The thighs, according to him, are kept separate, and so the abdomen cannot be contracted. Hence, this posture should not be used by the Elephant-type woman in 'low congress'. In 'equal union', however, it is practicable and quite popular.)

SUTRA 17. When a man lies on his side, he should always have the woman on his left (that is, she should be on her right side). This is the usual position and universally adopted. (However, the texts on the science of love say that in the case of the Elephant-type of woman, the man should arouse her passion by playing with her clitoris with his left hand.)

SUTRA 18. *Piditaka* or 'the pressing position', is acquired when the woman after congress through the clasping position, brings her thighs as close as possible and presses them against each other. (This also can be either (*a*) *Parshva* or sidewards, or (*b*) *Uttana* or supine. In this posture, the abdomen becomes even more contracted.)

SUTRA 19. *Veshtitaka* or 'the twining position' results when in 'the clasping position', the woman turns her left thigh to the right and the right one to the left. The mutual turning of the thigh contracts the abdomen even more than in 'the pressing position'.

SUTRA 20. *Vadavaka* or 'the mare's position' results when the man's phallus after congress is held very firmly by the woman, rather like a mare. It requires much practice. (An Elephant-type of woman is able to please a Rabbit-type of man by this posture.)

SUTRA 21. Generally speaking, this posture is popular with the women of one of the Eastern provinces.

These are, then, (seven) postures for congress, according to Babhravya and his followers. Suvarnanabha, however, describes the following in addition to those:

SUTRA 22. When the woman holds up both her thighs, it is called *Bhugnaka* or 'the rising position'. (This position is only recommended for the Elephant-type of woman. She can either choose from Babhravya's list or Suvarnanabha's.) It is called *Bhugnaka*.

SUTRA 23. When the man holds up her legs (and rests them on his shoulders before congress) it is called *Jrimbhitaka* or 'the yawning position'.

SUTRA 24. When the man bends the woman's legs and presses them down with his bosom it is *Utpiditaka* or 'the pressed position'. (It is so named because pressure is exerted on one's bosom.)

SUTRA 25. When only one of her legs is so stretched, it is named *Ardhapiditaka*, or 'the half-pressed position'. (After being stretched, it is turned towards the side of the other leg.)

SUTRA 26. When in the posture described above, one of her legs is stretched and the other is kept resting on the man's shoulder, it is called *Venudaritaka* or 'the splitting of the bamboo'. (There are two possibilities here: either the left leg is bent and the right is stretched, or the right leg is bent and the left is stretched. The name is self-explanatory.)

SUTRA 27. When one of the legs is held above her head and the other is stretched out, it is known as *Shulachitaka*. This posture is achieved after much practice. (Again, this posture is of two kinds, according to which of the two legs is involved. It is so named because it appears like a body speared into two.)

SUTRA 28. When the woman's legs are bent at the knees and wedged below the man's navel just before congress, it is named *Karkata* or 'the crab position'.

SUTRA 29. When the woman's thighs are raised and crossed one on the other, it is named *Piditaka* or 'the packed position' (since the abdomen is contracted and appears to be tightly packed).

SUTRA 30. When the thighs are crossed (so that the right foot is on the left thigh and the left foot is on the right thigh) it is named *Padmasana* or 'the lotus position'.

SUTRA 31. When a man after congress, turns around without leaving her, while the woman continues to embrace his back, it is named

Paravrittaka or 'the turned position'. This posture requires prolonged practice. (This posture is also possible when congress is effected by the man from the back of the woman and this also comes after continual practice.)

SUTRA 32. These postures for congress can, according to Suvarnanabha, be equally well employed in water as on the ground – in lying down, sitting or standing attitudes.

SUTRA 33. But according to Vatsyayana, this is not proper or commendable, since it is denounced by learned and cultured sages. (The writers of Smritis, the holy texts, have also condemned it.)

SUTRA 34. Apropos the enumeration of postures for congress, some amusing ones are now described. (These can also be adopted on the ground.)

SUTRA 35. When the man and the woman support themselves against each other, or against a wall or a pillar and then engage in congress, it is called *Sthita Rata* or 'the steady congress'.

SUTRA 36. When the woman embraces the man who is standing against a wall, by encircling his neck with her hands, and supports herself on both his hands, clasps his thighs with hers and places her feet against the wall, then swings from side to side after congress, it is called *Avalambitaka* or 'the suspended congress'. (Both these postures are described as 'Chitra' or amusing, since they are usually adopted in a jovial mood.)[1]

SUTRA 37. When a man is down on all fours and adopts the stance of a beast before uniting with the woman from behind her, like a bull, it is called *Dhenuka* or 'the congress of a cow and bull'.

SUTRA 38. In this posture, the different modes of arousing passion, like embracing, nail-marks and so on, should be done on her lips instead of her bosom.

SUTRA 39. A man can similarly adopt the postures peculiar to the dog, the deer, the male goat, the donkey, the cat, the tiger, the elephant, the boar, the horse, and so on. Even the peculiarities (of voice and sounds) may be imitated.

SUTRA 40. When a man unites with two women simultaneously, both of whom love him equally, it is called *Sanghataka* or 'the united congress'.

SUTRA 41. When a man unites with several women simultaneously, it is called *Gauyuthika*, or 'the congress of a herd of cows'.

SUTRA 42. Similarly, it is called *Varikriditaka* or 'the congress in a water pool'; *Chhagala* or 'the congress of a herd of goats'; *Aineya* or 'the congress of a herd of antelopes', and so on, according to the name of the animal which is imitated. (Just as it is possible for a man to unite with two or more women at the same time, so it is possible for the woman to unite with two or more men at the same time. When one woman unites with two men, it is named *Sanghataka* or 'the united congress'. When she unites with many men, it is called *Gauyuthika* or 'the congress of a herd of cows'. Similarly, the woman can also indulge in *Varikriditaka* or 'congress in a water-pool'.)

SUTRA 43. In the provinces of Gramanari, Strirajya and Bahlika, many young men enjoy one woman, either one after the other or all at once, according to which union she desires. (These women are intensely passionate, and keep a number of young men in their apartments.)

SUTRA 44. One young man holds her, another unites with her, a third one feels the hips, a fourth one kisses her, a fifth man holds her waist, and so they unite with her by turns.

SUTRA 45. In the same way, one courtesan can be enjoyed by several Vitas, and one queen by several noblemen. (The union with several women mentioned in Sutra 41 is in reference to one's wives when there are more than one.)

SUTRA 46. The people of the South also indulge in *Adhorata* or 'the congress in the anus'. (It can be indulged in by the man either with another man or another woman. It is described as 'Chitra' or 'artificial' because that part of the body is generally considered unsuitable for congress – Vimagra. Oral congress, similarly, is considered artificial when done by a woman, but not so when done by a eunuch.)

SUTRA 47. The movements of a man after he has united with a woman will be dealt with when we discuss the inverse posture of the woman.

SUTRA 48 (verse). A man should be able to gauge the inclinations of the woman he unites with, and select the postures for congress accordingly – the deer, the birds, the elephants and so forth. (He should also imitate their voices and physical movements, and resort to more and more animal acts.)

SUTRA 49 (verse). Thus a man succeeds in securing the love and gratification and admiration of the women he unites with only when he perceives their inclinations, recognises provincial customs and employs the postures for congress most desired by them, with all the intensity of passion at his disposal.

NOTES

1   Sculptures depicting these are at Khajuraho, Konarak, etc.

CHAPTER VII

ON STRIKING AND THE SOUNDS APPOSITE TO THEM

SUTRA 1. The union of the sexes, by nature, is a combat, offering plenty of scope for differences of opinion. In spite of its tender origin, such love leads to dizzy heights of intense passion which, in its culmination, becomes blind to the force, and even the pain, of the ways and means used.

SUTRA 2. Accordingly, in a state of high passion, striking or thrashing is considered one of the chief factors for arousing passion, the places most suitable for it being the shoulder, the head, the bosom, the back, the Jaghana and the sides.

SUTRA 3. Striking is of four kinds:
- *Apahastaka* – when it is done with the back of the palm and outstretched fingers.
- *Prasritaka* – which will be described later.
- *Mushti* – when the fingers are folded in the fist.
- *Samatalaka* – when it is done with the palm in a steady position. (This is called 'Mustaka' in popular parlance).

SUTRA 4. Thrashing and other such sadistic acts result in *Sitkrita* or shrieking, which again is of various kinds.

SUTRA 5. On the other hand, what results from intense passion and not pain, is *Viruta* or cooing, which is of eight kinds:

SUTRA 6

- *Himkara* which is a nasal sound resembling 'him'.
- *Stanita* which is a deep 'ham' sound.
- *Rudita* or sobbing.
- *Sutkrita* or 'Shvasia' which resembles the sound 'su-su'.
- *Kujita* or cooing.
- *Dutkritam* or the 'sound similar to that of a splitting bamboo.
- *Fu-fu* or the sound resembling the fall of a berry in water.

(All these are inarticulate sounds.)

SUTRA 7. Words like *Amba* are uttered to prevent the man from further indulgence, to get herself free or to convey to him that what is done is more than enough. Other words are also uttered, indicating pain, sufficiency, and so on.

SUTRA 8. A woman may also imitate the shrieks and calls of doves, koels, pigeons, parrots, bees, sparrows, swans, ducks and quails. (While thrashing is in progress, the woman should intersperse different calls at intervals.)

SUTRAS 9-10. When a man strikes the woman who is seated on his lap with his fists, she should, as if unable to bear pain, give out inarticulate sounds – *Stanita*, *Rudita* and *Kujita* and retaliate by striking him with her fists.

SUTRAS 11-12. During the actual union, the man should strike the woman's bosom in the *Apahastaka* way, slowly at first but gradually increasing in force until her passion is greatly aroused and finally allayed. (The woman should be lying down. Special mention is made here of the bosom since there are only three places in a woman's body which are the repositories of her passion, the head, the Jaghana, and the heart. When a man strikes any of these parts, even a long-time woman gets the orgasm soon.)

SUTRA 13. At such a time, the woman should utter the shrieks without any order of precedence, according to her habit (that is, when she is struck in the *Apahastaka* way).

SUTRA 14. When a man strikes the woman's head, with his fingers bent (like a hood), while she is protesting, and accompanies this with the *fu-fu* sound it is named *Prasritaka*. (This is to be done if she is not satisfied with the *Apahastaka* way, and desires another form of thrashing. The *fu-fu* sound tends to increase her passion.)

SUTRA 15. At such a time, the woman should alternately utter the cooing sound from inside her mouth and the *fu-fu* sound. (The *fu-fu* sound is almost the opposite of cooing sound, which is usually done with the mouth kept open.)

SUTRA 16. At the end of the union, the sounds usually emitted are *Shvasita* and *Kudita* (due to fatigue). *Dutkritam* is the sound produced by imitating the splitting of a bamboo.

SUTRA 17. The *fu-fu* sound resembles that produced by a berry falling in water. (It is made by the tip of the tongue touching the palate.)

SUTRA 18. When a man indulges in kissing and in other modes of arousing her passion, the woman should respond in the same way and utter *Sitkrita* and other shrieks. (This also makes him respond to her with similar shrieks.)

SUTRA 19. If the man, overcome by his passion, persists in thrashing the woman, she should utter sounds for preventing him from doing so and for setting her free; sounds showing that she has had enough – sounds like *Amba* and other similar inarticulate sounds or bird-calls, indicating pain. When the passion begins to wane after the culmination, he should strike the woman on her Jaghana and sides continuously. (A man knows this from the state of his organ, and when he is nearing the end he should immediately begin thrashing in the *Samatalaka* way and continue to do so. It is essential to time it correctly.)

SUTRA 20. When the man thus strikes the woman in the *Samatalaka* way, she should shriek like the quail and the swan.

So much for the description of shrieking, cooing, inarticulate sounds and bird-calls and sadistic acts.

SUTRA 21 (verse). The characteristic qualities of manhood are harshness and suddenness, while those of the feminine nature are helplessness, painfulness, shrieking, cooing, inarticulation and loss of strength. (This refers to the time of their union; the man has intense passion and the woman's nature is to suffer.)

SUTRA 22 (verse). At times, however, owing to intense passion or an unusual posture, the contrary may appear to be true, but this illusion does not last long, and ends in the natural way.

SUTRA 23. There are four additional types of thrashing also, making a total of eight including the four mentioned earlier in Sutra 3:
- ◆ *Kila* or the wedge, made on the bosom.
- ◆ *Kartari* or the scissors on the head.
- ◆ *Viddha* or the piercing instrument on the cheeks.
- ◆ *Samdamshika* or the pincers on the bosom and the sides.

These types of thrashing are largely favoured by the Southerners, specially *Kila* which is found done on the bosoms of young women according to the prevalent provincial custom. (*Kila* is done by keeping the thumb over the index and middle fingers; *Kartari* by keeping the thumb between the index and the middle and small fingers; *Samdamshika* by keeping the index finger and the thumb together, or the index and middle fingers together.)

(According to the Acharyas, however, only the first four forms of thrashing are to be recommended, though the Southerners specially favour the latter four, in spite of the fact that they sometimes disfigure the woman.)

SUTRA 24. Vatsyayana maintains that one should never indulge in acts which will cause pain to others: these are only done by wicked and uncivilized people.

SUTRA 25. Also, no person should practise habits peculiar to one province in another province. (For instance, *Prastara* and other similar types of thrashing are favoured by Southerners only and should only be practised in the South.)

SUTRA 26. Even in those provinces, carrying these practices .to excess should be totally avoided. (Acts which may disfigure or prove fatal must be totally avoided.)

SUTRA 27. Once, during congress, the king of the Chola country killed a courtesan named Chitrasena by striking her in the *Kila* way.

SUTRA 28. On another occasion, Shatakarni, the Shatavahana King of the Kuntala country, killed the crowned queen, Malayavati, by the *Kartari* way of striking.

SUTRA 29. Naradeva, whose hand was maimed, similarly struck a dancing girl in the *Viddha* way and blinded her in one eye. (*Samdamshika* is not illustrated here, but it is not very harmful.)

SUTRA 30 (verse). However, after all is said and done, in matters of love the ruling authority is the force of passion – not scientific treatises. (The force of passion is common to the ignoramus as well as to the learned man conversant with scientific treatises; the only difference is that the latter is backed by knowledge and is able to draw upon it freely.)

SUTRA 31 (verse). The inclinations which predominate and the modes which the lovers use to arouse each other's passion during a loving union on the spur of the moment, are so elusive as to be almost as undefinable as dreams. (No scientific treatise is followed here.)

SUTRAS 32-33 (verses). Like a horse at full gallop which is blinded by speed to any pillar, pit or cave that comes along his way, the uniting couple are utterly blinded by their intense passion and urge to any excesses or painful extremes, and unite in congress without another thought.

SUTRA 34 (verse). Therefore, when a man who knows the science of love arouses and unites with a woman, he should always consider his own strength and weakness, as much as his beloved's strength and delicacy.

SUTRA 35 (verse). One must not use all the postures for congress delineated here indiscriminately; the place, the province and the time should always be taken into account.

CHAPTER VIII

ON WOMAN ASSUMING THE MAN'S ROLE

SUTRA 1. When, during the union, the woman finds the man tired, but still full of passion, she may 'roll' him over and assume his role in order to help him. This she may do either with or without his consent, to satisfy his curiosity or for the sake of novelty. (The woman is at liberty to do this when she has gained her lover's confidence, or when she herself desires such a union, or when she knows that her lover desires it, or she may do it in spite of the fact that he is not tired.)

SUTRA 2. This union can be effected in one of two ways: either after the actual union, the woman can turn the man on his back holding him continuously, or by the woman assuming the man's natural position from the start. (There is no third type.)

SUTRA 3. With flowers dropping from her dishevelled hair, her laughter interrupted by her breathing, her breasts pinning down her lover's chest in kissing, her head bent down often, the woman should retaliate with all the tricks her lover had used on her, saying, 'I was down earlier, but now I will press you down', and thus, jokingly, poke and dig him with her fingers. Then, fatigued, she should display her bashfulness and show that she wishes to end the congress by acting the same way as the man did after congress.

SUTRA 4. Now we will describe how the man must make advances. (These are of two kinds: External and Internal.)

SUTRA 5. He should start by loosening the knot of the woman's lower garment, while she is lying in bed and pretends to be perturbed by his amorous words and obstructs him from untying the knot, but he should allay her fears by kissing her cheeks and other parts. When his phallus is erect, he should gently feel her body, and if he is uniting with his beloved for the first time, he should touch her in between the thighs which are kept close to each other. If she is a maiden, he should press her breasts together, feel her arms, sides, shoulders and neck and closed thighs before untying the knot. However, if she is a free woman (and has enjoyed congress with a man before), the procedure is usually according to mutual inclinations.

He should also forcibly grasp the locks of her hair before kissing her mouth, and pressing her chin with his closely held fingers. Usually a maiden without any previous experience in matters of love closes her eyes at the time of her first union. *Purushopasripta* is that congress in which a man starts the advances, while *Purushayita* is that in which the woman assumes the man's role. The man must act in different ways with a maiden, on the one hand, and the experienced woman, on the other.

When she is experienced, the man proceeds in four states:
- ◆ Untying the knot.
- ◆ Rubbing her parts with his hands.
- ◆ Widening her closed thighs and
- ◆ Holding her tightly by the locks while kissing her lips.

When she is a maiden and yet inexperienced the man should very gradually win her confidence by first pressing her breasts close together, stroking her sides, shoulders and neck, touching her closed thighs, and when she closes her eyes out of bashfulness, very gently untie the knot.

SUTRA 6. In any case, a man should find out which tricks arouse the woman's passion for congress and proceed accordingly.

SUTRA 7. According to Suvarnanabha, the secret of satisfying a woman's desire successfully lies in the man's perceiving where the woman turns her glance after congress, and pressing those parts with increasing movement and pressure. (Other learned men of the science of love have other theories, but since Suvarnanabha's is acceptable to Vatsyayana, it is mentioned here.)

SUTRA 8. The woman's fulfilment and complete satisfaction is indicated by the languor of the limbs, closing of the eyes, disappearance of her bashfulness and the pressure of her abdomen against that of the man. (The first two symptoms indicate the approach while the last two indicate the fulfilment of her satisfaction.)

SUTRA 9. She shakes her hands, perspires, bites, prevents him from getting up, kicks her legs, and continues the movements even after the man has finished.

SUTRA 10. The man should be familiar with the sequence, and always make it a point to soften her yoni by titillating it with his fingers before the actual congress. (The man shapes his fingers like an elephant's trunk; sometimes an artificial male organ may be used.)

SUTRA 11. There are ten varieties of strokes in congress:

SUTRA 12. When it is done mildly and naturally, it is *Upasriptaka*, meaning 'moving forward'. (This comes naturally even to cowherd women.)

SUTRA 13. When the man holds his phallus and turns it around on all sides in the yoni, it is *Manthana*, meaning 'churning'.

SUTRA 14. When the yoni is lowered and the man unites from a higher level, it is *Hula*, meaning 'piercing'.

SUTRA 15. When exactly the opposite is done (viz., the yoni raised and congress effected from a lower level by the man) suddenly and with some force, it is *Avamardana*, meaning 'rubbing'.

SUTRA 16. When the man thrusts his phallus in the yoni with some force and continues to exert pressure till the very end, it is *Piditaka* or 'pressing'.

SUTRA 17. When the man slightly withdraws the phallus, then again presses his abdomen against the woman's with some force, it is *Nirghata* or 'giving a blow'.

SUTRA 18. When only one side of the yoni is rubbed with the phallus it is *Varahaghata* or 'the biting of a boar'.

SUTRA 19. When both the sides of the yoni are so rubbed, it is *Vrisha-ghata*, meaning 'the blow of a bull'. (Like the bull thrusting its horns on all sides.)

SUTRA 20. When the man, without withdrawing his phallus, continues the strokes one after the other, it is *Chatakavilasita*, meaning 'the sporting of the sparrow'. It usually indicates the end of the passionate condition. This is natural when the man's fluid is about to flow.

SUTRA 21. When the union is effected without withdrawing the phallus and both the man and the woman lie united and press each other's thighs, it is *Samputa*. (This has been described before in Part II, Chapter 6, Sutra 15.)

SUTRA 22. The man has to decide which of these ten the woman would favour and unite with her accordingly.

SUTRA 23. When the woman assumes the man's role (i.e., in the case of *Purushayita*), there are three varieties of strokes:

SUTRA 24. When the woman, through assuming the *Vadava* pose for congress, holds the phallus in her yoni, tries to press it in further, and keeps it inside for a long time, it is named *Samdamsha*, meaning 'a pair of tongs'.

SUTRA 25. When the woman is on top of the man, holding his phallus in her yoni, and turning it, round and round in a circle, it is *Bhramaraka*, meaning 'spinning of the top'. This is achieved only after some experience. (Here the woman supports her own body with her hands placed on the man's body.)

SUTRA 26. The man must lift up his thighs to help the woman in circular movements and continuous congress.

SUTRA 27. When the woman swings her hips and abdomen on all the sides (back and forth and side to side, or in a circular movement), it is named *Prenkholita* or 'the swing'. (She should choose from these three according to her lover's inclinations and tastes.)

SUTRA 28. While still united with her lover, the woman should rest by placing her forehead on that of the man.

SUTRA 29. And when she has thus overcome her fatigue, the man recommences the union.

SUTRA 30 (verse). Though a woman may be reserved and try to hide her feelings and desire, she cannot successfully do so when she assumes the role of the man through intense passion.

SUTRA 31 (verse). At all times, a man must carefully observe every action of the one he loves, and so gauge her character and passion, and unite with her keeping them in mind.

SUTRA 32. (verse). A man must never allow the woman to act the man's part if she is menstruating, if she has recently delivered a child, if she is of the Deer-type, if she is pregnant and if she is too corpulent.

- Some say that in this position the woman is unlikely to conceive. If she does conceive, the progeny is likely to have similar nature.
- It may also result in prolapsus.
- In case the woman is of the Deer-type, the Bull and Horse types of men may suffer from the injury known as 'Avapatika', described in Part II, Chapter 6, Sutra 9.
- The pregnant woman may abort.
- The corpulent woman may be entirely incapable of any movement whatsoever.

CHAPTER IX

ON ORAL CONGRESS

SUTRA 1. Eunuchs are of two kinds: those who assume the male form and those who assume the female form. (Males imitate men's beards and so forth while females assume a bust and imitate dress and so forth. Both these types of eunuchs make oral congress their main business in life.)

SUTRAS 2-4. The female eunuch should use all the tricks of the trade of the courtesan, and imitate her dress, voice, gait, laughter, delicacy, timidity, loveliness, helplessness and bashfulness. She can thus derive pleasure as well as her livelihood from such oral congress with a man, which is otherwise named *Auparishtaka*.

SUTRA 5. When the male eunuch wishes to unite with a man, she should conceal her desire and undertake to massage him. (The oral congress in this case is similar to the female eunuch's, but the procedure towards it is different.)

SUTRA 6. She should massage the man's thighs with her limbs, as if embracing him, and with growing familiarity, she should touch the thigh joints over and over again, leading on to the phallus.

SUTRA 7. When she finds his phallus has stiffened, she should play with it with her hands and jest with him about his fickle-mindedness.

SUTRA 8. If, after this, she find that the man does not ask her to proceed, she should commence the oral congress herself. But if the man does ask, she should feign bashfulness and consent to do it after prevarication. (Whenever ordered to do oral congress by the man, whether he shows his desire or not, the male eunuch must invariably feign hesitation. In the case of the female eunuch, however, the man does not order it at all, since her desire is obvious from the start.)

SUTRAS 9-10. There are eight types of oral congress in order of precedence, and the eunuch should pretend to stop after each one and show that she does not wish to do more. (This is simply to arouse the man's curiosity and make him solicit her for more.)

SUTRA 11. The man should order her to do the second after the first, the third after the second and so on. (However, when the eunuch indulges in oral congress from her own desire, she can choose any order she likes.)

SUTRA 12. *Nimita* or 'the nominal congress' results when the eunuch places the man's erected phallus between her lips, and holding it with her hand, moves it about in her mouth.

SUTRA 13. *Parshvatodashta*, or 'biting the sides' takes place when the eunuch grasps the phallus in her hands and with her lips forces it to one side without biting, saying the while, 'This is enough – no more!'.

SUTRA 14. *Bahih-Sandamsha* or 'pressing outside' is done when, on being urged again, the eunuch presses the tip of the phallus with her lips as if drawing it in, and then lets it go. (These three are grouped as 'Bahya', that is, dealing with the external part.)

SUTRA 15. *Antah-Sandamsha* or 'pressing inside' is done when the eunuch on being entreated to do more, takes the phallus into her mouth as far as the man allows, presses its tip with her lips, and then ejects it. (This is specially done when the eunuch desires the oral congress more than the man.)

SUTRA 16. *Chumbitaka* or 'kissing' results when the eunuch grasps the phallus in her hands and kisses it as if she were kissing the man's lower lip.

SUTRA 17. *Parimrishtaka* or 'rubbing' is done in the same way as kissing but, is more extensive, and the eunuch kisses the phallus on all sides with the tip of the tongue and strikes its end similarly.

SUTRA 18. *Amrachushitaka* or 'sucking a mango fruit' results when the eunuch, in high passion, takes in and forcibly sucks the phallus with the skin up, and after pressing it over and over again, with the lips and tongue, releases it.

SUTRA 19. *Samgara* or 'swallowing up' takes place when the eunuch, with the man's consent, takes the phallus into her mouth as far as it goes and presses it until the man's fluid falls. (The eunuch must realise when the man's culmination is imminent, and help the man with movements of her lips and the tongue.)

SUTRA 20. Shrieking and cooing and thrashing and other sadistic acts may be resorted to during oral congress, as the occasion demands. So much for oral congress. (In this love-sport, embracing and kissing and so forth have no place.)

SUTRA 21. Oral congress is practised only by unchaste and immoral women, quite free from any inhibitions, or by female attendants and masseurs. (In other words, by women without morals, or by those who were once attached to someone before, 'but subsequently freed'.)

SUTRA 22. The Acharyas (learned sages) advise men against this practice of oral congress, since the holy texts forbid it and declare it as abhorred and detested by all good men. Moreover, the man himself is likely to suffer from a mental aversion if he allows himself to come in contact with the mouths of these 'Kulata' or unchaste women during the oral congress.

SUTRA 23. Vatsyayana, however, argues that what the holy texts say does not affect the thoroughly immoral man who, as a consequence, does not consider oral congress sinful. Besides, there are ways of avoiding the unhealthy consequences arising from contact with the mouths of these women. (For instance, the mouth may be covered. In some places, oral congress is quite a popular practice.)

SUTRA 24. The people of the Eastern provinces avoid uniting with those women who indulge in oral congress. (They do unite with other types of women with whom they do not find fault.)

SUTRA 25. The men of Ahichhatra do not usually unite with courtesans, but when they do, they avoid oral congress.

SUTRA 26. The men of Saketa, however, unite indiscriminately, without any regard to the purity or impurity of the women.

SUTRAS 27-28. The people of Pataliputra do not indulge in oral congress, but those of Shurasena indulge in all the acts without any reservations.

SUTRA 29. They argue, 'Since by their very nature, women are unclean, who can believe in their natural purity, good conduct, inherited status, promises or speech?' Yet, they are not to be abandoned on that account. Religious texts (Smritis)[1] consider women to be pure. (The cow's udder is pure, though the calf feeds on it; the deer is pure, though the dog hunts it; the fruit is pure, though the bird has dropped it; similarly, the woman's mouth is pure for purposes of congress.)

SUTRA 30. Vatsyayana, however, recognises a difference of opinion among knowledgeable men on this topic, and admits an alternative interpretation of the texts, and therefore enjoins a man to follow the accepted local conventions and the dictates of his own conscience and judgment.

SUTRA 31 (verse). Young masseurs, usually wearing ear ornaments, do allow some men to have oral congress with them. (Sometimes young actors or dandies allow undersexed, or old or inexperienced men to have oral congress with them.)

SUTRA 32 (verse). It is also practised by some citizens who know each other well. (Sometimes citizens who are effeminate indulge in oral congress with each other simultaneously, by lying alongside one another inversely. Some women also do the same, specially in harems, where there is a dearth of virile men.)

SUTRA 33 (verse). In some cases, oral congress is indulged in by a man and woman together, in which case, it should be done in the same way as kissing. When the woman does this with a man, it id described as *Sadharana* or 'ordinary', but when she does it with her maid, it becomes *Asadharana* or 'extraordinary'.

SUTRA 34 (verse). Oral congress between a man and a woman who lie alongside each other inversely and kiss each other's organs, is technically named *Kakila*. (This term is also applied to oral congress between two men and two women.)

SUTRA 35 (verse). It is for this reason that courtesans avoid enticing virtuous, intelligent and generous men, and instead become attached to servants, elephant-drivers and others of low standing.

SUTRA 36 (verse). Oral congress should never be indulged in by a Brahmin learned in sacred books, an official governing a state, or by any other person in whom confidence is reposed by other men. (If they do, their reputation will be marred.)

SUTRA 37 (verse). A thing should not be done merely because there is a text in support of it; the injunctions of the Shastras are general, and have to be selected from for particular application in the right context.

SUTRA 38 (verse). For instance, in medical treatises, dog's meat is recommended for helping the sense of taste and for strength; does that mean, however, that wise men should eat it?

SUTRA 39 (verse). Similarly, in the case of oral congress, all that may be said is that in some cases, on some occasions, in some places, some persons may find it useful or satisfactory.

SUTRA 40 (verse). Eventually, before a man decides to act one way or the other in this matter, he must consider the time, the place, the means at his disposal, religious sanction, his own inclination, and similar other factors, and act accordingly.

SUTRA 41 (verse). Yet, since these things are done secretly, and as the minds of men and women are generally fickle, who can tell how or when or why things will or will not be done?

NOTES

[1] Vasishtha Dharma Sutra, 28-8; Baudhayana Dharma Sutra, 1-5-49; Manu Smriti, 5-130; Vishnu Smriti, 23-49.

CHAPTER X

ON THE BEGINNING AND ENDING OF CONGRESS. THE DIFFERENT TYPES OF CONGRESS AND ON LOVE QUARRELS

SUTRAS 1-12. In his well-furnished house and in the privacy of his bedroom, which has been made fragrant with incense, the citizen, bedecked with flowers and attended by servants, should receive the woman, bathed and decorated, and ply her with drinks, converse with her, and request her to join in the revelry. Seating himself on her right, he should then caress her hair and hands, touch the hem of her garment and the knot of her undergarment, and embrace her with his left hand, thereby preparing her for the congress. They should then jest with each other and cajole, as indicated in previous chapters. He may then talk suggestively about things which would be fit for this occasion, but which at others would be considered coarse and vulgar.

Then amidst singing and music played on instruments, with or without dancing, and amidst discussions on the finer points of art, he should make further suggestions and arouse greater passion in the woman. He should then offer her flowers, sandal paste and betel leaf: she is now fully aroused, and seeing this, he should dismiss the attendants and continue with the embraces described earlier, and gently untie the knot of her undergarment. So much regarding the beginning of congress.

SUTRAS 13-22. After congress, when both lovers are gratified, they go to different washrooms avoiding each other's glances, and acting like strangers: this is technically named 'Ratavasanika'. On returning from the washrooms, their bashfulness disappears, and they sit normally, sharing betel leaves. The man applies sandal paste on his beloved's body, and embracing her with his left hand, offers her his drink to appease her. They may both then partake of water and sweetmeats and other eatables to their taste. These eatables should include mutton soup, broth, fried meat, mixed vegetables, juices, mango fruits, dried meat, circular slices of glazed citron, or any other dish liked in different provinces, and known to be sweet and delicious. Seating themselves either on the floor of the room or on the terrace so as to enjoy the moonlight, they should regale each other with pleasantries, while he may take her on his lap and describe the various constellations planets and satellites – the morning star (Arundhati), the polar star (Dhruva), the seven Rishis (Saptarshi) or the Great Bear. In this way congress should be rounded off.

(Stimulants may be either internal, such as food and the various delicacies, or they may be superficial, such as sherbets, liquor, juices, and so forth. Soup may be also of two kinds – that made from mutton or that made from rice. Sitting on the terrace floor is recommended because of the fresh and cool air.)

There are some verses in this context:

SUTRAS 23-27 (verses). Lovers will find that if they dally with each other in pleasing ways and so create confidence in each other, both at the commencement and at the end of congress, they will heighten the love between them. These acts please both their tastes, dispel anger and enhance love; acts such as Hallisaka and other dances, songs, dramatic performances, women moving in a circle and singing, gazing at the moon and the stars with love-laden eyes, glistening with emotion. If the lovers are reminiscent of the pleasure of their first meeting, the pain of separation, they find they become passionate and express their passion through embraces and kisses.

SUTRA 28; The different kinds of *Rata* or congress are:
- *Ragavat* or 'loving congress'.
- *Aharya* or 'congress of subsequent love'.
- *Kritrima* or 'congress based on artificial love'.
- *Vyavahita* or 'congress based on transferred love'.
- *Pota* or 'congress similar to that of eunuchs'.
- *Khala* or 'degrading congress'.
- *Ayantrita* or 'congress of unfettered love'.

SUTRA 29. It is called *Ragavat* when a man and woman feel passion for each other at first sight and then unite
- after some attempt
- after returning from a separation forced by a journey
- after a lover's quarrel and reconciliation

SUTRA 30. This congress is carried on at will till both the lovers feel fully satisfied

SUTRA 31. It is named *Aharya* when lovers unite while their love is still young and untried

SUTRA 32. *Kritrima* is descriptive of a congress of lovers who come together in spite of loving other persons in reality. They excite themselves with the help of the sixty-four arts laid down in the texts of the science of love.

SUTRA 33. In this case, the lovers are not naturally in love with each other, and also when they avail themselves of the sixty-four arts, they must choose from them discriminatingly.

SUTRA 34. It is called *Vyavahita* when a man unites with a woman and indulges in the various modes of love-play with her, but privately thinks of quite another who is really his beloved.

SUTRA 35. A man is said to indulge in *Pota Rata* when he unites with
- a woman lower than him in status
- a woman lower than him in caste
- a servant maid

(The word 'Pota' really denotes a eunuch, namely, a woman who can assume either a male's or a female's characteristics.)

SUTRA 36. If the man unites with a eunuch, he must eschew some love-sport for arousing passion.

SUTRA 37. *Khala Rata* results when a courtesan unites with an uncultured and uneducated rustic till her desire is satisfied. (When she cannot attract a citizen, she has to resort to a villager to allay her passion, and this she has to conceal from others as it is quite low and degrading for her.)

SUTRA 38. Similarly, when a citizen (out of sheer passion), is forced to unite with a village-woman or unworthy woman, it is also known as *Khala Rata*.

SUTRA 39. It is termed *Ayantrita* when a man and woman entertain mutual love and confidence and unite with each other spontaneously.

(These seven types of *Rata* or 'congress' are collectively termed as *Chitra Rata*, since they are noted for the complete absence of any restraint on the part of the lovers.)

SUTRA 40. Now regarding love-quarrels.[1]
A woman who has grown to love a man, should not tolerate
- his mentioning the name or names of his other wives,
- his praising their virtues, or
- his calling her by the name of another whom he loves, or
- his continued attentions to another of his wives.

(The first three are considered to be his faults in speech, while the last is designated a fault in action.)

SUTRA 41. The offended woman usually displays her anger by crying, forcing physical discomfort and pain on herself. She will shake her head so that her hair is dishevelled, beat her own limbs, fling herself on the ground, tear off her flowers and ornaments and prostrate herself on the floor. (Some commentators, however, differ from this interpretation and say that the woman strikes the man and not herself, by grasping his locks of hair, and that sleeping on the floor signifies that she wishes to sleep alone.)

SUTRA 42. Remaining cool and unperturbed, the man must placate her and falling at her feet, he should persuade her to get up and occupy the bed.[2]

SUTRA 43. She, on her part, must reply by grasping his hair, kicking his hands, his head, his chest repeatedly, thus showing her increasing anger.

SUTRA 44. Finally, she must proceed to the door and sit there weeping.

SUTRA 45. Here Dattaka gives a warning that no matter how angry she is, the woman must not step outside the door, since that gesture will be misunderstood. (On this occasion, the woman, kicking her lover on the head, is not objected to: on the contrary, some citizens of old consider it a sign of her strength.)

SUTRA 46. Thus persuaded, the woman should still keep on taunting him and hurting him, but should now start expecting favours from him. She may allow her lover to embrace her tightly and allow herself to feel passionate. (The man must recognise that kicking him is the sign of the woman's ultimate anger, and she must realise that falling at her feet is the limit to which the man will go in persuading her. She must begin to give in then, though she may continue her taunting: otherwise her lover will be annoyed if her anger remains unabated.

This approach applies to highborn maidens and widows.)

The approach of a courtesan and of a woman who is married to another man should be patterned thus:

SUTRA 47. The woman, who in her own house has had a quarrel with her lover due to any of the causes mentioned above, should display her anger in the natural way (such as show her jealousy and frown and knit her eyebrows).

SUTRA 48. The lover tries to pacify her through the good offices of either the Pithamarda, the Vita or the Vidushaka, and when she is thus pacified, she should go to her lover's house and spend the night there. (Falling at the feet of such men is forbidden, hence the need for these messengers. She must, on her part, go to the man's house to retrieve her lost dignity and to eventually satisfy her lover.)

SUTRA 49 (verse). To conclude: When a man is well versed in all the sixty-four arts of love and can command their use when winning over women who are also accomplished in those arts, he may be sure of success. (If he is ignorant of these, no matter how well acquainted he may be with the other sciences, he will not be respected by others.)

SUTRA 50 (verse). If he is not conversant with these sixty-four arts of the science of love, he will never be respected among learned men, never be able to fulfil the three Aims of Life, though he may be quite competent to explain the theory and application of other sciences.

SUTRA 51 (verse). On the other hand, simply by a thorough knowledge of these sixty-four arts, a man commands a leading position among men and women who discuss these topics, although he may be ignorant of other sciences. (For instance, when men and women discuss topics such as the various postures for congress, other topics have no place there.)

SUTRA 52 (verse). Who does not respect these sixty-four arts which are respected universally by the learned and the cunning, and revered by all the guilds of courtesans?

(Learned men who propound the ways and means of attaining the three aims of Dharma, Artha and Kama, consider these sixty-four arts as essential for the protection of women; the crooks find that they help them materially, while the courtesans depend on them for their very living.)

'Nanda' or 'Nandana' means 'Puja' or adoration. 'Nandini' thus means that science which includes 'Nanda'.

SUTRA 53 (verse) The great scholars of the science of love mention this 'Nandini' as having four aspects:

♦ 'Subhaga' as it is practised by all householders.
♦ 'Siddha' because it also brings other things in its wake – knowledge, feeling, etc.
♦ 'Subhagankarani' because it achieves physical loveliness and moral wellbeing.
♦ 'Naripriya' because it largely benefits women.

SUTRA 54 (verse). A man who is expert in these sixty-four arts is much respected by maidens, other men's wives and by courtesans. ('Punarbhu' or 'widow' is included in 'other men's wives'. The word 'Ganika' should have been replaced by the word 'Veshya', but here it is used as signifying 'other women'.)

NOTES

1   Cf. Amarushataka, 51-52, 151, 22, 29.
2   Cf. Amarushataka, 26, 38, 39.

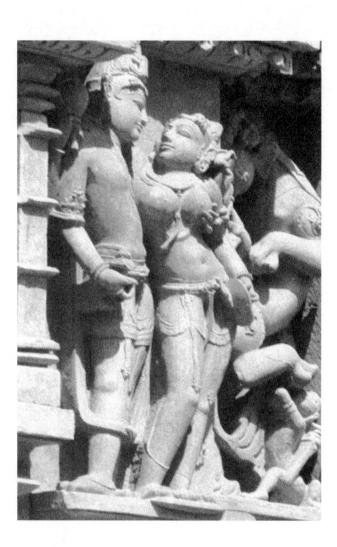

PART III

ON ACQUIRING
A WIFE

CHAPTER I

ON SELECTION AND ACCEPTANCE OF THE BRIDE

SUTRA 1. When a marriage with a maiden of one's own caste, who is also a virgin, is arranged in compliance with the holy texts, it is conducive to the aims of Dharma and Artha, progeny, relatives, more friends, and a pure and natural love between the married partners.

SUTRA 2. When a man, therefore, on completing his studies, selects a bride, he should see to it that she is a virgin, at least three years younger than himself, born in a well-to-do family, whose parents are experienced guardians still alive, and whose way of life is praiseworthy. She should have and cherish many relatives, both on the paternal and the maternal side. She must possess beauty and character, good health and proportionate limbs, and have good teeth, nails, ears, hair, eyes, and breasts, and suffer from no ailment. Of course, the man must also possess the same qualities which he expects in his bride.

SUTRA 3. If, says Ghotakamukha, a man should select such a maiden for his bride, he will have done the right thing and none of his equals would be able to criticize him.

SUTRA 4. In selecting the bride, parents and relatives and mutual friends of the two partners should exert themselves (usually at the instance of the man himself).

SUTRAS 5-6. Friends should indicate to the parents of the maiden the deficiences of other aspiring candidates, which may or may not be visibly proved, and warn them of future dangers; but in the case of their friend, on whose behalf they are negotiating, they should praise his excellent ancestry, his (literary and artistic) accomplishments, and such other praiseworthy qualities and traits which may help to build a favourable opinion (in the minds of the maiden's parents). They should also patiently recount the man's qualities most admired by the maiden's mother, and demonstrate those benefits already present and those which may accrue in future (from the proposed marriage).

SUTRA 7. Then the astrologer should be sent for by the citizen, and his help should be sought in forecasting future benefits such as greater wealth and other happy events from the position of the planets, sounds of birds and from the particular signs and marks on the body.

SUTRA 8. The maiden's mother should be convinced by the astrologer beyond all doubt that greater advantages should accrue to the girl if she married that particular citizen whose cause the astrologer was advocating, than to any other man. (The astrologer may further add that the parents of other marriageable daughters have also shown him their horoscopes and consulted him about that particular citizen.)

SUTRA 9. A maiden should be selected for marriage and given in marriage according to the compatibility of horoscopes.

SUTRA 10. Ghotakamukha warns that the decision about the marriage must not be exclusively that of the citizen and of the maiden's parents respectively but other members of the family must also be consulted. (This opinion of Ghotakamukha is not contradicted by others and may therefore be considered acceptable to them.)

SUTRA 11. While selecting a bride, a citizen should take care to avoid one who is asleep, or who is crying or who is going out of the house (sleeping forebodes early death, crying denotes misery, while going out of the house presages desertion).

SUTRA 12. The following also should be avoided:

One who has an inauspicious name.
One who is concealed.
One who is already married to another.
One who has brown blemishes.
One who has white blemishes.
One who has a manly build.
One who stoops at the shoulders.
One who is bow-legged.
One whose forehead is too wide.
One who has lighted her father's funeral pyre.
One who has committed adultery.
One who has fully acquired puberty.
One who is dumb.
One who is already friendly with the citizen.
One who is comparatively too young for the citizen.
One who is always perspiring or her hands and on her feet.
'Kapila' causes the death of her husband.
'Prishata' destroys both husband and wealth.
'Rishabha' is one who has a weak character.
'Vinata' is one who is of loose morals.
'Vikata' brings misery.
'Vimunda' destroys the husband.
'Raka' is no more a virgin.
'Phalini' fails in any communication.
'Varshakari' is one who sweats profusely.

SUTRA 13. Similarly, a maiden who bears the name of a Nakshatra (star), river, tree, or whose name ends in either 'i' or 'r', or one whose reputation has suffered, should be avoided while selecting a bride.

SUTRA 14. In the opinion of some sages of old, marriage with a maiden who at first sight pleases the mind and delights the eye always results in the fulfilment of the three aims of life; it is not so with those who don't, and they must therefore be avoided.

SUTRA 15. The functionaries on the maiden's side should dress her in attractive and decent clothes at the time of the 'Varana' (i.e., on the occasion of choosing a bride), and carry on the ceremony till the afternoon.

SUTRA 16. A marriageable maiden should be smartly dressed when playing with her women friends every day, and when she attends religious or marriage ceremonies, other people would make an effort to see her. She should be seen at festivals as a marriageable commodity and be able to arouse people's curiosity. Having maidens in attendance at public gatherings adds to the girl's prestige, as she is not then seen very easily. A girl who is seen too easily is not appealing.

SUTRA 17. During the 'Varana' ceremony, the bridal party should welcome the bridegroom's party who should conduct themselves with dignity and conformity, with offerings of auspicious rice and curds.

SUTRA 18. Then the maiden, who has been decked out in all her finery on some pretext or the other, is shown to them.

SUTRA 19. The members of the bridal party would then leave it to Prajapati or the divine ordainer to bring about the bride's marriage and in that hope would consider the matter with their friends and relatives and appoint a time limit for the bridegroom's reply.

SUTRA 20. Then the members of the bridegroom's party are invited to bathe and dine. They should take care not to commit themselves about anything on the day, but merely to say, 'Everything will be done at the proper time'.

SUTRA 21 When the marriage is thus subsequently arranged, the ceremony may be selected according to the prevailing provincial custom, or from that of Brahma, Prajapatya, Arsha or Daiva forms of marriage.

There are some verses in this connection:

SUTRAS 22-24 (verses). The games which are to be played collectively, marriages and friendships, should all be between persons of the same age group – not with too elderly persons nor with the too young.

Wise husbands avoid the relationship with their bride's family whereby they have to behave like their servants. This is technically the 'Uchcha' relationship. (Only the helpless resort to it.)

SUTRA 25 (verse). That relationship is the most acceptable which enables both partners in marriage to take pleasure in each other's activities.

SUTRA 26 (verse). Even if the citizen has been forced into the 'Uchcha' relationship, he should return to his own home (and so make a break from it).

On no account should he enter into the 'Heena' or the low type of marriage relationship, which has been condemned by the wise and the learned.

CHAPTER II

ON CREATING CONFIDENCE IN THE BRIDE

SUTRA 1. The newly-wedded couple should sleep on the floor for the first three nights, observing celibacy (until the fourth day, when proper oblations are offered), partaking of food (at night) which is free from jaggery and rock-salt. For the next seven days, they should continue their celibacy as before, but should indulge in ceremonial baths to the accompaniment of pipe music, bedeck themselves with ornaments and suitable clothes, eat together, attend dramatic festivals and honour their relatives (with perfumes and garlands). This applies to members of all the four castes. (Alternatively, this is termed 'the vow of ten nights'.)

SUTRA 2. After this period, the bridegroom may commence his amorous advances to his wife in a delicate manner, in a secluded chamber at night. (Brides are of two varieties, those who have attained puberty and are therefore fit for the union; and others who are still immature. Advances of the first type are for creating confidence in the bride, leading to the actual union; those of the other type are for removing fear, and distrust and suspicion from the immature bride's mind.)

SUTRA 3. Followers of Babhravya opine that these advances are necessary in as much as the maiden, seeing her bridegroom silent and inactive like a pillar, during the first three days, may become worried and confused, and may take him to be a eunuch.

SUTRA 4. Vatsyayana's contention is that although the bridegroom should make advances to induce confidence in his bride, he should, however, abstain from the actual union and not transgress the vow of celibacy.

SUTRAS 5-6. During his advances, he must avoid doing anything rashly, for women are like flowers, and can only bear a delicate approach. Rashness in advances not only fails to create confidence, but engenders a disgust towards the ultimate union in the mind of the bride. At all times, therefore, the bridegroom must be gentle and considerate.

SUTRA 7. The man should gain his bride's confidence by availing himself of any of the following advances:

SUTRAS 8-9. He should start with a short and pleasant embrace, usually on the upper part of her body, since there it is more easily endured.

SUTRA 10. If the maiden is grown up or if the man has known her for some time, the embracing may be done in lamplight; in case the maiden is still very young or the bridegroom has not known her before, these embraces must take place in the dark.

SUTRA 11. When she has acquiesced in this embracing, the man should offer her a betel leaf from his own mouth. If she does not accept it, he should make her take it with pleasing words, oaths, beseeching, and then fall at her feet. However bashful or angry a maiden may be, she can never utterly disregard her husband falling at her feet; this is common experience.

SUTRA 12. While the betel leaf is being offered, the man should imprint a soft, touching and silent kiss on her mouth.

SUTRAS 13-14. Once she is thus won over, the man should attempt to engage her in conversation and draw her out by asking her short questions and pretending not to know the answers.

SUTRA 15. If she still remains silent, the man should persevere with sweet and pleasant conversation without however annoying her.

SUTRA 16. If she remains silent even after this, the man should further importune her.

SUTRA 17. Ghotakamukha says, all maidens hear the man's words, without sometimes uttering a word themselves.

SUTRA 18. When the maiden is thus engaged in conversation, she may reply silently by a nod of her head. If she wishes to disdain her lover, she should not even nod.

SUTRA 19. When the bridegroom asks her: 'Do you desire me or not? Do I appeal to you?' She should pause as if to think it over, and on being further pressed for an answer she should say exactly the opposite of what she had intended (e.g., 'You do not appeal to me,' 'I do not like you,' etc.).

SUTRA 20. If the man has known his bride for some time, he may converse with her in this manner in the presence of her chosen friends and confidantes.

SUTRA 21. She should smile with her face down during this conversation.

SUTRA 22. Then, if any of her friends should transgress certain limits, the bride should chide her and rebukingly exchange words.

SUTRA 23. The friend, on her part, should argue that what was said was said jokingly, although this may not have been the case.

SUTRA 24. Then the bride, dismissing this conversation, should remain silent when spoken to by her bridegroom.

Sutra 25. If pressed for a reply, she should say haltingly and inaudibly, 'I do not say this'.

Sutra 26. Sometimes she should cast sidelong glances at him in a jesting manner. These are the tricks to be employed by a couple who have known each other for some time.

Sutra 27. Thus a bride who has cultivated sufficient familiarity with her husband, should prepare betel leaves, sandal paste and garlands for him without his having to ask for them, and then proceed to tie them up in his upper garment.

Sutra 28. While she is engaged in doing this, he should embrace her small and growing bosom in the *Achchhuritaka* manner.

Sutra 29. When she tries to avoid him, he should request her to embrace him. Then, gradually, he should extend his hand towards her navel and withdraw it, saying all the while that he has no intention of doing anything more. Very gradually, he should proceed to take her on his lap and press his advances further.

Sutra 30. (If she does not respond, he should then intimidate her thus); 'I will make teeth-marks on your lips and nail-marks on your bosom. I will make similar marks on my own body and then tell your friends that you made them. What will you then say to them?' Thus resorting to tricks which would frighten children and force them to acquiesce, the man must win over his bride's confidence, subtly and gradually.

Sutra 31. On the second or the third night, after she has acquired greater confidence, he should make further advances with the help of his hands.

Sutras 32-33. The man should then proceed to kiss all parts of her body and shampoo her thighs, pressing them many times.

Sutras 34-35. If she does not permit him to do this, he should question her about the objections, but slow down the shampooing all the same. When he finds that she can endure it, he should touch her pubic region, loosen her lower garment and put it aside, and continue to press her thighs. These are the various ways of approaching the bride.

SUTRA 36. After the fourth day, when oblations are offered, and on being united in congress, he should promise to please her every moment. Till then, however, he must not break the vow of celibacy.

SUTRAS 37-38. After that, the bridegroom should initiate her into the sixty-four arts, treat her with loving care, describe to her the desires he had before, take an oath before her that he would, in future, do whatever she wishes him to do. He should remove her fears about his co-wives, and continue uniting with her who is now no longer a young maiden, in the most considerate and pleasing manner. So much for creating confidence in a woman.

There are some verses on this subject:

SUTRA 39 (verse). The man acting according to his bride's inclination, should so win her confidence that she grows more and more attached to him and becomes his trusted companion.

SUTRA 40 (verse). He is never able to win over maidens by either doing exactly as they wish or by going too much against their wishes. The best way to win them over is by striking the golden mean.

SUTRA 41 (verse). He who knows the secret of obtaining greater pleasure, who respects and honours the dignity of maidens and who knows the art of creating confidence in them, becomes the most endearing of men.

SUTRA 42 (verse). The man who neglects a maiden thinking her to be too bashful, is despised by her as ignorant of the working of her mind, and usually comes to grief, like other animals.

SUTRA 43 (verse). The man who approaches a maiden suddenly,

precipitately, without regard to her feelings, engenders fear, disgust, dejection and detestation in her mind.

SUTRA 44 (verse). When the maiden is not aroused properly, she harbours resentment against her husband whom she hates, and resorts to other men.

CHAPTER III

ON WAYS OF COURTING AND WINNING THE HEART OF THE BRIDE

SUTRA 1. A poor citizen, though he may be blessed with virtues, or one of low birth, though he may possess mediocre qualities, or one who is a neighbour, though he may be wealthy, or one who has to depend for this livelihood on his parents and brothers, or one who looks like a child even though he has easy access to the girl's house – such a man should not himself select a girl for marriage, since he will find it impossible to win her over on his own.

SUTRA 2. (If he must, however, do so) he should win her over from her very childhood.

SUTRA 3. A citizen in Southern India, who suffers from any of the handicaps mentioned above, or who is a penniless orphan living at his maternal uncle's home, may thus strive to win over the latter's daughter, even though she be betrothed to another, from her very childhood; otherwise he may find her inaccessible owing to his maternal uncle's wealth and pride.

SUTRA 4. Similarly, he may try to win over any other girl. In the opinion of Ghotakamukha, when unstinted and pure contact with the maiden is established from her childhood, the wooing of her by the man is above reproach.

SUTRAS 5-6. The man should then collect flowers and make garlands in her company, and in keeping with their ages and mutual acquaintance, indulge in such games as making (wooden or mud) toy houses, dolls (of rags, threads, etc.); in cooking (with sand and pebbles); in weaving long strips of wool or thread; in guessing what is in closed fists, or the game known as Panchasamaya; in espying the middle finger when jumbled with the others and closed into a fist; in the game of six pebbles and in many similar games popular in her province and favoured by her. He may play these games either alone with her or in the company of her relatives and attendants.

SUTRA 7. Other games which he should play with her with the help of her friends involve some exertion:

◆ Blind man's buff.
◆ At a hand clap from the umpire, one person runs in search of another.
◆ The game called Lavanavithika.
◆ Stretching hands, and turning round in a circle as if with wings.
◆ Finding out hidden coins from heaps of rice and grain.
◆ A blindfolded player points out any other player who taps lightly on his own forehead.

And other games which happen to be popular in that province (games like Mandukika, Ekapadika, etc.).

SUTRA 8. The suitor should always be on very cordial terms with the woman whom he thinks to be the girl's confidante, and as their acquaintance grows, he should consolidate their friendship.

SUTRA 9. Above all, he should obligate the daughter of the girl's nurse with little acts and kindnesses which benefit her both momentarily and permanently. If she is pleased, this nurse's daughter will not say anything against him, even if she is aware of his designs; on the contrary, she may sometimes become instrumental in bringing the two together, even though she is not told to take a leading part in bringing about their union.

SUTRA 10. Even if the nurse's daughter is not aware of the man's intentions, she will nonetheless praise his excellent virtues to the girl in such a way that the maiden will be irresistibly drawn to the man.

SUTRA 11. The suitor should find out if the girl is curious about anything in particular: if she is, he should enlighten himself on the subject and then satisfy her curiosity.

SUTRA 12. He should obtain and present her with new dolls and toys of original designs which other young girls find difficult to obtain.

SUTRA 13. He should show her a ball decorated with various colours and. designs all around it, and several other playthings and toys made of threads, wood, horn, ivory, wax and clay.

SUTRA 14. He should show her the work to be done in the kitchen to enable her to cook meals for the family (after her marriage). He should show her figures of a man and a woman united and carved from one wooden piece; similar figures of rams and goats, miniature temples and houses made of clay and bamboo chips; cages made of clay and other materials and containing birds such as parrots, koels, Madanasarika, Lavaka, cocks and partridges; water pots of different shapes and designs; mechanical devices; toy Veenas; a stand for keeping dolls and toys; a casket or basket (for keeping cosmetics and manicure aids); the red paint, Manahsila, Haritala, red mercury oxide (Sindoora), powdered Rajavarta, sandal paste, kumkum, betel nuts and betel leaves. Whenever she requires anything at any particular moment, he should give it to her either secretly or openly, according to the circumstances. In short, he should act in such a way as to make the girl feel that he is able to fulfil all her wants.

SUTRA 15. When he wishes to see her, he should plead with her for a secret meeting, and regale her with anecdotes (about other people in such a way as would make her feel attracted to him).

SUTRA 16. If she questions about some of his gifts being secret, he should point out his fear of elders and indicate that such things are also liked by others.

SUTRA 17. If her imagination is stimulated by tales and anecdotes, he should please her by narrating them to her.

SUTRA 18. If she is fond of seeing conjuring tricks, he should demonstrate these to her and see her wonderstruck. If she is curious about objects of art, he should display them to her. If she is fond of music, he should please her with melodious songs.

On the eighth night of the waning phase of the moon, and on other moonlit nights, during festivals and gatherings, on the days of lunar and solar eclipses, or when the girl visits him at his own house – on all these occasions he should please her with different kinds of garlands for the head, leaf cuttings, wax, clothes, rings and ornaments, provided there is no harm done in presenting these to her.

SUTRA 19. The nurse's daughter, knowing that this suitor is superior to others in as much as he possesses certain qualities, should pass on the knowledge of the sixty-four skills of the art of love to the girl, after learning them first from the suitor who has had experience in these matters.

SUTRA 20. Under the pretext of instructing the nurse's daughter, the suitor would be able to show his chosen maiden his skills in the art of love.

SUTRA 21. He should attire himself in attractive clothes and often be seen by her without any obstruction.

SUTRAS 22-23. His growing attraction for her will become apparent to her, for young women usually love the first man with whom they become acquainted and whom they see very often; but though they feel attracted to that man, they will not proceed further themselves and become united with him. This is the general rule, and therefore these advances to a young maiden have been recounted above.

SUTRA 24. We will now describe the gestures mentioned above (which reveal the attraction the girl feels for the man).

SUTRA 25. She does not look him straight in the face. If seen, she becomes bashful.

SUTRA 26. She will expose one or other of her beautiful limbs on some pretext or the other (while actually making a show of covering that part).

SUTRA 27. If the man is inattentive or alone or distant, she keeps on looking in his direction.

SUTRA 28. When questioned, she speaks but little with a smile, inaudibly and indistinctly, haltingly, and keeping her face down.

SUTRA 29. She likes very much to be with him for a long time.

SUTRA 30. Even though she stands far away, she expects him to notice her, and believing this, she speaks to her attendants with expressive mien, and does not leave the place.

SUTRA 31. She laughs if she notices anything there, and spins out some yarn (to her attendants) in order to remain in that place.

SUTRA 32. She embraces and kisses a child sitting in her lap, and makes the mark on the forehead of the maidservant.

SUTRA 33. Surrounded by her attendants she performs all those feminine acts[1] (such as plaiting or parting her hair, bending or stretching her limbs, yawning and so forth).

SUTRA 34. She places confidence in his friends, respects their opinion and is guided by it.

SUTRA 35. She treats his servants kindly, talks with them and even plays the game of dice with them.

SUTRA 36. She orders them to perform their respective duties attentively as if she were their 'master'.

SUTRA 37. When they talk among themselves about their master, she listens attentively.

SUTRAS 38-39. Encouraged and escorted by the daughter of her nurse, she enters her suitor's house and expresses her desire to play games with him or to converse with him with the help of her chaperon.

SUTRA 40. If she is at any time not properly bedecked or well attired, she avoids being seen by him.

SUTRA 41. When she asks him for a ring or a garland or an ear ornament made from a leaf, he slowly and gracefully removes it from wherever he has worn it and places it in the hand of her friend; and since it is given by him, she puts on the ornament every day.

SUTRA 42. When she hears anything relating to other suitors, she becomes dejected and shuns the company of any members of their families.

SUTRA 43 (verse). When the maiden's love for a man becomes apparent to him through such expressions and gestures, he should proceed to explore the various possibilities of eventually uniting with her physically.

SUTRA 44 (verse). A young girl is won over by dolls and toys; a young maiden by a show of artistic talent; and a fully mature woman by winning over her own confidante.

NOTES

1 Vatsyayana has used the word 'lila'. Yashodhara perhaps did not clearly understand the meaning of this word. It does not mean combing and plaiting the hair as given by him. It means imitation of the acts of one's lover. 'Ishta Janasya Anukrithi'. Cf. Bharata, Natyashastra, 24-14. See also, Nagarasarvasva, 13-16.

CHAPTER IV

ON HOW A MAN MUST BEHAVE FOR THE POSSESSION OF THE BRIDE. HOW THE WOMAN CAN WIN A DESIRABLE MAN AND SUBJUGATE HIM

SUTRA 1. When a man observes through the various expressions and gestures mentioned in the earlier chapter that the maiden loves him, he should endeavour to secure physical union with her thus.

SUTRA 2. First, regarding superficial advances. While arguing in games, he should hold her hand as if to indicate his selection and final acceptance of her.

SUTRA 3. He should then indulge in the four types of embraces (*Sprishtaka*, etc.) with her as described in an earlier chapter.

SUTRA 4. He should cut out two figures on a leaf and show them to her, suggesting his own desires (this sport is known as 'Patrachchhedya').

SUTRA 5. Other designs may also be cut and shown from time to time.

SUTRA 6. While engaged in water-sport, he should dive at a distance from her but emerge near her, and having touched her, should once again dive into the water.

SUTRAS 7-8. While playing with her such rural games as 'admiring new foliage' (Navapatra), he should reiterate his sentiments towards her and tirelessly emphasize the torment he suffers on her account.

SUTRA 9. He should relate to her his dreams of love with reference to other maidens.

SUTRAS 10-11. At a dramatic performance or among family gatherings, he should sit next to her and touch her on one pretext or another, and press his foot on hers in order to finally rest his body against hers.

SUTRAS 12-13. Having done so, he should feel each of her fingers slowly, and scratch his toenail against her fingernails.

SUTRA 14. After this much is accomplished, his advances should proceed upwards (towards the abdomen and the posterior, rather like climbing the steps of a ladder).

SUTRA 15. The man should persevere with these embraces until she gets used to them.

Now regarding deeper embraces.

SUTRA 16. When she offers her feet to him for washing, he should press her fingers between his fingers (as if held by tongs).

SUTRA 17. When he offers her things (like betel nut), or when he accepts things from her, he should do it by making nail-marks on her hands.

SUTRA 18. When she offers him water for rinsing (Achamana), he should sprinkle some of it on her after Achamana.

SUTRA 19. Seated beside her in a lonely place or lying down beside her on a bed in the dark, he should observe her reactions (to the advances described above).

SUTRA 20. He should make his feelings known to her without in any way distressing her.

SUTRA 21. He should say, 'I have something to say to you in private'; but when she questions him about it, he should keep silent, and only observe her feelings, through her gestures, as will be described later in Chapter V.

SUTRA 22. After making sure of her feelings towards him, he should feign a sickness (such as headache), and cause her on that pretence to be brought to his house.

SUTRA 23. When she comes there, he should describe his ailment to her and make her press his head on all sides. While she is doing this, he should grasp her hand and express his feelings by bestowing kisses on her eyes and forehead.

SUTRAS 24-25. He should ask her to get him the required medicine, saying, 'Only you can do this. This should not be done by anybody else except a maiden.' Thus, while she is going, he should request her to return to his house once more.

SUTRA 26. This device of feigned illness may be practised for three days and three nights.

SUTRA 27. At every visit, he should try to engage her in discussions on art or narrate stories to her for prolonging her visit.

SUTRA 28. In order to induce her confidence, he should press his advances further in the company of other women, but should avoid speaking about his love on these occasions.

SUTRA 29. Ghotakamukha contends that however hard a man tries to gain the confidence of the girl he loves, he can never successfully win her over without a great amount of exertion on his part.

SUTRA 30. Only after he has won her over completely in this fashion, should he try to have union with her (by the Gandharva Vidhi).

SUTRA 31. Generally speaking, women have very little fear of being seen at nightfall, during the night itself or wherever there is darkness. It is then easier to arouse their passion and achieve union with them, since they do not discountenance a man's advances. It is therefore generally agreed that women should be approached at such a time.

SUTRA 32. When a man finds that his single-handed efforts are not enough, he should engage the help of his beloved's nurse or her woman companion, both of whom can persuade her to do certain things, without divulging his real intentions. In this way, the man can keep approaching the girl and proceed with his advances.

SUTRA 33. Alternatively, he should depute one of his own maid servants to befriend his beloved.

SUTRA 34. In conclusion, a man should first ascertain his beloved's inclinations from her gestures and general behaviour, and when he attends various functions with her, like sacrificial rites, marriages, excursions, festivals or other public engagements, he should make his advances to her when others are not looking. He may, after that, press his advances further when she is alone. (He should try to win her by the Gandharva Vidhi.)

SUTRA 35. Vatsyayana contends that if a woman is well inclined towards a man and reveals that to him through her gestures, she will not resist his advances if properly timed and placed.

SUTRA 36. A maiden, even though endowed with outstanding womanly virtues, but whose relatives are of a low caste, or a maiden who is highborn but without wealth and hence not sought after by her equals, or a maiden who is an orphan and dependent on a relative, should each seek a young man's hand in marriage herself when she comes of age.

SUTRA 37. She should approach a young man of strong qualities, one who is capable and good-looking, with fondness similar to that which she had in her games in her childhood

SUTRA 38. When she finds a man making advances to her because of his inability to control his natural impulses and without parental intercedence, she should try to win him over with her loving ways and the means at her disposal, so that they meet each other frequently.

SUTRA 39. The maiden should be encouraged in this by her mother (when alive or by her foster-mother) and by her women-friends and nurses.

SUTRA 40. The maiden should select the place of rendezvous with her lover in a secluded spot and at odd times take with her perfumes and betel leaves.

SUTRA 41. She should at other times display her accomplishments in the various arts, and shampoo and press his head – but all these she should show him with all due propriety.

SUTRA 42. The maiden should employ all the ways and means described in earlier chapters which a man employs to win over his beloved. This includes the narration of stories congenial to her lover's temperament.

SUTRA 43. However, the old sages maintain that a maiden should never begin the advances herself, no matter how strong her passion, for then she loses her grace and charm.

SUTRA 44. She should confine her advances to those 'superficial' expedients which her lover would have employed had he wanted to approach her.

SUTRAS 45-46. When she is sitting on his lap or being embraced, she should not betray any agitation or disapproval, but on the contrary, welcome his advances and feign ignorance of his real intentions.

SUTRAS 47-48. When he holds up her face for a kiss; she should behave as if it were being done by force, and when he requests her to rouse his passion, she should touch his phallus reluctantly.

SUTRA 49. Despite his requests, she should not expose too much of her body, since there is no certainty of marriage on his part.

SUTRA 50. If, on the other hand, he becomes completely attached to her and she feels sure that he would not go back on his word, she should encourage him in his advances towards a final consummation.

SUTRA 51. When she is thus ravished, she should confide this fact only to her confidantes.

So much for the description of the ways and means of winning over the beloved.

SUTRA 52 (verse). When a maiden has to choose her husband from among young men making advances to her, she should select one who is the most agreeable, and who in her opinion is likely to carry out whatever she would ask him to do, and thus add to the marital happiness.

SUTRA 53 (verse). If she is avaricious, she may marry a wealthy man in spite of his co-wives, in utter disregard of his accomplishments, good looks or the fitness of things.

SUTRA 54 (verse). A maiden should not reject a young man who is accomplished, capable, obedient and honest in his intentions, who makes advances to her by all the means at his disposal.

SUTRA 55 (verse). A man who is capable of supporting his own family and blessed with a docile nature, even though poor and without any accomplishments is to be preferred to a man who maintains several wives although he be accomplished.

SUTRA 56 (verse). Generally, the wives of such rich men are without any discipline or self-control, and though they enjoy material pleasures, they do not experience the deeper pleasures (arising from a happy marriage).

SUTRAS 57-58 (verses). A man of low caste, or an aging man, or one who is given to much travelling is not fit to be married; nor is the man who comes to his wife only when he wishes it, or who pretends much or who gambles and wastes his wealth, or who has many wives and several children. (Any one of these is enough to disqualify a man as a suitable husband.)

SUTRA 59 (verse). Of all suitors of a maiden, who are equally accomplished, he alone should be preferred who is the most gentlemanly and the most loving of them.

CHAPTER V

ON THE DIFFERENT FORMS OF MARRIAGES

SUTRA 1. When a man finds that frequent meetings with the maiden in secluded places are difficult, he should befriend the maiden's nurse with presents and, through her, press his advances further.

SUTRAS 2-3. Pretending not to know the young man too well, the nurse should praise the qualities of the man which she knows are prized by the maiden.

SUTRAS 4-5. At the same time, the nurse should criticize and disparage the other suitors for whom the maiden does not care, and explain that her parents and relatives favour them out of greediness alone, without really getting to know her beloved's accomplishment; citing examples of Shakuntala and other maidens, she should convince her that they attained conjugal happiness because they selected their own husbands.

SUTRA 6. (In contrast), she should point out how maidens married into influential families generally come to grief through the manoeuvres of the co-wives, and eventually, are abandoned and hated; while her future happiness with the man of her choice would be secure.

SUTRA 7. The advantages of being the one and only wife of the suitor who loves her should be brought home to her.

SUTRA 8. (Finding the maiden gradually persuaded in favour of the man) the nurse should proceed to remove from her mind all thoughts of danger and fear and bashfulness.

SUTRA 9. She may employ all the means open to a female messenger to bring the maiden around.

SUTRA 10. Reassuring the maiden that her beloved would take her out and with some force try to win her over, she should make her agree to this arrangement.

SUTRA 11. Thus, when the maiden awaits her beloved at a lonely place, he should spread the Kusha grass and light it with the sacred fire brought from a Brahmin learned in the Vedas, and having offered oblations according to the Smriti texts, he should walk around it three times with the maiden.

SUTRAS 12-14. He should then disclose this ceremony to her parents, for according to the convention, accepted by the Acharyas, marriage vows taken before the sacred fire are irrevocable. Thereafter, he should unite physically with his betrothed, and tactfully reveal this to his own relatives (in order that she may come to be accepted by his family).

SUTRAS 15-16. He should so arrange it that the brothers of the maiden seemingly may give her in marriage only to him; this would free them from the stigma on the family and punishment in the form of a fine. Then with gifts and loving attention, he should win over her brothers.

SUTRA 17. (In this manner) the man should marry the girl according to the Gandharva form of marriage.

SUTRA 18. If, however, the maiden does not agree to the marriage, he should employ another woman of a good family who has easy access to his beloved's house; she should be known to him before, should also be affectionate and loving by nature, and should succeed in arranging a rendezvous under some pretext or other along with his confidential servants.

SUTRA 19. He should then arrange to bring the sacred fire from the house of a Brahmin, learned in the Vedas, and perform the marriage rites as explained above.

SUTRA 20. If the maiden is to be married to another young man shortly, the suitor's friend should describe to her mother the limitations of the chosen man, and let her repent for her selection.

SUTRA 21. Then, having conducted the suitor to a neighbouring house, with the maiden's consent, she should cause the sacred fire to be brought at night from the house of a Brahmin, learned in the Vedas, and proceed with the ceremony as described above.

SUTRA 22. For a long time he should befriend and please the brother of the maiden who is about his own age, and oblige him with presents; he should exert himself on his behalf in matters requiring skill, and eventually should let him know his intention (of marrying his sister).

SUTRA 23. Generally speaking, young men of equal ages are capable of sacrificing their lives for the sake of their friends who share similar habits and a similar way of life. In this way it should be easy for him to arrange a meeting with his beloved, through her brother, in a sequestered spot accessible to both of them.

SUTRA 24. Paishacha Marriage: (In this form of marriage) the nurse should allow the maiden to inebriate herself on the eighth night of the waxing moon, and feigning work of her own, she should bring her to a secluded and easily accessible spot (where the suitor would await them).

SUTRA 25. There, while the maiden is still not herself, and unaware of what is happening, he should ravish her and proceed with the ceremony as described before (in this, the Paishacha variety of marriage, the sacred fire is not to be brought).

SUTRAS 26-27. Rakshasa Marriage: (in this form of marriage) the man must arm himself adequately, and on hearing that the maiden is going to a garden or a neighbouring village, should abduct her, either by terrorising or belabouring the guards (accompanying her). (In this Rakshasa type of marriage also the sacred fire is not to be brought.)

These are the different forms of marriage.

SUTRA 28. The forms of marriages described above are in the order of precedence, each preceding the other being better suited for practising the religious way of live. The other forms should be employed only if the man finds the preceding one impossible to adopt.

SUTRA 29. The ultimate object of the different ceremonies is after all the mutual love between couple. In this respect, the Gandharva form is considered the best, although it is not enumerated as the first. This ceremony does not require too much effort, nor does it involve the various stages of wooing and is based entirely on mutual love. For these reasons also, the Gandharva is said to be the best form.

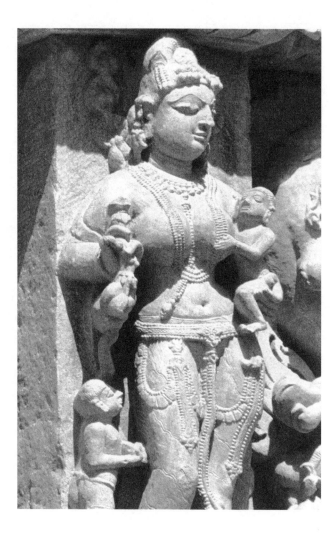

PART IV

ON THE DUTIES AND PRIVILEGES OF A WIFE

CHAPTER I

ON THE CONDUCT OF THE DEVOTED WIFE, AND HER BEHAVIOUR DURING HIS LONG ABSENCE

SUTRA 1. The woman who is a man's only wife, and who has deep and genuine affection for her husband, should adore him as a divine being and behave in accordance with his likes and dislikes.

SUTRA 2. With his consent, she should take upon herself the cares and anxieties of maintaining their family.

SUTRA 3. She should keep their home clean and properly dusted, with flowers at various places; the floor of the worship room should be smooth and pleasant, and oblations offered to the deities three times a day.

SUTRA 4. According to Gonardiya, there is nothing more pleasing to a man than a pleasant residence.

SUTRA 5. The wife should behave in a fitting manner towards her elders, servants, the sisters of her husband, and their husbands.

SUTRA 6. In the vacant plots around the house, she should plant coriander and ginger, vegetables, sugar cane, Jiraka, Sarshapa, Ajamoda, Shatapushpa and Tamala plants.

SUTRA 7. In the plots near her house she should plant creepers, such as Kubjaka, Amalaka, Mallika, Jati, Kurantaka, Navamalika, Tagara, Nandyavarta, Japa, coral trees, Balaka, and others, such as Ushiraka, Patalika, and prepare pleasant pieces of land levelled and squared for religious use.

SUTRA 8. In the centre of the garden, she should have a water pool or a step-well constructed.

SUTRA 9. She should abjure the company of a beggar woman, a recluse, a woman who has renounced the world (and donned red garments), a debauch, a woman practising jugglery, an inquisitive woman (or a fortune teller), and a woman adept in the arts of Muladeva (witchcraft).

SUTRA 10. In the matter of food, she should try to know what her husband likes and dislikes, what is wholesome and what is harmful.

SUTRA 11. When on his return, she hears his voice outside, she should come to the centre of the house (in the porch), ask him what he needs and see that he is satisfied.

SUTRA 12. She should not allow the female attendants, but should herself wash his feet.

SUTRA 13. Even when she is alone with him she should not appear before him unadorned.

SUTRA 14. When she finds that her husband is overspending, or squandering money, she should speak to him in private.

SUTRA 15. She should obtain his consent for visiting her parents, attending marriages, sacrifices, excursions, feasts, social gatherings, or religious festivals.

SUTRA 16. She should not take part in community games and amusements without his consent.

SUTRA 17. She should sleep only after he has slept, and wake up before he wakes up. She should not disturb him in his sleep (till it is morning).

SUTRA 18. The kitchen should be situated well inside the house (so that no intruder can come in) and it should be well ventilated and properly lighted.

SUTRA 19. If she is offended or displeased by lapses on the part of her husband, she should not remonstrate with him or make a scene.

SUTRA 20. She may reproach him sometimes when he is alone or in the company of his friends, but she should never resort to the use of the arts of Muladeva.

SUTRA 21. Gonardiya opines that a husband has no cause for distrusting his wife except when she uses these arts to her advantage.

SUTRA 22. She should avoid harsh words, never lose charm, never talk with her face turned away. She should never stand at the entrance of her house and gaze at the road; she should not indulge in whispering to her friends in the garden, nor should she stay alone for any length of time in a secluded place (standing in the porch or gazing at the road indicates that she is easily available; talking privately in the house garden or standing alone in a lonely place for a long time, indicates that her love for her husband is on the wane).

SUTRA 23. She should realise that sweat, tartar on teeth, offensive odour, etc., cause disaffection in the husband.

SUTRA 24. For inviting and attracting her husband, she should dress up and make up properly by putting on various ornaments, decorating herself with coloured blossoms, perfumes, fragrant paste and colourful garments (red garments particularly attract men's attention).

SUTRA 25. On excursions, the wife's outfit should consist of thin and sparing clothes having a fine texture. Ornaments may be used, but moderately, and the same applies to scents and cosmetics and white flowers.

SUTRA 26. She should take vows and undertake fasts for his good fortune and if he tries to dissuade her she should request him to desist from doing so.

SUTRA 27. For domestic use it is her duty to buy vessels made of clay, bamboo, wood, leather and iron at a proper rate. (This includes copper and pewter vessels, etc.)

SUTRA 28. Similarly, she should keep a stock in her house of rock salt, oil (ghee), essences, bitter gourds, medicines and so forth – generally things which are not available easily.

SUTRA 29. She should also collect seeds of the following plants and sow them during the proper season: Mulaka, Aluka, Palanki, Damanaka, Amrataka, Ervaruka, Trapusa, Vartaka, Kushmanda, Alabu, Surana, Shukanasa, Svayamgupta, Tilaparnika, Agnimantha, garlic, onion, etc. (These include radish, potato, common beet, Indian wormwood, mango, cucumber, eggplant, Kushmanda, pumpkin gourd, Surana, sandalwood, garlic plant and so forth.)

SUTRA 30. Whatever her husband confides in her about their wealth and other secrets should never be divulged to others.

SUTRA 31. She should try to excel other women in proficiency in the arts, cookery, dignified bearing, good grooming, and devotion to her husband.

SUTRA 32. She should budget her annual income and spend it with discretion.

SUTRA 33. She should know how to extract and prepare ghee from curds left over after a feast (of the Brahmins engaged in performing sacrifices), oil from sesamum seed, jaggery from sugar cane, thread from cotton, weave cloth from threads, ceiling brackets, ropes, noose or sling, preserve barks for making other things. She should supervise the pounding and grinding of rice, give away (to maid servants) the small grain and chaff (Achama and Manda), make use of husk for smearing the floor (with cow dung), collect small grains of rice (for cocks and other birds), collect useless and broken grains of rice (for cows and sheep), and also use live coals after they have cooled down. She should know the wages of her servants and look after their lodging, she should also acquaint herself with various agricultural processes, such as ploughing (this includes sowing, planting and transplanting), animal husbandry, knowledge of conveyances and their upkeep (such as saddling a horse, etc.) and knowledge of the eating habits and proper maintenance of rams, cocks, quails, mynas, cuckoos, peacocks, monkeys, and deer. Finally she should know how to total and tally her income and expenditure of the day.

SUTRA 34. Worn-out garments should be mended and rewashed and recoloured, and should be given away as presents to the servants who have served the family faithfully and for a long time; or they may be used for other purposes (such as making lamp wicks, etc.).

SUTRA 35. She should preserve (privately) pots of Sura and Asava, and supervise their use. Accounts of purchases and daily income and expenditure should also be maintained by her.

SUTRA 36. She should welcome and honour the friends of her husband with garlands, fragrant paste and betel leaves.

SUTRA 37. She should be at the beck and call of her parents-in-law, refrain from retorting, talk moderately and in a hushed voice, and never indulge in loud laughter in their presence.

SUTRA 38. She should behave with the people he likes or dislikes as if she herself liked or disliked them.

SUTRA 39. Wealth and material comforts should never lead her to snobbishness.

SUTRA 40. Politeness to the servants and the dependants of the family should be the order of the day.

SUTRA 41. Any gifts (that she may choose to give to anyone) may not be done without her husband's consent (even if she has sons, she is not free to give them anything she likes without her husband's consent).

SUTRA 42. She should entrust particular duties to particular servants and during festivals she should honour them (with gifts of clothing, food, etc.). This comprises the duties of the one and only wife who is devoted to her husband.

The wife's duties when the husband is away from home:

SUTRA 43. When the husband is away from home on his travels, the wife should wear only the auspicious ornaments (such as conch-shell bangles). She should observe religious fasts, obtain as much information about her husband as possible, and keep herself occupied with housework.

SUTRAS 44-45. At night, she should sleep near her mother-in-law, and during the day, she should act in accordance with her wishes.

SUTRA 46. She should try to collect objects which her husband is fond of, and look after them until her husband returns.

SUTRA 47. Expenditure should be restricted to her daily requirements or periodical needs.

SUTRA 48. She should also complete any work that her husband has left unfinished.

SUTRA 49. She should not visit her parents (without any ostensible reason), except when there is either a festival or a death.

SUTRA 50. At this time she should not discard the simple clothes she wears to indicate her husband's absence, nor should she stay too long, and at all times be surrounded by servants.

SUTRA 51. She should observe fasts which are approved of by her parents-in-law.

SUTRA 52. She should curtail her expenses and exercise utmost economy in the sale or purchase of commodities, by entrusting it to honest and faithful servants.

SUTRA 53. When her husband returns home[1] she should first meet him in the same simple dress worn by her during his absence; then, after performing the daily worship of family deities, she should offer him presents. So much for the duties of the wife while the husband is away.

SUTRA 54 (verse). In this way, the one and only wife who cherishes the welfare of her husband, whether she be married or a widow remarried, or a courtesan, should conduct herself, at all times, in a virtuous and unblemished fashion.

SUTRA 55 (verse). It is said that wives who follow a virtuous path usually obtain religious merit, material wealth, social position, good reputation and a husband who has no other wives.

NOTES

[1]   Cf. Aniarushataka, 45; Sarasvatikanthabharana, Parichchheda, 3; Gathasaptashati, 2-40, 3-61.

CHAPTER II

ON THE DUTIES OF THE ELDEST AND YOUNGEST WIFE

(IN THE CASE OF MORE THAN ONE); ON THE CONDUCT OF THE WIDOW REMARRIED; ON THE CONDUCT OF THE ESTRANGED WIFE; ON THE WOMEN IN THE ROYAL HAREM; ON THE CONDUCT OF THE HUSBAND WHO HAS MORE THAN ONE WIFE

SUTRA 1. A man marries another wife, either out of foolishness, immoral character, misery, barrenness of the first wife, successive births of daughters, or through his own sensuous weakness.

SUTRA 2. The wife, should, from the very start, take precaution against these by exhibiting her devotedness, character and cleverness.

SUTRA 3. If she finds herself barren, she should encourage her husband to marry again.

SUTRAS 4-5. In this event, she should employ all possible means at her disposal to maintain her status and dignity in the household.

With the new wife she should behave with tact, much like her elder sister.

SUTRA 6. She should supervise the evening toilet of the new wife in spite of the latter's unwillingness, and she should make this known to her husband.

SUTRA 7. If the new wife blurts out her happiness at her own fortune, or makes faces out of perverseness she should try to ignore these things.

SUTRA 8. If she finds the newcomer negligent to her husband, no further attention need be paid to her.

SUTRA 9. If, however, the newcomer realises her own mistake and tries to do the proper thing, she should affectionately guide her.

SUTRA 10. She should instruct her in the arts, not yet known to her husband, either privately or in the presence of her husband.

SUTRAS 11-12. If the new wife bears a son, the first wife should show much love towards him. She should be charitable to the servants of co-wives.

SUTRAS 13-15. Friends of the new wife should also become her friends, and she should guard against too much affection for her own relatives while to the relatives of the new wife she should display great friendliness.

SUTRA 16. When there are several co-wives, the senior wife should keep in close touch with the wife next to her in seniority.

SUTRA 17. When the most senior wife finds that her husband favours the new wife too much, she should instigate the wife who was lately his favourite against the newcomer and cause a quarrel.

SUTRA 18. Then she should pacify the wife with whom the husband has quarrelled.

SUTRA 19. Without herself quarrelling she should set all the other co-wives against the newcomer and cause her to lose her husband's favour.

SUTRAS 20-21. She should take up cudgels for the wife with whom the husband has quarrelled recently and so add fuel to the fire.

SUTRA 22. If she finds that the quarrel has abated, she should recommence it herself.

SUTRA 23. If, on the other hand, the husband perseveres in pacifying all his wives, she should take it upon herself to make peace with all of them.

So much for the behaviour of the senior wife.

SUTRA 24. The youngest wife should think of the seniormost co-wife as her mother.

SUTRAS 25-26. When she makes use of gifts, given by her relatives, she should consult the senior co-wife, and in general, conduct all her affairs with the guidance of the senior co-wife.

SUTRA 27. Even when her turn comes to sleep with her husband, she should not do so without her co-wife's permission.

SUTRA 28. It is also her duty to guard the senior wife's instructions and not divulge them to any of the other co-wives.

SUTRAS 29-30. The children of the senior or other co-wives should be treated with greater consideration than her own children, while to her husband, she should show even more consideration (but in private so that his affection for her may increase).

SUTRA 31. She must never complain (to her husband) about the ill-treatment meted out to her by the other co-wives. (She may, however, convey it to him subtly through others.)

SUTRAS 32-33. She must endeavour, in her own way, to create respect for her husband and at all times make it clear to him that her object in life is to receive his favours and his respect; this is the life-giving medicine for her.

SUTRA 34. She must learn never to show her hatred towards the other wives or to indulge in self-praise.

SUTRA 35. A married woman who divulges secrets usually displeases her husband.

SUTRA 36. Gonardiya contends that the youngest co-wife should try and obtain her husband's respect to arm herself against the senior co-wife.

SUTRA 37. But she should show sympathy and pity for the senior co-wife who is unfortunately childless, and should try and engender the same feelings in her husband.

SUTRA 38. In spite of the senior co-wife, the youngest wife should adhere strictly to the conduct of the one and only wife described earlier.

So much for the description of the youngest co-wife.

Now regarding the widow (not a virgin) remarried to another person.

SUTRA 39. The widow who seeks to enjoy married life once again because of uncontrolled passion, is named Punarbhu. She must, however, possess the qualities, required of a wife. (This is the opinion of Gonardiya.)

SUTRA 40. According to Babhravya, however, the Punarbhu is at liberty to leave her husband if she finds him devoid of gentlemanly qualities, and to seek another person as her husband.

SUTRA 41. If she is not satisfied even then, she may choose yet another husband (without the necessary qualities) in order to secure happiness.

SUTRA 42. Gonardiya argues that such a woman achieves real happiness only when she marries a man having qualities described earlier, and combines these with a satisfactory physical union with him.

SUTRA 43. Vatsyayana however thinks that a widow may marry any person she likes who she thinks will suit her.

SUTRA 44. With the help of her relatives, she should seek such work from her husband as would be sufficient to meet the expenses of social parties, toilet requirements including flowers and garlands, alms for religious ceremonies and receptions for friends and so forth.

SUTRA 45. She should wear ornaments given to her by her new husband, or have new ones made from the money he gives her.

SUTRA 46. There is no compulsion for her to wear ornaments presented to her by her relatives.

SUTRA 47. In the event of her leaving her husband's house, she should return of her own free will all things given to her for her use, except permanent gifts from him. However, in the event of her being driven out of the house, she need not return anything.

SUTRAS 48-49. During the time she is at the house of the husband, she should assert herself as the mistress of his household, but she should behave affectionately towards his legally-married wives.

SUTRA 50. She should behave with consideration towards the members of his household and receive and welcome friends cordially.

SUTRA 51. She should display her mastery over the arts and her knowledge of other crafts (not known to her husband).

SUTRA 52. If her husband makes mistakes which may lead to quarrels, she should herself reproach him.

SUTRA 53. During her physical union with him, she should utilize her knowledge of all the sixty-four arts (including *Purushopasripta*).

SUTRAS 54-55. Whenever occasion arises, she must oblige her husband's legally-married wives, and present ornaments, garlands and flowers to their children.

SUTRA 56. At all times, she should behave like their master (or as the husband behaves with them).

SUTRAS 57-58. Whenever she dresses them up, she should do so with affection, and towards the members of the household and towards friends she should be more hospitable than the other co-wives.

SUTRA 59. She should cultivate a taste for social gatherings, garden parties and excursions.

So much for the duties of the Punarbhu.

Now regarding the unfortunate wife.

SUTRA 60. The wife who is unfortunate (in being unloved and being altogether neglected by her husband), oppressed and worried, should cultivate friendship with the most favourite wife of her husband.

SUTRAS 61-62. She should exhibit her skill in the arts, which may be worthy of display. (She may do so with the favourite wife's help.)

SUTRAS 63-64. She should nurse the children of her husband, win over all his friends (with sweet words and presents) and with their assistance convey her devotion to her husband.

SUTRAS 65-66. She should take the lead in religious ceremonies, vows and fasts, display great consideration for the members of the household, but never show herself as excelling the other wives or members of the family in any sphere of activity. (This comprises her behaviour in public.)

Now regarding her behaviour in private.

SUTRA 67. When she is in bed with her husband she should respond to his passion equally (even if she is unwilling).

SUTRA 68. She should not show her unwillingness or reproach him.

SUTRA 69. If her husband has quarrelled with one of his wives, she should volunteer to effect reconciliation.

SUTRA 70. She should assist him in all his love affairs without speaking about it to anybody.

SUTRA 71. In this way her husband would recognise her faithfulness and acknowledge her sincerity.

So much for the behaviour of the neglected wife.

SUTRA 72. The conduct of the other co-wives in the harem should follow the pattern of the conduct of the wives described in the foregoing Sutras.

The conduct of the king will now be described.

SUTRA 73. The female attendants in the harem (called severally, Kan-chukis, Mahattarikas) should, while bringing garlands, scents and robes to the king, tell him that they are sent by his consorts.

SUTRA 74. The king, having accepted these, should in return present them with garlands worn by himself.

SUTRA 75. In the afternoon, when his toilet is complete, the king should visit all the members of the harem and eventually assemble with all of them in a royal chamber.

SUTRA 76. He should accord them the status and respect according to time and propriety, and make jovial conversation with them (this only refers to his married wives).

SUTRA 77. Thereafter, he should meet the Punarbhus in his harem and behave with them similarly.

SUTRA 78. Finally, he should meet the courtesans and actresses in his harem (those who entertain him with dramatic performances).

SUTRA 79. The apartments of all these members of the harem are arranged in their order of preference (first, the consorts, then the Punarbhus, then the courtesans, and finally the actresses).

SUTRAS 80-81. After the king awakes from his midday rest, the chambermaids and the servants of the respective consorts should inform him whose turn it is to keep him company, who is in her period, and so forth, and should then give him the ring (with the seal), perfumes and robes sent by those wives. The king chooses the gifts from one particular consort, and in this way indicates her turn.

SUTRA 82. During festivals, the king should participate with his consorts according to their status, and should honour them all. He should act similarly during musical parties and dramatic performances.

SUTRA 83. Those who are confined to the harem are not permitted to come out, nor do outsiders have access to it, except those whose character and morals are known to be unimpeachable.

SUTRA 84. In the matter of physical unions, the king need not exercise any restraint.

This completes the description of the behaviour of the members of the harem.

Now for the behaviour of the husband who has many wives.

SUTRA 85 (verse). A husband who secures many wives should be fair to all of them and see that he neglects none; but he should not tolerate any lapses on their part (otherwise they will continue to commit lapses).

SUTRAS 86-87 (verses). He should not confide in one wife the physical blemishes of another, nor should he praise before one wife the enjoyment he has had from another,[1] and he should certainly not convey the confidential reproaches of one wife to another. If one of his wives speaks ill of another wife to him, he should not permit her to do so, and point out her own faults in return.

SUTRAS 88-89 (verses). He should learn to please all his wives in different ways. One he should make his confidante; another he should treat with deference; a third he should honour and cherish; a fourth, he should entertain with outdoor excursions; a fifth, by joyful union; a sixth, by heaping gifts and presents; still another by honouring her relatives, and yet another by loving caresses.

SUTRA 90 (verse). Ultimately, the young wife who can conquer her anger (and command a good temper), conducting herself with due regard to instruction in the scientific texts on love stands above all the co-wives and controls them.

NOTES

[1]   Yashodhara interprets the word 'Vaikrita' differently in K. S. 4-2-7 from what he does herein

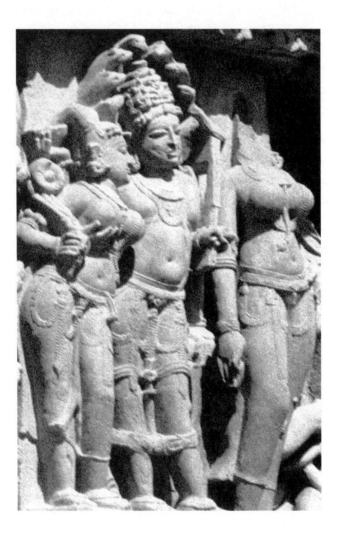

PART V

ON RELATIONS WITH WIVES OF OTHER MEN

CHAPTER 1

ON THE CHARACTERISTICS OF MEN AND WOMEN IN LOVE;

ON REASONS FOR KEEPING FREE FROM TEMPTATION; ON MEN WHO ARE NATURALLY ATTRACTIVE TO WOMEN; ON WOMEN WHO CAN BE WON OVER EASILY

SUTRAS 1-2. The circumstances under which a man may resort to the wives of other men have already been enumerated earlier (Part I, Chapter V), but from the very beginning, he should ascertain these points: how accessible she is, whether there is any danger in securing her, whether she is fit to be secured and united with, whether she is likely to bring him good fortune, whether it is going to affect his own livelihood, and so on.

SUTRA 3. When a man finds that his love for another woman becomes stronger and stronger in intensity, he should proceed to win her over for the sake of saving himself from further harm.

SUTRAS 4-5. The intensity of love grows with each of the following ten stages:

- ◆ Love at first sight.
- ◆ Mental attachment.
- ◆ Lingering thoughts.
- ◆ Loss of sleep.
- ◆ Physical emaciation.
- ◆ Indifference to other affairs.
- ◆ Absence of a sense of shame.
- ◆ Mental imbalance.
- ◆ Physical debility leading to fainting, etc.
- ◆ Death.

SUTRA 6. Learned sages maintain that a man should recognise from the start the woman's disposition, truthfulness, purity, strength or weakness of passion, accessibility, and so forth, from her anatomical signs and features.

SUTRA 7. However, Vatsyayana is of the opinion that merely anatomical signs and features are not enough to go by, but that a woman's conduct and bearing should also be observed from her gestures and taken into account while assessing her character.

SUTRA 8. Gonikaputra argues that although a woman may feel attracted to every handsome man she sees, and a man also desires every beautiful woman he sees, they do not always go deeper than to fulfil their desires. (There are various reasons why, in some cases, physical union is not striven for.)

SUTRA 9. (Although the morals of both are equally good), there is a difference in the woman's approach in this matter.

SUTRA 10. Although she feels love for such a man, she will not unite with him physically, not so much out of religious considerations as out of other sundry factors.

SUTRAS 11-12. By her very nature, she shrinks from the act when the man approaches her, although she is not really averse to the idea;

but she is finally won over only through patient and continuous overtures.

SUTRA 13. On the other hand, the man who is attracted to a beautiful woman refrains from physical union in spite of desiring it, more from religious and social considerations than from others.

SUTRA 14. Even when the woman approaches him with love-sport and little flirtations, he restrains himself from being won over because of his mental attitude.

SUTRA 15. At times, he makes an attempt to win over the object of his affections without any deep reasons but if she does not respond, he does not press his attentions and usually leaves her alone thereafter. Similarly, after a woman is won over, he becomes indifferent to her.

SUTRA 16. A man detests a woman who is gained over too easily, longs for one who is not – this is a generally recognised truth in the world.

SUTRA 17. A description of the causes of refraining from the act:

SUTRA 18. Love for her – own husband (prevents the woman from physical union with another man).

SUTRA 19. Consideration for family and children.

SUTRA 20. Owing to her advanced age.

SUTRA 21. From mental grief or bereavement in the family due to death (of some close family relative).

SUTRA 22. Inability to separate from her husband.

SUTRA 23. Owing to her anger when she realises that the other man desires her, not out of love, but for other reasons.

SUTRA 24. Owing to the difficulty or the impossibility of fathoming the man's sentiments or inclination towards her, resulting in her hesitation to harbour kindly thoughts for him.

SUTRA 25. Because of the doubt lingering in her mind that he would go to another woman; that there would be no future for them together; and because of a suspicion that he may already be attached to some other woman.

SUTRA 26. Fear of his proneness to a public scandal.

SUTRA 27. His intimacy and frankness with his own friends, resulting in the fear that she may possibly be neglected.

SUTRA 28. Her suspicion that he might approach her without purpose, more out of wantonness.

SUTRA 29. Her fear arising from his powerful position in society.

SUTRA 30. If the woman is of the Deer-type and she thinks that he has a powerful sexual urge, she will fear the use of force in their union. (She may have a suspicion of his being the Horse-type.)

SUTRA 31. Her complex at realising that, he being a cultivated citizen, would be expert in the arts. (This applies to a rural woman, and not one well versed in the arts.)

SUTRA 32. The thought of having once lived with him, but purely on friendly terms. (Hence her hesitation for a new relationship.)

SUTRA 33. An absence of a sense of propriety on his part (for physical union as well as in other things).

SUTRA 34. In the likelihood of her being ridiculed by her friends (because of his low birth) and hence her shyness and hesitation towards him.

SUTRA 35. The absence of response on his part, even after she has shown him her inclination.

SUTRA 36. If the woman is of the Cow-elephant-type and she suspects the man to be the Hare-type, she concludes that their physical union will not be satisfactory.

SUTRA 37. Her anxiety to see that he does not come to any harm because of her.

SUTRA 38. A realisation of her own insufficiency – hence she does not encourage him.

SUTRA 39. Her fear that if their physical union comes to light, she may be excommunicated by her people.

SUTRA 40. Her hesitation at noticing his advanced age, betrayed by his greying hair.

SUTRA 41. Her suspicion that he may have been commissioned by her husband to test her faithfulness, resulting in her cautious approach.

SUTRA 42. Purely religious considerations.

SUTRA 43. Whichever causes the man detects as applicable to him, should be removed from the start.

SUTRA 44. He should increase her passion for him and see that her hesitation, arising out of her noble upbringing, does not interfere with their affair.

SUTRA 45. He should recognise other obstructions and suggest ways and means of remedying the difficulties.

SUTRA 46. He should remove fears arising from her doubts and suspicions, by cultivating greater intimacy with her.

SUTRA 47. By displaying his manliness and dexterity in the arts, he should prove to her that he is conscious of proprieties regarding time and place.

SUTRA 48. If she suspects him to be fond of publicity, he should set her mind at rest by falling at her feet (and requesting her favour privately).

SUTRA 49. With the help of a sympathetic attitude, he can remove all the causes responsible for her hesitation.

SUTRA 50. The following are the types of men who generally obtain success with women:

One who is conversant with the Kama Sutra or the art of love.

One who is expert in narrating episodes and tales.

One who is intimately known to her from childhood.

One who is mature.

One who has secured her confidence through his expert knowledge of games and so forth.

One who is obedient to her.

One who is soft spoken.

One who does all the things that she likes.

On who has already played the part of the love-messenger once.

One who knows her secrets.

One who is already sought after by another woman superior to her.

One who is secretly wooed, by a woman friend.

One who is known for his good fortune and comfortable circumstances.

One who is brought up with her.

One who is a neighbour and is well versed in matters of sex.

One who is a servant and also well versed in matters of sex.

One who is a lover of the daughter of her nurse.

One who is a newly-married son-in-law in the family.

One who is fond of dramatic performances and garden parties, and who is liberal in his gifts to others.

One who is recognised as the Bull-type.

One who is adventurous.

One who is brave.

One who excels her husband in knowledge, good looks, capacity for enjoyment, and other similar qualities.

One who dresses and behaves in an aristocratic manner.

SUTRA 51. Just as a man thinks to himself as to how liable he is to be won over, so also he should see how other women are likely to be won over.

SUTRA 52. The following types of women are likely to be won over easily by merely approaching them:

One who loiters about the entrance of her house, gazing along the highway.

One who arranges group discussions at a neighbour's house.

One who is given to continuous staring.

One who turns her glance sideways when she is noticed.

One over whom a co-wife has been brought into the house.

One who hates her husband.

One who is hated by her husband.

One who has no discrimination (for the type of male in physical unions).

One who is childless, always sheltering in her parents' house.

One whose children have died.

One who is always busy arranging parties and gatherings.

One who displays passionate tendencies.

One who is the wife of an actor or a dancer.

One who is a child-widow.

One who is poor.

One who seeks enjoyment continuously.

One who is a senior wife and has many young brothers-in-law.

One who is high-born and proud and whose husband is low-born (and unworthy of her).

One who is proud of her own cleverness.

One who is discontented with the folly of her husband.

One who is dissatisfied with her husband's inadequacy and covets to gain more.

One who has been betrothed with great effort during her maidenhood, but who has not consummated her marriage, and is now approached.

One who has many things in common with another man – intelligence, disposition, strength of character, common pursuits, similar provincial traditions, and mutual attraction.

One who is humiliated without provocation or fault of her own.

One who is ridiculed by her equals in beauty and
accomplishments.
One whose husband is away from home for long periods.

Wives of the following types of men are also easily won over:
One who is jealous.
One who is dirty.
One who is the wife of a Choksha. (A caste, married women of
which are profligate.)
One who is a eunuch.
One who is given to procrastinating.
One who is not brave.
One who is hunch-backed or deformed.
One who is stunted.
One who is ugly.
One who is the wife of a setter of precious stones.
One who is rustic (in his manners).
One who is foul-smelling.
One who remains sickly.
One who is old and haggard (therefore unable to indulge in
physical pleasures).

SUTRA 53 (verse). It is said that love born naturally and nurtured
through mutual regard becomes steadfast and survives many crises
when once the causes of fear and suspicion are recognised and
removed.

SUTRA 54 (verse). A man, confident of his abilities in matters of love,
and perceptive about the signs and gestures of women, is generally
successful in his affairs with women.

CHAPTER II

ON MAKING THE ACQUAINTANCE OF THE WOMAN AND THE EFFORTS TO WIN HER OVER

SUTRA 1. According to the sages, a maiden is not as easily won over by approaches through a messenger as she is by one's own personal efforts; but wives of other men, who necessarily conceal their sentiments, are more easily gained over through messengers than through personal efforts.

SUTRA 2. Vatsyayana opines that in all cases (of maidens and of others' wives) self-approach is better than approaches through a messenger. However, in some cases, a messenger has necessarily to be employed.

SUTRA 3. As a general rule, where women are to be won over for the first time and with whom communication by speech is restricted, they should be beguiled by personal efforts; in other instances a messenger's services have to be enlisted in the adventure of winning a woman's mind and body.

SUTRAS 4-5. A man who is bent upon approaching a woman personally should in the beginning glance at her naturally, and cultivate some intimacy.

SUTRA 6. He can do this near his own house; alternatively, he can make a deliberate attempt to view her, and this he can do near the house of either a friend or a kinsman, or an officer of high rank or of a physician, on various occasions like marriages, sacrifices, festivals, sorrowful occasions (like funerals), garden parties, and so on.

SUTRA 7. Whenever the man catches sight of her, he should look at her steadily, and observe her when she is tying up her loose hair or when she is scratching with her nails, or when she jingles her ornaments, or when she is pressing her lower lips, and indulging in other acts of a similar sort. He should so arrange it that he is seen by her when he is surrounded by his friends, and converse about her under the guise of conversing about another person. He should make it known to others that he has many pleasures of life and lives liberally. When he is seated beside a woman friend, he should yawn and stretch his limbs, listening to her words in a bored way. When he is next to his object of affection, he should address the boy seated in her lap and tell him a story relating to her, but ostensibly concerning another person. He should declare indirectly his own cherished desires while narrating this story and kiss the young lad as if he would kiss her, embracing him, offering betel leaf to him as if he would offer it to her, press his finger against his chin, and indulge in such other actions on other parts of the boy's body with an eye to propriety and fitness of time. (These actions are covertly directed towards the woman.)

SUTRA 8. He should fondle the lad sitting in her lap, bestow gifts of toys for his playing, constantly be near her and commence small talk with her. Having befriended her close friend, he should try to find out some excuse for some work which will take him near her, and he should frequently make use of this excuse. Out of sight, but within her earshot, he should discuss topics of sex and love.

SUTRA 9. When thus such intimacy has been established he should leave certain belongings at her house on trust, saying that he would take them away afterwards one by one.

SUTRA 10. Objects such as perfumes and betel nut should be taken by him frequently, if not every day.

SUTRA 11. Then in order to create confidence in her, he should invite her over to have confidential talks with his wives and arrange for them to sit together in secluded places.

SUTRA 12. In order to have some excuse for seeing her, he should arrange either by himself or through servants, to engage the services of goldsmiths, gem-setters, artisans of precious stones, dyers of blue and red garments and so forth.

SUTRA 13 In this way he will keep himself occupied on her behalf while also have occasions to see her for long periods and become well known to the people as a hard worker.

SUTRA 14 While engaged in this work, he should pay particular attention to any odd jobs she may want to have done. If she is at a loss for having these done he should show her a way to do it, demonstrate to her the way to acquire knowledge of the subject, and thus prove his capabilities in these matters.

SUTRA 15. He should conduct long discussions with her and her attendants about the merits and defects of precious stones and articles and divert them with episodes (from the old epics).

SUTRA 16. In some of these matters, he should fake a difference of opinion and appoint the woman as adjudicator for deciding the truth.

SUTRA 17. However, when he disagrees with her on certain points, he should appoint one of her closest attendants as adjudicator.

So much regarding the means of cultivating intimacy with another woman.

SUTRA 17A. The woman with whom a man has cultivated some intimacy should be approached with the same care and solicitude with which a maiden is approached – once the woman has made her sentiments known through definite signs and gestures.

SUTRA 18. In the case of a maiden, however, the approaches are made very carefully and not quite so openly since the maiden is not familiar with the concept of a physical union.

SUTRA 19. But in the case of other women, since they are experienced in physical union, the approaches are made somewhat more openly.

SUTRA 20. When once the woman has expressed her sexual inclinations through certain signs, the man should make use of her belongings in the same way as she would use his things. This results in mutual enjoyment.

SUTRA 21. Among the things that he should give her are costly perfumes, upper garments, flowers, rings and betel leaves, and he should beg her to give him a flower from her hair when he is on his way to attend social gatherings. (Begging a flower from her hair is likely to bring good fortune to the lover.)

SUTRA 22. When he bestows these gifts of scents and other things (through others), they should bear his nail- and teeth-marks, but (when given personally) they should merely express his sentiments.

SUTRA 23. Thus with gradual approaches, step by step, he should rid her of her timidity.

SUTRA 24. In the course of time he should take her to a secluded spot, embrace and kiss her, offer her the betel leaf, exchange cherished gifts, and arouse her passions physically. These are named the Bahya and Abhyantara approaches. (Touching of the armpits and abdomen should be by the Utkshipta mode.)

SUTRA 25. When a man is engaged in gaining power over one woman he should not make overtures to another woman in the same house. If there is an old lady in the house, experienced in sexual matters, she should be won over by presents.

SUTRA 26 (verse). A man should not approach a woman whose husband goes out for physical satisfaction, even though she be won over easily.

SUTRA 27 (verse). An intelligent man, knowing his own capacity, should not even think of approaching a suspicious woman, or one who is too well guarded, or one who is afraid of her husband, or one who has a mother-in-law.

CHAPTER III

ON TESTING THE WOMAN'S INCLINATIONS

SUTRA 1. When a man makes overtures to a woman (as if to a maiden) he should put her behaviour to the test and thereby gauge her sentiments.

SUTRA 2. The woman who does not reveal (her inclination for physical union) should be won over through a messenger.

SUTRA 3. If, at the first approach, she fails to respond, but at the second approach, is at least accessible, he should consider her hesitation as a favourable sign and attempt to win her over gradually.

SUTRA 4. If, at his first approach, the woman fails to respond, but takes the initiative and meets him a second time decked out in her finery, he should take her to be approachable and forcibly unite with her in a lonely place.

SUTRA 5. A woman who passes over many approaches and fails to respond to them even after a long time, should be considered as a trifler in love, but even she can be won over by the man keeping constantly in touch with her.

SUTRA 6. Because the human mind is fickle and unsteady he should decline, for a time, to have intimate relations with her. (When intimacy is interrupted by estrangement, there is a natural inclination for another attempt at continuation.)

SUTRA 7. When a woman, even though approached, tries to avoid the man, and does not respond to him out of pride and self-respect, and respect to the man, she can be won over only with the greatest of difficulties and only after a long friendship. Such a woman should be won over with the help of a mediator who knows her secrets.

SUTRA 8. If she tries to reject the man's advances with harsh words he should ignore or overlook them.

SUTRA 9. If, in spite of the harsh words, the man thinks that she is desirous of love, he should continue in his efforts to win her over.

SUTRA 10. For instance, if she tolerates the touching of her limbs, but for some reason or other, does not know the true intentions of the man, she shows her wavering mind and the man should win her over patiently with sustained effort.

SUTRA 11. For instance, if she is sleeping nearby, he should also pretend to be asleep, keeping his hand over her; if she does not lay the hand aside, while pretending to sleep, but does so on awakening, he should construe this as an encouragement for further approaches.

SUTRA 12. In a similar way, one of his legs should be kept over hers.

SUTRA 13. When this is allowed to continue for a long time he should undertake to embrace the sleeping woman.

SUTRA 14. If, on being unable to bear the close embrace, she suddenly wakes, but on the next day is found as unperturbed as on the previous day, he should finally realise that she desires his approaches. However, if he does not see her the next day, he should know that she is likely to be won over through a messenger.

SUTRA 15. If he does not see her for a long time, but after that is still approachable in the natural way, he should renew his efforts since she has already expressed her sentiments through signs and gestures.

SUTRA 16. When a woman, without being approached by the man, invites him to a lonely spot, she shows herself as being accessible. She manifests this in the following ways :

SUTRA 17. She trembles and talks in a faltering voice.

SUTRA 18. She perspires at her hands, fingers, face and feet.

SUTRA 19. She offers to press his head and massage his thighs.

SUTRA 20. While massaging, her passion rises and while she shampoos him with one hand, with the other she touches his limbs one by one and finally embraces him.

SUTRA 21. Pretending to be tired, she rests herself half asleep against him, cooing with pleasure, and embracing him with her arms and thighs.

SUTRA 22. She rests her forehead against his thighs.

SUTRA 23. When he asks her to massage his thigh joints she does not resent it or desist from it.

SUTRA 24. She keeps one hand in that place quite steadily.

SUTRA 25. When the man embraces her quite closely with his thighs, she lingers and extracts herself only after a long time.

SUTRA 26. Having thus accepted the approaches of the man she goes to him once more the following day in order to massage him again.

SUTRA 27. She does not approach him blatantly; nonetheless, she does not hesitate when approached.

SUTRA 28. She voices her sentiments in a lonely place. When she meets him in public places she behaves normally and does not reveal her sentiments.

SUTRA 29. She behaves in the same way if she is approached by a servant on behalf of the lover. But she is won over through a messenger who knows her innermost secrets.

SUTRA 30. If she retracts (while being approached through a messenger) he should see whether she does it genuinely or merely pretends. In this way he can test her sentiments.

SUTRA 31 (verse). A man should first get himself introduced to a woman, and then he should start conversing with her, and eventually find out her inclinations in matters of love. (While he is engaged in talking to her he should present her with perfumes and betel leaves and so forth intending to take them away later.)

SUTRA 32 (verse). If he is able to ascertain her inclinations by her response, he should set all fear aside and press on with his approaches.

SUTRA 33 (verse). If a woman expresses her sentiments through signs and gestures she should be approached at once, at first sight.

SUTRA 34 (verse). When a woman is invited by a man, not too emphatically or ardently, and she responds favourably, she should be considered as immediately won over and desirous of physical union.

SUTRA 35 (verse). These minute details of procedure are for the benefit of those men who find some women either slow to respond or timid or those whose sentiments require to be tested. Other types of women (who do not hide their inclinations) are easily gained over.

CHAPTER IV

ON THE DUTIES OF A MESSENGER

SUTRA 1. When a man wishes to approach a woman with whom he is not acquainted, and whom he does not see very often, he should seek the help of a woman messenger, and through her make his advances. (There are three kinds of women messengers, but their duties are collectively described.)

SUTRA 2. The woman messenger who is on intimate terms with the woman who is sought after, should display her good character, show her painted scrolls depicting well-known tales, ply her with hints and recipes for various types of make-up and toilet for beautifying her body, regale her with popular stories, recite poems, indulge in gossip relating to other wives, and generally entertain and flatter her by praising her beauty, affable nature, adaptability and other virtues.

SUTRA 3. She should make her repent by explaining, 'How can such an accomplished woman like you have such a husband?'

SUTRA 4. 'O fortunate one he is not fit even to be your servant!'

SUTRA 5. The woman messenger, having in this way secured the woman's confidence, should privately dilate upon her husband's weak passion, jealousy, cunning, ungratefulness, apathy, miserliness, fickle-mindedness, unfitness for physical pleasures and other such defects.

SUTRA 6. She should dilate on the faults of her husband and by degrees gain intimacy with her. (This results in mental disturbance in the woman's mind.)

SUTRA 7. If the woman belongs to the Deer-type and the husband belongs to the Hare-type, this fact should not be mentioned since it is not a defect. (But if he belongs to the Horse-type, the disparity between them should be emphasised.)

SUTRA 8. If the woman belongs to either the Mare- or the Cow-elephant-type, and the man belongs to the Horse- or the Bull-type, the combination is not objectionable, but if the man belongs to the Hare-type the combination will not be satisfactory.

SUTRA 9. Gonikaputra has the following theory. He theorises that when the man wishes to approach a woman who is embarking on her first sexual adventure and whose sentiments are undefined, he should seek the help of the woman messenger.

SUTRA 10. (It becomes the duty of the woman messenger) to describe to the other woman the good life of the man – his fitness and aptitude for a physical union with her. (This involves the three stages – the beginning, middle, and end of the union as described in earlier chapters.)

SUTRA 11. When the woman messenger has gained the other woman's confidence she should fulfil her mission by speaking plainly thus:

SUTRA 12. 'O fortunate one, listen to this strange truth. Having seen you here, this man, nobly born, experiences instability of mind. Since he is by nature weak, and since he has never experienced such mental agony before, the miserable man may now possibly die!'

SUTRA 13. When on the next day, the man finds that the woman messenger had a patient hearing, he should start with common gossip and try to find out through her manner, speech, expression, and sympathetic hearing, whether she finds this agreeable.

SUTRA 14. While the woman is listening, the messenger should narrate the anecdotes of Ahalya, Avimaraka, Shakuntala and other popular tales relating to the wives of others.

SUTRA 15. Thereafter, she should praise his abilities in matters of love, his knowledge of the sixty-four arts and of the sixty-four Panchalika modes, his good fortune, praiseworthiness, his past love-life and his fresh adventures. She should carefully take note of her reactions.

SUTRA 16. Having noted her reactions, the woman messenger begins to talk smilingly.

SUTRAS 17-18. She invites the other woman to a seat, asks her questions about where she spent the day, how she slept, ate and dallied and whatever else she did.

SUTRAS 19-21. She conducts her to a lonely place to relate anecdotes, pretending to be engrossed in contemplation (as if thinking of something else), heaving sighs of desire.

SUTRAS 22-24. The messenger gives her presents (such as bracelets or upper garments), remembers her on festive or joyful occasions, and lets her depart only after pressing her to consent to another meeting.

SUTRA 25. When the messenger conveys the feelings of the lover to the woman she exclaims: 'Oh friend – you who always speak the truth, how is it that you speak so cruelly to me?'

SUTRA 26. After this interjection, she continues the conversation. She enumerates the faults of the lover – his roguishness and fickle-mindedness.

SUTRA 27. The other woman, on her part, has a desire to relate certain things to the messenger after she has seen her lover, but refrains from doing so, wishing to be asked about it.

SUTRA 28. When the cherished desire of the lover is conveyed to her, she ridicules it but does not pass any definite remark.

SUTRAS 29-30. However, when the woman messenger is able to gauge the woman's reactions fully, she should make further attempts to press the cause of the lover. She should refer to her meetings with him in the past, but if they have not been acquainted at this stage, she should praise the qualities and loving nature of the man and thus win her favour.

SUTRA 31. According to Auddalaki, when a man and a woman have not been acquainted before and the woman has not shown her inclination through signs and gestures, the woman messenger is useless.

SUTRA 32. Followers of Babhravya, however, think the woman messenger becomes necessary in such cases.

SUTRA 33. According to Gonikaputra, the woman messenger is necessary for the man and woman who are acquainted but whose love for each other has not been expressed.

SUTRA 34. Vatsyayana maintains that the woman messenger is indispensable for a man and woman who are unacquainted and whose mutual affection has yet to be expressed.

SUTRA 35. The woman messenger begins with gifts pleasing to the woman – betel leaves, perfumes, garlands, rings and garments sent by her lover.

SUTRA 36. They should bear significant nail- and teeth-marks and any other marks the lover considers proper on them (these marks are expressive of a desire for union).

SUTRA 37. The garments should bear the marks of his palm smeared with red dye (this signifies the man's intention to win the love of the woman).

SUTRA 38. There should also be carved designs of Bhurjapatra signifying his longing. Love letters written on leaves should be enclosed with ear ornaments and flower ornaments for the head.

SUTRA 39. All these gifts are designed to convey his love and the woman should similarly return these.

SUTRA 40. In this way, through mutual exchange of gifts, personal contact is established through the services of the female messenger.

SUTRA 41. Followers of Babhravya contend that the lovers' meeting can be arranged while going to a temple for worship, or during a gathering in honour of a deity, or during games in a garden, or during swimming contests, or during marriage ceremonies, sacrifices, funerals, festivals; or in the event of dacoities, national wars or during theatrical performances.

SUTRA 42. According to Gonikaputra, the places convenient for the rendezvous are the houses of a woman-friend, a beggar woman, a recluse or a woman practising penance.

SUTRA 43. In the opinion of Vatsyayana, the place convenient for such meetings is the woman's own house where secret entrance and exit are made known to the lover. In the event of trouble the remedy is ready at hand, and since the entry and exit are usually timed secretly, any trouble is forestalled. (This is not possible at a friend's house.)

SUTRA 44. There are different types of female messengers:
1. One who accomplishes her mission by her own intelligence.
2. One who merely executes particular duties.
3. One who carries a letter.
4. One who undertakes to do her duties with selfish motives.
5. A messenger commissioned by the neglected wife.
6. One who acts as a messenger for her own husband, enjoying his full confidence.
7. One who is a silent messenger.
8. One who gives the message in code.

SUTRAS 45-46. (1) This type of messenger, who knows the intention of both parties and who uses her intelligence, is useful only to those lovers who are acquainted and between whom some oral communication has already taken place.

SUTRA 47. If she is commissioned by the woman, she becomes useful when the lovers are acquainted, but where no oral communication has taken place.

SUTRA 48. On occasions, she may even act out of sheer bravado and curiosity, thinking them to be fit for each other even though unacquainted.

SUTRA 49. (2) This woman messenger, knowing that some approach has already been made and part of the work done, completes the remaining part of her mission.

SUTRA 50. Her services are used when the lovers have seen each other, but meet very rarely.

SUTRA 51. (3) This type of messenger, i.e., Patrahara, merely carries the oral message (sometimes a written message or a letter).

SUTRA 52. She is useful when there is great intimacy between the lovers. She then only has to inform the one or the other of the place and time of their next meeting.

SUTRA 53. (4) This type of messenger, i.e., Svayamduti, when on a mission to the man, tries to corner him for herself. She conveys to him her desire for union as if speaking in ignorance of her real mission, lazily and seductively. She derides his wife, shows her jealousy, gives him a present bearing her teeth- and nail-marks, informs him that, in the first instance, she was to be given to him in marriage, questions him in private as to who is fairer – she or his wife.

SUTRAS 54-55. She should be seen by him in a lonely place and it is only there that he should approach her. Under the pretext of being a messenger of some woman whose love message is to be conveyed to him, the Svayamduti tries to win him for herself, attributing some deficiency to the woman who actually commissioned her, and thus letting her down.

SUTRA 56. The male messenger, acting on behalf of a man who follows the Svayamduti's example and who does everything for his own advantage, is also here mentioned.

SUTRA 57. (5) The Mudhaduti tackles the neglected wife of the husband – young and innocent. Having taken her into her confidence, without causing her any anxiety and knowing, in her heart, that she is in love with her husband, the Mudhaduti should question her about her husband's affairs, teach her the various modes of union, adorn her with jewels and ornaments, instruct her to follow certain seductions, herself inflict nail- and teeth-marks on the young wife's body and in this way attract the attention of the husband for his wife and arouse his passion.

SUTRA 58. Even the replies of the husband should be conveyed to the wife through the Mudhaduti.

SUTRA 59. (6) The Bharyaduti – when a man commissions his own foolish wife to gain the confidence of another woman whom he wishes to enjoy, he exhibits his own abilities through her. The other woman's sentiments should also be known to the man through the help of his own wife.

SUTRA 60. (7) Alternatively, the man may send a young maidservant who is inexperienced in matters of love to the woman's house, with some plain excuse (such as toys). He should hide his love letter in the garland or the leafy ear ornament, after having made nail- and teeth-marks on the letter. The young maidservant should also request the woman for a reply. This type of messenger is named Mukaduti.

SUTRA 61. (8) This type of messenger, the Vataduti, conveys a man's love message to the woman in a manner which is unintelligible to others but full of meaning for the lovers. The message has common expressions but double meanings. The Vataduti should also request the woman for a reply.

SUTRA 62 (verse). A widow, a fortune-teller, a maidservant, a beggar woman, a woman artisan – each of these is able to create confidence in a woman and usually succeeds as a love messenger.

SUTRA 63 (verse). She can create hatred in the mind of the wife against her husband, relate to her his other romantic affairs, tell her about the many pleasures of love, and recount original modes of physical union.

SUTRA 64 (verse). She can describe the man's love for her, praise his abilities in matters of love, show her the attractions he has for several other women, and finally convey to her his determination to possess none but herself.

SUTRA 65 (verse). A woman messenger has the ability to bring back to the woman some things left out due to her lover's oversight – things which her lover may not have even thought about. She can do this with her skill and speech and artfulness.

CHAPTER V

ON THE LOVE OF PERSONS IN AUTHORITY TOWARDS OTHER MEN'S WIVES

SUTRAS 1-2. Neither kings nor ministers have occasion to enter the house of ordinary persons. The common people can see their actions and follow them from a distance, just as the threefold living world seeing the sun rise, wake up after that, watch him traverse the heavenly path, and then shape their actions accordingly.

SUTRAS 3-4. It follows, therefore, that kings and ministers should not do anything that can be censured; they will find this impossible to do and quite reprehensible. If it becomes absolutely essential to act in a certain way, there are ways and means of doing so.

SUTRA 5. The women of the villages can be won over by a mere word of the village headman, the village revenue officer, or the agricultural officer's sons. Such women are named Charshanis by the Vitas. (These women do not expect even an overture or an approach.)

SUTRA 6. These Charshanis may be won over while they are engaged in pounding grain, cooking food, entering a granary, taking things out of or into the house, cleaning or tidying up the house, sowing seeds or transplanting, purchasing raw cotton, wool, flex, hemp, and thread for spinning, or when receiving these yarns, or while selling and purchasing other material or while engaged in other similar acts.

SUTRA 7. In the same way the officer in charge of cattle is able to win over the wives of shepherds.

SUTRA 8. The officer in charge of yarn is able to win over widows, destitute women, or those who have renounced worldly life.

SUTRA 9. The city office is able to win over unattached women through his knowledge of their secrets during his night tours.

SUTRA 10. The market officer is able to win over the wives of buyers and sellers in the market while he is engaged in his work of buying and selling articles for the royal household.

SUTRA 11. Generally speaking, women living in Pattana, Nagara and Kharvata indulge in playing games with the women in the harem of a chieftain on moonlit nights, on the eighth night of the waxing moon, and during the festival of Suvasantaka in the spring.

SUTRA 12. When the play is over, these women from the cities (with the other women) should separately enter the palaces of the different queens on the strength of their acquaintance with them, and having exchanged gossip and tales and after being honoured (with gifts and refreshments), and having drunk sufficiently should be made to leave the ruler's palace at dusk.

SUTRAS 13-14. On such occasions, a female attendant of the king, who is already acquainted with the woman whom the king desires, should accost her when she is on her way to her house and induce her to see the beautiful things around the palace.

SUTRA 15. At the appropriate moment she should say,

SUTRA 16. 'In this game I will show you beautiful things in the royal palace.'

SUTRA 17. 'I will show you the emerald flooring, tiles studded with rubies, the garden, vine-creepered bowers, the house with shower baths and the palaces with secret passages between the walls, the murals, the royal pastimes, mechanical devices, birds, caged tigers and lions, and other such things.'

SUTRAS 18-19. Then, privately, she should relate the king's love for her, praise his competence in the sport of love.

SUTRA 20. Finally she should arrange a rendezvous with the king, assuring her that it would be a secret known only to the three of them.

SUTRA 21. In case the woman does not consent, the king should personally go to her, please her with gifts and loving approaches, and permit her to go in the company of other women ungrudgingly.

SUTRA 22. Or, having made the acquaintance of the husband of the woman he desires, the other wives of the king should get the wife to visit the harem daily as if they were conferring a favour upon her. Thereafter, the royal woman-messenger should be sent to her and should act in the same way as described above.

SUTRA 23. Or, one of the queens should befriend the woman who is to be won over through the help of a maidservant. When some contact is established, the queen should see her under some pretext. Afterwards, when the woman has visited the harem, a woman confidante of the queen should be sent there and should act in the same way as described above.

SUTRA 24. Or, the woman who is to be won over, being well known as being exceptionally talented in one of the arts, should be invited to the royal harem by the king's wives and requested to display her talent. After this, she should be rewarded respectfully with gifts and put in contact with the woman confidante of the king. The woman confidante's approach has already been described above.

SUTRA 25. Or, a woman beggar, in league with the king's wife, should say to the woman whom the king desires and whose husband may have lost his wealth, or who is afraid of the king for some reason or other, thus, 'This particular queen, who is a favourite of the king and whose every wish is attended to, pays me a great deal of attention (and listens to my advice). She is by nature benevolent, so I will tackle her in this way. I will get you admitted into the harem and she will do away with all cause of danger and fear from the king.' Having thus won her over and got her admitted into the harem, twice or three times, through the efforts of the beggar woman, the favourite queen should then afford her every protection. After this, when the woman is delighted and pleased with the queen's favour, she is approached again by the woman confidante of the king and tackled in the same way as described earlier.

SUTRA 26. What has been said above regarding the wife of a man who has reason to fear the king applies also to the following persons:
- Wives of persons seeking employment.
- Wives of persons oppressed by high ranking officials.
- Wives of persons, who, are forcibly arrested.
- Wives of persons whose activities are illegal.
- Wives of persons who are discontented.
- Wives of persons who desire royal favours.
- Wives of persons who are ambitious.
- Wives of those oppressed by their kinsmen.
- Wives of those who desire to supersede other members of their caste.
- Wives of persons who are informants.
- Wives of those whose very nature of work forces them to seek royal favours.

SUTRA 27. If the woman who is to be won over is attached to another person, she should be arrested by the king and eventually employed in the harem and thus, gradually, be made a permanent slave there.

SUTRA 28. Her husband should be accused by the king as a traitor with the help of his spies, after which the wife can easily be taken into custody as punishment and gradually admitted into the harem. These are the secret ways of winning over other men's wives, open to the king.

SUTRA 29. Under no circumstances should the king ever enter the abode of other persons.

SUTRA 30. Abhira, the king of Kotta, who had entered the house of another person (a merchant prince) was killed by a washerman commissioned by the brother. And similarly Jayatsena, king of Kashi, was killed by the superintendent of horses.

SUTRA 31. When the king makes advances to other men's wives openly, he may do so according to the custom of the place.

SUTRA 32. (For instance), in Andhra province, newly-married village girls usually enter the harem on the tenth day of their marriage carrying presents, and after they are deflowered, they are allowed to return home.

SUTRA 33. In Vatsagulma province, the women in the harem of the ministers make it a practice to go to the king at night and attend to his comforts.

SUTRA 34. In Vidarbha province, the women in the royal harem allow the beautiful village women to enter and stay with them for a fortnight or a month, for the same reason.

SUTRA 35. In Aparanta province, beautiful wives are actually presented to the king and ministers.

SUTRA 36. In Saurashtra province, the women, whether they belong to villages or towns, visit the royal harem for the king's pleasure, either separately or in groups.

SUTRA 37 (verse). These are the various ways and means adopted by different kings (and persons in office) characteristic of different provinces. In these ways they can gratify their desires.

SUTRA 38 (verse). But a king who has the welfare of his people at heart should not resort to these ways and means, for it is said that a king who can control the six enemies of mankind (the six passions) can conquer the world.

CHAPTER VI

ON THE WOMEN OF THE ROYAL HAREM AND ON PROTECTING ONE'S OWN WIFE

SUTRA 1. Since the women of the harem are not allowed to see other men, being very well guarded, and since they have only one husband common to all of them, they are physically dissatisfied, and they therefore give pleasure to each other in the various ways described below.

SUTRA 2. They dress up the daughter of a nurse or a woman friend or a maidservant like a man, and equip that person with unnatural aids, such as a part or whole of roots and fruits (Kanda: Aluka and Kadali; Mula : Tala and Ketaki; Phala: Alabu and Karkati).

SUTRA 3. They may unite with persons who look like men, but who have no moustache or beard.

SUTRA 4. Kings who are kind to passionate wives, go to many wives in one night, even though their own desire has abated; they use unnatural aids for indulging in union until their wives are satisfied.

But to those whom they really love and whose turn it is on that particular night, after being duly cleansed after the monthly period, they go with genuine passion. This custom is prevalent in the East.

SUTRA 5. Like the women in the harem, men who are unable to satisfy their desires try to do so unnaturally by manipulating with the hand, by indulging in bestiality and pygmalianism.

SUTRA 6. The women in the harem, sometimes with the help of the maidservant, smuggle in refined men disguised as women (after sunset).

SUTRA 7. The daughters of the nurses who are acquainted with the secret desires of the women in the harem, should try to win over the refined men to visit the harem by pointing out to them future advantages.

SUTRA 8. They should confide certain relevant information to them regarding easy access, safe exit, the lie of the palace, lack of vigilance of the guards, and carelessness and irregularities of the attendants.

SUTRA 9. They should not, however, force this on a man if he is not inclined that way, nor should they arrange it if entry and exit to the place is not easy. This would endanger the man's safety.

SUTRA 10. Vatsyayana maintains that a man should not enter the harem in spite of easy access, since the whole undertaking is fraught with other dangers.

SUTRAS 11-13. However, if he is invited over and over again he must consider the material gain accruing, and after having taken all necessary precautions, enter those pleasure gardens in the harem alone which have proper exits, long side-enclosures guarded by just a few guards who are not too vigilant. He must do this only when the king is out of the capital and taking proper note of the side-entrances, he should contact the guards with some excuse or the other every day as far as possible.

SUTRA 14. He should pretend to be in love with one of the maid-servants of the harem. She should be made aware of his true intentions, and when she is not able to meet him, he should feign to be sorrowful.

SUTRA 15. He should guide his actions towards all the messengers who have access to the harem according to instructions, mentioned in an earlier chapter.

SUTRA 16. He should get himself acquainted with all the spies of the king.

SUTRAS 17-18. If the messenger is unable to enter the harem to carry out the mission to the woman to be won over, he should wait at the palace gate, provided the woman has expressed her inclination, and engage the guard in conversation, pretending to wish to see one of the maidservants.

SUTRA 19. While doing so, he should catch the eye of the woman who desires him, and express his own sentiments by signs and gestures.

SUTRA 20. The spot where she happens to be should be chosen by him as suitable for placing a portrait of hers beside his, poems with double meanings (inscribed on leaves), playthings bearing marks made by him, and head ornaments made of blossoms, also bearing his marks, and a ring.

SUTRA 21. He should carefully note her reply to these tokens and then attempt to enter the harem.

SUTRA 22. When he knows that a certain place is frequented by his beloved, he should hide himself there earlier.

SUTRAS 23-24. At night, he should enter the palace disguised as one of the guards with the guard's connivance, and make hidden entry and exit after being covered with sackcloth and blankets.

SUTRA 25. Or he can make himself and his shadow invisible by the use of magical tricks such as Puta and Aputa.

SUTRA 26. The recipe for this is: The beard of a mongoose, seeds of Choraka and gourd, eyeballs of a serpent, all these should be cooked together without allowing them to smoke, and then converted into a paste by mixing with an equal quantity of water. A person who applies this to his eyes can render himself and his shadow invisible.

SUTRA 27. At night or on moonlit nights he should enter and exit from the palace in the company of maidservants bearing torches, or by way of a subterranean passage.

SUTRAS 28-30 (verses). Generally speaking, a young man can enter a palace when goods are being taken out, or when vehicles enter the palace, or during social parties and festivities, or when maidservants leave one palace gate to enter another one, or when abodes are changed or when guards change their stations, or during garden parties, or when pilgrimages are undertaken, or when returning from pilgrimages, or while the king is abroad or has gone on a long pilgrimage.

SUTRAS 31-32 (verses). The women of the harem, knowing one another's secrets and having one object in common, become united, and the harem which was erstwhile impregnable, ceases to be so. In this way, the women can enjoy the fruits of their efforts without spoiling one another's pleasure.

SUTRA 33. In the Aparanta province, only the women have access to royal harems and are in a position to allow or disallow any persons inside, since the harems in this province are not adequately guarded.

SUTRA 34. In the Abhira province, the women fulfil their desires with the help of the Kshatriya guards who stand guard outside the harem.

SUTRA 35. In the Vatsagulamaka province, the women who have access to the harem smuggle into the harem young men dressed like maidservants.

SUTRA 36. In the Vidarbha province, the royal princes who have unrestricted access to the harem, freely unite with the members, excepting with the mother.

SUTRA 37. In the Strirajya province, the women in the harem unite only with those who have access to their palace and only with their kinsmen and men from their own community.

SUTRA 38. In the Gauda province, they unite only with Brahmins, friends, attendants, slaves and errand boys.

SUTRA 39. In the Sindhu province, they unite with doorkeepers, servants and such other menials who have easy access into their harems.

SUTRA 40. In the Himalayan terrain, the men are adventurous and, bribing the guards with money, they enter the harem and unite with the women.

SUTRA 41. In the Banga, Anga, and Kalinga provinces, the educated Brahmins obtain royal permission to enter the harems with the excuse of offering flowers, and holding conversation with the women. Although there is usually a curtain between them they contrive to unite with the members.

SUTRA 42. In the Eastern provinces, the women in the harem conceal one young virile man between every batch of nine or ten women.

So much about approaching the wives of others.

SUTRA 43. For these reasons also one should protect one's own wife.

SUTRA 44. The ancient sages are of the opinion that guards, when chosen, should be free from excessive passion.

SUTRA 45. Gonikaputra argues that since guards can be coerced by other men if they are cowardly or liable to corruption they should be carefully chosen so that they may not succumb to these temptations.

SUTRA 46. According to Vatsyayana, guards must possess the one quality of faithfulness, and only those who are fearless and averse to bribes should be employed, since they alone will be found to be faithful.

SUTRA 47. Followers of Babhravya contend that a man should allow his wife to associate with a young woman who would inform him about the secrets of other people, and in this way, test his wife's chastity.

SUTRA 48. Vatsyayana, however, says that faults are natural to young women, and they should not, therefore, be charged with them without proper reasons.

SUTRA 49. The following things are usually said to ruin women, and should be avoided:
- Excessive talking.
- Absence of restraint.
- Independence from her husband.
- Too much mixing with other men.
- Continued and long absence of her husband while on a journey.
- Living in another province for some length of time.
- Unemployment or loss of livelihood on the part of her husband.
- The company of loose women.
- Jealousy of her husband.

SUTRA 50 (verse). The man learned in the science of love, conversant with the various ways and means of winning over the wives of others as described in this chapter, is not likely to be deceived in respect of his own wife.

SUTRA 51 (verse). However, he would be ill-advised if he resorted to these himself, since they are not quite natural; moreover, they are fraught with danger for himself, besides going against the precepts of Dharma and Artha.

SUTRA 52 (verse). This chapter is intended for the wellbeing of men and for guiding them in the ways of protecting their wives. It is not to be used for the seduction of other men's wives and thus spoiling their own future.

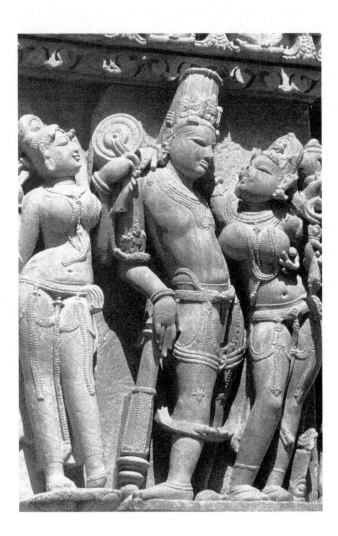

PART VI

ON COURTESANS AND THEIR WAY OF LIFE

CHAPTER I

ON SELECTING THE RIGHT MAN AND ON THE METHODS OF BEGUILING HIM

SUTRA 1. The courtesans court their paramours partly for physical pleasure but basically for their own livelihood.

SUTRAS 2-3. The first of these is a natural instinct, but the second is certainly not natural, yet they have to make it appear natural.

SUTRA 4. Men become attached to those courtesans who are attractive towards them physically since they inspire a feeling of confidence in them.

SUTRA 5. The courtesan must make an effort to impress upon him the fact that her love for him is genuine and not a means to satisfy her want.

SUTRA 6. Since she has to maintain her hold on him the extraction of remuneration should be done intelligently and thoughtfully.

SUTRA 7. She should always adorn herself with ornaments and look out on the road without exposing herself too much, as if she were a commodity for sale.

SUTRA 8. She should brief her agents to help her in drawing the young man towards her. They should be in a position to separate the young man from other women, and protect her from harm, assist her in her mission, and in case she is overpowered by those who approach her, they should be able to save her.

SUTRA 9. These persons are:
- Officers, who maintain law and order.
- Senior executive officers .
- Fortune-tellers.
- Desperados.
- Powerful men.
- Artists or instructors of the sixty-four arts.
- Pithamardas.
- Vitas.
- Vidushakas.
- Florists.
- Perfumers.
- Owners of liquor-shops.
- Washermen.
- Barbers.
- Beggars.

And others who may be able to help her.

SUTRA 10. The following persons should be courted only for the purpose of obtaining money:
- A young man who is unattached.
- A very young man.
- A wealthy man.
- One who has secured his livelihood in the same place.
- An officer.
- One who has inherited wealth or has had a windfall.
- One who has a competitor in business.
- One who has a steady income.
- One who is vain and considers himself very handsome.

- One who is given to boasting.
- One who has little brains but pretends to show much.
- One who has no manliness.
- One who gives money and wishes to be considered manly.
- One who is a rival of another person.
- One who is by nature generous.
- One who has great influence with the king and his ministers.
- One who is a fatalist.
- One who does not attach much importance to money.
- One who disobeys the orders of his elders.
- One who is a cynosure of his equals.
- A man of property.
- An only son.
- An ascetic who is internally troubled by passion.
- A dexterous man.
- One who knows the uses of medicine.

SUTRA 11. However, certain men should be won over for their excellent qualities (and accomplishments) so that the courtesans may obtain their love and fame and material prosperity.

SUTRA 12. Qualities which make a man approachable: Being of noble family, learned, familiar with the different faiths, endowed with a poetic nature, expert narrator, eloquent speaker, dignified, expert in the various arts, respecting sages and learned men, ambitious and aspiring to greater things, zealous, faithful, free from jealousy, generous-hearted, devoted to friends, religious and social enthusiast, theatre-goer, actor and player of games, healthy, unblemished, physically strong, manly, virile, kind, gallant to the ladies, not enslaved by women, independent, broad-minded, and so forth. These qualities in a man should be fully considered by the courtesan.

SUTRA 13. The qualities desirable in a courtesan herself are: Beauty, youth, marks on the body proving her good fortune, sweet speech, appreciation of virtues and accomplishments of the young man, not undue fondness of material gain, desire for love and physical union, consistency of mind, honesty and frankness in her dealings, ambition for acquiring extraordinary accomplishments, generosity, and appreciation of the arts and of social gatherings. But the most common qualities which courtesans actually possess are:

SUTRA 14. Intelligence, character, good behaviour, honesty, gratitude, foresightedness, absence of inconsistencies, awareness of the proprieties of time and place, refined way of life, absence of begging, loud laughter, speaking ill of others, citing faults of others, anger, covetousness, disrespect for the things to be respected, fickle-mindedness, interrupting others' speech, and expert knowledge of the science of love and its ancillary arts.

SUTRA 15. When one (a courtesan or a man) has the very opposite qualities of those mentioned above, they become defects. (They do not then deserve the name Nayaka or Nayika.)

Defects which make a man unapproachable:

SUTRA 16. Infection of some wasting disease (like tuberculosis or leprosy), where the presence of germs makes physical union dangerous, foul mouth odour, too great an attachment to his own wife, harshness in speech, miserliness, cruelty, being abandoned by elders, practising thieving, hypocrisy, addicted to secret formulas for practising seduction, having disregard for honour, insulting, befriending even enemies for the sake of material gain, and having excessive shyness.

SUTRA 17. The motives for courting are as follows: The sages say that a person is motivated by passion, fear, desire for money, rivalry, revenge, sheer curiosity, partiality, sorrow, religious duty, fame, compassion, friendly advice, shyness, familiarity with a friend, good connections, inevitable decrease of passion, proximity of birth and caste and neighbourhood, continued intimacy, and dignity.

SUTRA 18. According to Vatsyayana, the principal reasons for courting are: Material gain, escape from dangers (physical, financial, etc.) and love for the particular person.

SUTRA 19. The consideration for material gain is not incompatible with real love, as the former becomes necessary for a courtesan's livelihood.

SUTRA 20. If the reason is escape from danger of some sort of fear, she should weigh the importance of material gain and love according to the circumstances.

Now about the proper person to be approached.

SUTRA 21. Even if invited, the courtesan should not immediately proceed to the person concerned nor accede to his request too quickly, since men dislike women who are too easily gained over.

SUTRA 22. However, she should commission one of her own helpers, such as those engaged in shampooing, musicians, and jesters, or any such person who attends to the man's requirements, to gauge his inclinations. If such persons are not available, she should employ Pithamardas and others.

SUTRA 23. Through them she should find out if the man behaves well or ill, if he is inclined towards a physical union with her or not, whether he is attached or unattached and his generosity or lack of it.

SUTRA 24. (Only after this is done) should she send the Vita in advance and then begin her affair with him.

SUTRA 25 Then the Pithamarda should fetch the man to the courtesan's place or, alternatively, should take her to the man's place on the pretext of showing her cockfights, ram-fights, quail-fights, or listening to parrots and mynas, or for attending musical or theatre parties.

SUTRA 26. On his arrival she should present him with some token of her love. This creates in his heart a good and favourable impression, especially when she tells him that no ordinary person ever receives that token.

SUTRAS 27-28. She must entertain him with discussions (on poetry and the arts), and please him by offering him betel leaves, garlands, etc. When he returns to his house she should send him some gift or other frequently through her maidservant who is adept in pleasant conversation and jokes. Whenever she can, on one excuse or another, the courtesan herself should accompany the Pithamarda to his house.

SUTRA 29 (verse). Whenever he arrives at her house, she should receive him lovingly with betel leaves (full of various ingredients), perfumed sandalwood paste, flower garlands neatly threaded, and arrange discussions on poetry and the arts.

SUTRA 30 (verse). As their mutual love grows they should exchange presents frequently – she should offer him various presents and he should offer her rings and upper garments, and in this way they should demonstrate to each other their desire for physical union.

SUTRA 31 (verse). She should then please him more and more by showering on him gifts and presents with loving care and inviting, alluring and suggestive requests (made by the Pithamarda or herself), until she becomes united with him. (The Pithamarda should do his bit by saying, 'Why do you not sleep here', and so forth.)

So much for approaching and inviting the proper person.

CHAPTER II

ON THE BEHAVIOUR OF A COMPLIANT COURTESAN

SUTRAS 1-2. When a courtesan is finally united with her lover she should conduct herself like the one and only wife. She should so arrange it that he feels attracted to her, but not absolutely tied to her; she should however show by her actions that she, on her part, is in fact attached to him.

SUTRA 3. She should show obedience towards her own mother who is usually avaricious and cruel by nature. If she is motherless, she should behave equally obediently to her foster-mother.

SUTRA 4. The latter should not show any great affection for her daughter's lover. In fact, under certain circumstances, she is in a position to take away her daughter from one lover and place her at the disposal of another, even by force.

SUTRA 5. This usually results in the young courtesan becoming averse to love, subject to mental depression, timidity and nervousness, yet she is not in a position to disobey her mother's orders.

SUTRA 6. Sometimes, in such a case, the courtesan may pretend to suffer from one or another affliction which her lover may possibly construe as being accidental. Without actually detesting her for it and without his own conviction about her illness, he may believe that she is to be temporarily avoided. (Ailments such as a headache or a pain in the stomach, which need not have visible effects, are all temporary.)

SUTRA 7. (As she is under orders to go to another lover) this pretended illness becomes sufficient cause for not uniting with her previous lover.

SUTRA 8. In such a case the courtesan should send her maidservant to bring back to her the used flower garlands and the remaining betel leaves (after he has availed himself of them).

SUTRA 9. To her new lover she should display her feeling of wonder and admiration for his cleverness in love, and show her own readiness to learn the sixty-four ways and modes of the love-sport from him as a pupil. She should then practise the various postures taught by him, behave in the way he likes, confide in him all her aspirations, conceal the deficiencies of her body, overlook it if he has the habit of sleeping in the bed with his face turned away from her, allow him to fondle her, kiss him while he is asleep, until finally, she can embrace him.

SUTRA 10. She should look at him when his mind is engrossed in something else. When he passes by along the main road, she should watch him from her own house, and if she is detected, she should become bashful, which after all, is a cunning expedient. She should pretend to hate the things that he hates, like the things which he likes, be pleased with things that please him, be happy when he is happy, dejected when he is dejected. She should be curious to find out if he is attached to another girl, and in case it is so, she should feign a fit of temper and suspiciously tell him that the nail- and teeth-marks which she has herself made on his body are inflicted by the other woman.

SUTRA 11. She should never directly express her love for him, but signify it to him merely through signs and gestures. At times, she can express it while in a pretended delirium, and praise him for the good actions which he has undertaken (such as building temples, digging wells and tanks).

SUTRA 12. She should always be attentive to what he has to say, praise him after properly understanding the meaning, counter it by showing him that she also knows a great deal about certain matters, and reply to his questions intelligently, provided she is sure that he really loves her.

SUTRA 13. She should prove to him that she follows him with attention when he is narrating some tales, except when they relate to one of his other wives.

SUTRA 14. She should show concern when he heaves a sigh or when he yawns or interrupts his narrative due to forgetfulness or if he falls down.

SUTRA 15. If he happens to sneeze during conversation or laughter, she should exclaim, 'May God bless you! long life to you!' (out of sheer love for him).

SUTRA 16. Whenever she herself feels depressed (through hearing some bad news about another lover) she should excuse herself with some feigned illness which afflicts her like an enemy.

SUTRA 17. She should never praise the good qualities of one lover to another, never pass adverse remarks against a person who suffers from the same faults as her lover, always accepting and using whatever is offered to her by him.

SUTRA 18. Whenever her lover is afflicted with a calamity, she should refrain from wearing any ornaments, and if he falsely accuses her, she should desist from eating.

SUTRA 19. She should sympathise with him in his misfortune, show her willingness to leave the place with him. If she is retained by the king she should show her willingness to be redeemed (on payment of the fine).

SUTRA 20. She should always express how fortunate she has been in obtaining his love. Whenever he recovers from any illness or when one of his cherished wishes have been fulfilled or when her lover has a stroke of luck and a resulting increase in his wealth, she should offer worship in thankfulness, in response to the vow she had previously taken.

SUTRA 21. Under normal circumstances, she should deck herself with ornaments and partake of nourishing food in moderation.

SUTRAS 22-23. When she sings she should personally name her lover and his family. In the event of his getting fatigued, she should hold his hand against her forehead and bosom, and after noticing the soothing effects of these, she should sleep; but if she does not feel like sleeping, she should sit in his lap as if asleep, and follow him if he goes out of the room.

SUTRA 24. She may express her desire for a son through the union, but she should never crave for a long life.

SUTRA 25. She should not let him know anything that has been confided to her in private by other persons.

SUTRA 26. She should not allow him to observe fasts and vows, but take upon herself the sin for not observing those fasts and vows. However, if he cannot be dissuaded, she should join him in observing those fasts and vows.

SUTRA 27. In case of dispute concerning some other person, she should interfere by saying that even an able person like her lover is unable to give a final decision in the matter.

SUTRAS 28-30. She should look after his wealth as carefully as she looks after her own; never attend gatherings and social functions without him; express pride, and pleasure in using flower garlands worn by him, and in partaking of food only after he has eaten.

SUTRA 31. She should praise his family, good bearing, proficiency in the arts, nobility of birth, deep learning, natural complexion, wealth, his neighbourhood, the good qualities of his friends, his youth, and his smart speech.

SUTRA 32. If he already knows music and is familiar with the other arts, she should encourage him to add to his artistic achievements.

SUTRA 33. She should go to him in the face of danger, winter or summer, or rain.

SUTRA 34. Whenever she is distributing alms to the poor for securing happiness in the next life, she should express her wish to get the same lover in the life to come.

SUTRAS 35-36. She should imitate his tastes, his sentiments and his actions; show suspicion at his having adopted the magic rites pointed out by Muladeva (for winning over women).

SUTRAS 37-38. She should always pretend to have an exchange of arguments with her mother for being loyal to her lover, and if she is being led away forcibly by her mother to another person, she should threaten to poison herself or fast herself to death or kill herself with a weapon or hang herself.

SUTRA 39. Her secret helpers should convey to her lover that it was not the courtesan's fault but her mother's in her approaching another lover.

SUTRAS 40-42. She should be critical of her own profession; she should never argue; in matters regarding money, never do anything in the absence of her mother.

SUTRA 43. If her lover sets out on a journey she should take serious oaths on her own life and thus request him to return quickly.

Now for her behaviour during his absence.

SUTRA 44. When her lover is away from home, the courtesan should restrict her make-up to cleanliness alone. She should desist from wearing ornaments, except the Mangala ornament (signifying that her lover is living), and one conch-shell bangle only.

SUTRA 45. She should recollect (the pleasant times she has enjoyed in the company of her lover), visit female astrologers, go out into the squares and streets to observe good omens at midnight and envy the positions of the sun, moon, stars and constellations.

SUTRA 46. When she has a good dream at night, she should declare to her friends and relatives that she would soon be reunited with her lover.

SUTRA 47. But when she gets a bad dream she should become anxious and perform ceremonies to appease the deities so that no evil may befall him.

SUTRAS 48-50. When he returns safely, she should offer thanksgiving to the god of love and to the other deities and fetch home the vessel of fortune (covered with a cloth) and in the company of her friends.

SUTRA 51. She should feed crows as a token of her oblations (thus fulfilling her vows).

SUTRA 52. While the worship to the god of love and others should be done immediately after her reunion with the lover, the feeding of crows must be done subsequently.

SUTRA 53. When she is convinced that he has become completely attached to her, she should say that she would follow him into death.

The characteristics of the lover who is completely attached to a courtesan are:

SUTRA 54. Placing his full confidence in her, making himself agreeable to her in every respect, fulfilling all her wishes, never suspecting her in any way, and never coveting any monetary gain from her.

SUTRA 55. Whatever is laid down here is according to the sage Dattaka. Whatever the courtesan finds missing she should observe and practise from the way other people act and from a study of the nature of the persons concerned.

SUTRA 56 (verse). Since the sentiment of love is subtle, and women are avaricious, and since their actions are deceptive and misleading, even persons expert in the science of love are sometimes not able to gauge the true nature of their love correctly.

SUTRA 57 (verse). Sometimes women show attachment to their lovers, sometimes aversion, sometimes they have a mind to please them and sometimes to abandon them, and sometimes they may extract from them all the wealth that they may possess.

CHAPTER III

ON THE WAYS OF OBTAINING MONEY; INDICATIONS OF WANING ATTACHMENTS; HOW TO GET RID OF THE LOVER

SUTRA 1. There are two ways open to a courtesan for extracting money from the person attached to her – the natural way and the deliberate way.

SUTRA 2. The learned sages assert that when a courtesan is able to extract the amount already agreed upon, or sometimes more than that, she should not try to obtain any more.

SUTRA 3. According to Vatsyayana, if the lover is properly tackled he will usually give her double the amount that has been fixed by them beforehand.

SUTRA 4. The artifices to be used for obtaining moneys from the lover are: When the time comes for her to settle accounts with dealers from whom she has purchased articles, she should make the payment in his presence with her own articles such as ornaments, sweetmeats, food (cooked or otherwise), drinks, flowers, garments, perfumes, etc. (This is to show him that she is not avaricious in spite of her taking money from him.)

SUTRA 5. Praising his riches.

SUTRA 6. Performing of some religious rites, or planting trees, starting to build a grove, erecting a temple, constructing a tank, arranging garden parties or festivals, and presenting gifts to her friends.

SUTRA 7. Complaining to him that she is being robbed of her ornaments by guards and dacoits on the way to his house.

SUTRA 8. Reporting a fire in her house and the consequent loss of money, or a theft contrived by entering through a hole made in the wall or loss of money through (her mother's) negligence.

SUTRA 9. Through secret agents she may report to her lover details of ornaments possessed by others (but deposited with her), and which are now required back by them. She can use the same artifice relating to his own ornaments deposited by him with her, and in addition, mention to him the expenses incurred for visiting his house.

SUTRA 10. Bringing to his notice debts incurred by her on his account, and mentioning to him her quarrel with her mother over the latter's extravagance.

SUTRA 11. If one of his friends arranges a festival she should tell him that she cannot attend it as she has no presents to offer him.

SUTRA 12. Reminding the man that his friends had brought several expensive and valuable presents.

SUTRA 13. Curtailing expenses of even the necessary items of expenditure.

SUTRA 14. Getting the things she desires prepared by artisans if the bill is being paid by her lover.

SUTRA 15. Obliging physicians and ministers for selfish ends.

SUTRA 16. Assisting friends and benefactors in time of misfortune.

SUTRA 17. Making excuses for repairs or renovations to be carried out in her house, arranging festivals on happy occasions, such as the birth of a son to one of her women friends, satisfying her friend's desire when she is pregnant, or excuses of illness or alleviating her friend's misfortune, etc.

SUTRA 18. Selling of some ornaments for the sake of her lover.

SUTRA 19. Showing some ornaments and household utensils greatly valued by her to a dealer for the purpose of disposing of them. Purchasing new and larger utensils.

SUTRA 20. These have great value since all courtesans possess similar utensils, and there is possibility of a great deal of interchange.

SUTRA 21. Reminding him of the loans and gifts given to her in the past and praising them (when he gives her another one).

SUTRA 22. Informing him that he knows, with the help of her agents, how much more money several other courtesans have received from him.

SUTRA 23. When other courtesans visit her she should shyly relate to them, in the presence of her lover, her greater monetary gains and those that are likely to come from him.

SUTRA 24. She should refer to her flat refusal of higher offers made by previous lovers for regaining her love (in the presence of the present lover so that he might offer more thinking her to be, firmly attached to him).

SUTRA 25. Describing in his presence the liberality of his rivals.

SUTRA 26. If the courtesan finds out that he would not return to her, she should beg of him to do so like a child.

These are various ways of obtaining money.

SUTRA 27. A courtesan should always find out and keep herself informed about the state of her lover's mind – whether he has lost interest in her or not. She should gauge this from his behaviour, change in his temper, and expressions on his face.

The signs of a lover becoming indifferent are:

SUTRA 28. He offers her neither more nor less (than the amount agreed upon).

SUTRA 29. He contacts those who are against the courtesan.

SUTRA 30. He engages in activities concerning something else, giving some lame excuse.

SUTRA 31. He even stops giving her her daily allowance (towards her expenses).

SUTRA 32. He forgets to honour his promises to her, or deliberately tries to misinterpret them to suit his own purpose.

SUTRA 33. He speaks to his friends in an unintelligible manner through gestures and signs.

SUTRA 34. He sleeps elsewhere (at the house of another courtesan) giving an excuse of some urgent work undertaken on behalf of one of his friends.

SUTRA 35. He talks in private to the servants of his former mistress (about her behaviour, etc., as compared to the present one).

The courtesan should guide her actions in the following manner when she feels sure that her lover is becoming indifferent.

SUTRA 36. When she observes that her lover is becoming indifferent to her, she should herself take out, with her own hands, the gold and silver ornaments that he has given her, and making some excuse return to him some of the money, before he asks for the same.

SUTRAS 37-38. Her first creditor (with her connivance) should forcibly take these away from her hands, and if she finds that the lover is disputing the creditor's right to take these things away, she should take the matter up to judicial officers. This is the attitude the courtesan should adopt when she finds her lover becoming indifferent.

SUTRA 39. The courtesan should always continue to maintain friendly relations with her lover who has presented money, etc., to her generously in the past; even if he gives her little now, but remains attached to her, she should remain friendly with him despite this state of affairs.

SUTRA 40. But if she has accepted another lover, she should expel her previous lover who has become poor and has no means to maintain himself (and the courtesan).

Now we will describe the ways and means open to a courtesan for expelling such a lover.

SUTRA 41. Doing things whole-heartedly which he does not like; in his presence occupying herself with things he detests; pouting her lips (on seeing him); stamping on the ground with her feet; discoursing on topics of which he is ignorant; not being surprised or shocked by his knowledge of her secrets; passing adverse remarks; hurting his pride; mixing with his superiors; treating him with complete indifference; censuring those who suffer from the same faults as he does; hiding in a concealed corner (or having private talks with others).

SUTRA 42. Showing aversion to his gifts (of betel leaves, etc.); preventing him from kissing; concealing her body; showing distaste for his nail- and teeth-marks; adopting the position of crossed hands while embracing; keeping her limbs motionless and dispassionate; bending the knees; pretending sleep; pressing him to continue (with the physical union) even when he is tired; jeering at him when he cannot do so; not praising him even when he is able to continue the union; going away to another important personage during daytime for uniting with him when she knows his disinclinations from various signs and gestures. (She should get out of the sleeping chamber during daytime, leaving his desire unfulfilled.)

SUTRA 43. Pinpointing his faults while he converses; laughing even when the matter may be serious; laughing at quite another matter during a hilarious conversation; glancing at servants, or beating them with hands while he is talking; talking of quite other things during this time; alleging dissatisfaction on account of his misadventures and vices which cannot be overcome; divulging his secrets; accusing him indirectly by accusing the maidservant of some misdemeanour.

SUTRA 44. She should not show herself when he comes to meet her, nor ask for anything that he may not be able to give her and finally she should herself leave the man.

This procedure regarding the courtesan's behaviour towards her lover has been laid down by Dattaka.

SUTRA 45 (verse). From the beginning to the end the behaviour of a courtesan should be towards uniting, with the proper person after due and full consideration of his requirement and capacity, then to please her lover when she is physically united with him, and when he becomes attached to her she should extort money from him and finally abandon him when he is reduced to poverty.

SUTRA 46 (verse). If a courtesan follows the code of behaviour described above, she can never be cheated by the persons who approach her, nor can she be stopped from making a fortune.

CHAPTER IV

ON THE REUNION WITH A FORMER LOVER

SUTRA 1. When a courtesan is in the process of discarding a lover whose wealth she has exhausted, she should reconcile herself with her former lover with whom her affair has for one reason or another been disrupted.

SUTRA 2. This former lover should be approached only if he has not become attached to another courtesan, only if he shows some inclination towards being reconciled and only if he is sufficiently sound financially (to pay her dues).

SUTRA 3. However, if he is already attached to some other courtesan she should ponder the matter and arrive at a decision only after considering to which of the following six categories he belongs:

SUTRA 4. One who has left her of his own accord and in the same way left any other courtesan also.

SUTRA 5. One who has been discarded and therefore has left her, and similarly has been discarded by a second courtesan and has also therefore left her.

SUTRA 6. One who has left her, but who has been discarded by the second and has therefore left the second.

SUTRA 7. One who has left the first courtesan and got himself attached to another.

SUTRA 8. One who has been discarded and has therefore left her.

SUTRA 9. One who has been discarded and therefore left the first courtesan, subsequently getting himself attached to another courtesan.

SUTRA 10. If a man has left the first courtesan and subsequently a second one also, and if then he sends messages (through Pithamardas and others), he should be considered a fickle person – one who does not value the qualities of the beloved. (Considering him to be of unsteady mind, the courtesan should not have a reconciliation with him.)

SUTRA 11. A man who has been discarded by the first courtesan and has therefore left her, and met with a similar fate at the hands of the second and also left her – even in these circumstances, if the courtesan finds him to be of a steady mind, still financially sound, and if she discovers that he has been discarded by the second courtesan after she has obtained a great amount from him and therefore angered him, such a man is likely to give the first courtesan due regard, and therefore is fit for a reconciliation.

SUTRA 12. A man who has been discarded either because he is found to be wanting in money or because he is found to be miserly is not to be associated with.

SUTRA 13. If a man has left the courtesan of his own accord, becomes discarded by the second, and has therefore left her, and if he pays the first one extra money in advance, he should once more be accepted.

SUTRA 14. If the lover who has left the first courtesan of his own accord has become attached to another courtesan, but still continues to send messages to the first one, she should consider his offer after weighing the pros and cons as follows:

SUTRA 15. 'He has come to me expecting to get some more (pleasure); he desires to come back to me since he has not experienced any great pleasure with that other woman; he wants to find out for himself which of the two he prefers (while he is still attached to the other woman); he is likely to give me a great deal of money because of his passion for me after he is won over again.'

SUTRA 16. 'Having observed the other woman to have greater defects than me, he now appreciates my many good qualities; since he will come to admire me, he will give me a great deal of money.'

Now regarding the other type of lover, unworthy of reconciliation:

SUTRA 17. She may consider him to be too young and immature, or she may find him paying attention to several courtesans at once, or she may discover him to be intent on cheating her, or having a wayward and temporary infatuation with her. In these cases she may or may not become reconciled with him.

SUTRAS 18-19. A man who has been discarded by the first courtesan and who has therefore left her, and subsequently become attached to the second one and left her of his own accord, if then he continues to send messages to the first one, his case should be considered in the following manner: 'He desires to return to me because of his passion for me; he is likely to give great wealth to me, since he is now impressed by my qualities; he is enamoured of me, and shuns the company of the other woman.'

SUTRA 20. 'I have previously discarded him unjustly; perhaps he desires to avenge himself by courting me again; perhaps he desires to win back his wealth for me which I had earned professionally; perhaps he is taking me back into his own confidence; perhaps he desires some service in return for this; perhaps he desires merely to disrupt my relations with my present lover and then to just leave me.' She should not reconcile herself with this type of former lover, whose intentions are not honourable.

SUTRA 21. A vacillating lover should not be approached too suddenly but only after the lapse of a long time.

SUTRA 22. In this way a lover who has been discarded then becomes attached to another courtesan, but continues to send messages to the first one, should be considered and handled thus:

SUTRA 23. She should herself send replies through his messengers to her former lover who has now become attached elsewhere. Her reason should be:

SUTRA 24. 'He has been discarded by me on account of certain lapses; he has therefore been forced to go elsewhere, and should therefore be brought back to me.'

SUTRA 25. 'As soon as he starts contacting me, his relations with the other woman will be automatically disrupted.'

SUTRA 26. 'I will then make him swallow his pride.'

SUTRA 27. 'This is the proper time for his income; his social status has improved; he has acquired a higher office; he has lost his wife; he has become independent; or he has separated from his parents.'

SUTRA 28. 'By reconciling myself with this man, I will secure a rich lover for myself.'

SUTRA 29 '(Having been once discarded by me), he is now humiliated by his own wife (with whom he has reunited); I will set him against her (by reconciling myself with him).'

SUTRA 30. 'A friend of the discarded lover (who is powerful and wealthy) is enamoured of the woman who was as it were my co-wife. I will estrange that friend (of the discarded lover) through him by his meeting that woman (so that she would not gain materially from that friend).'

SUTRA 31. 'I will make him appear cheap (in the estimation of others) by encouraging his fickle-mindedness (in running after courtesans).'

The following ways are open to her in sending messages:

SUTRA 32. Pithamardas and other messengers should inform the rejected lover that the courtesan had been forced to reject him in spite of being really attached to him because of the difficult temperament of her mother.

SUTRA 33. (They should further add that) the contact of the courtesan with her present lover is really against her own desire. They should describe to him her distaste for her present lover.

SUTRA 34. They should remind him of his love for her in the past, by showing him tokens of love which he had in the past presented to her. They should recount love scenes that had taken place between them.

SUTRA 35. The tokens should relate to one or another act of gratitude done by the lover to the courtesan.

Here ends the description of ways and means of reconciliation with the discarded lover.

SUTRA 36. According to the old sages, if a courtesan is faced with a choice between a rejected lover and a lover who is a stranger, the rejected lover is to be preferred since his behaviour is known to her, his attachment for her has also been demonstrated, and since it is altogether easier for her to approach him.

SUTRA 37. According to Vatsyayana, however, since the rejected love would presumably be financially impoverished by her, he would be unable to give her much wealth, and it is therefore difficult for her to have confidence in him again; whereas the new lover may come to be pleased very easily.

SUTRA 38. However, the differences in the nature of the two men should also be duly considered.

SUTRA 39 (verse). There are three reasons why a courtesan should reconcile herself with a discarded lover: For disrupting his attachment to a new courtesan, or to separate a particular man from a particular woman, or for the reason of expelling her present lover.

SUTRA 40 (verse). The lover, when excessively attached, is usually afraid of contact with a new person; he overlooks the lapses of the courtesan with whom he is attached even at the cost of parting with a great deal of money.

SUTRA 41 (verse). A courtesan should congratulate the lover who is attached to herself and not attached elsewhere; but she should deride the lover, who is attached to herself and to another person.

SUTRA 42 (verse). When there is a message from a new lover, she should accept him if he is in a position to pay her a great deal. If an old lover who has been discarded sends messages to her again, she should wait for some time before accepting him. She should prolong her reconciliation without actually abandoning her present lover.

SUTRA 43 (verse). She should speak to her present lover who is attached to her and whom she can command before going to a new lover. She should, however, obtain money from the new lover, but at the same time please the lover who is attached to her at the moment.

SUTRA 44 (verse). The wise courtesan should renew her association with a rejected lover only if she is satisfied that good fortune, monetary gain, love, and friendship are likely to accrue as a result of such a reunion.

CHAPTER V

ON GAINS OF SEVERAL KINDS

SUTRA 1. A courtesan who can attach herself to several lovers at once can obtain great wealth every day and she should not rest content by being attached to a single lover.

SUTRA 2. She should fix her rates every night considering the place, the time, the position, her qualities and outstanding merits, her excellence or otherwise, as compared to the others.

SUTRA 3. When she finds that a particular man is fit to be approached, she should send messages to him. She should herself convey the messages to such men who are his regular associates.

SUTRA 4. Once she knows his inclinations the man should be approached twice, three or four times for getting some more money. She should use all the ways and means of winning him over and extorting money from him.

SUTRA 5. According to the old sages, the courtesan who wishes to obtain a great deal of money from the person whom she accepts can do so when she has many lovers at once. What she gains from each of them sets the value for the other.

SUTRA 6. However, according to Vatsyayana, that lover who gives her gold is to be preferred, since gold coins once given are never taken back, and also since gold coins are the basis of all commercial transactions.

SUTRA 7. The following list shows the value of payment in order of precedence: gold, silver, copper, bronze, iron, bedstead, blankets, silk cloth, perfume or sandalwood, chillies, furniture (big bench or cot), ghee, oil, corn and cattle.

SUTRA 8. When more than one person offers this to the courtesan, and the things offered are of equal value, she should choose that person first who comes from her own town; second preference should be given to that person who is recommended by her friend. She should consider also the possibility that the offer may not be renewed, their comparative large-heartedness and dignity, their comparative qualities and virtues and her preference for any of them.

SUTRA 9. The old sages say that one who is generous is to be preferred to the one who may be passionately attached to her. His generosity must take the shape of generous payments and gifts.

SUTRA 10. According to Vatsyayana, however, it is possible for a courtesan to induce generosity in the person passionately attached to her. If the person happens to be a miser he can be induced to part with some money in the shape of gifts, but a person who is not really devoted to her, though he may be generous, cannot be forced to any great generosity.

SUTRA 11. According to the old sages, a wealthy man is to be preferred to a poor man; and from among the wealthy men, one who fulfils her desires is to be preferred.

SUTRA 12. Vatsyayana argues that the lover who carries out the courtesan's wishes thinks himself indebted to her, but the generous man does not look at the first gift or payment as indicative of his indebtedness (since he is generous by nature).

SUTRA 13. From among these again, one who is the most dignified deserves to be chosen.

SUTRA 14. The old sages say that if there is a choice between one who thinks himself indebted to the courtesan, and one who is generous on the other hand, the latter is to be preferred (as she is sure to gain money from him).

SUTRA 15. Vatsyayana argues that a generous lover does not overlook her troubles, despite certain lapses in the past on her part. This is true even if he is given false reports against the courtesan by other rival courtesans. On the whole, generous lovers are by nature noble-minded, honest and considerate. The lover who considers himself indebted to the courtesan usually considers the past relationship, and is not easily prejudiced against her by false accusations since he has been favourably impressed by her conduct in the past.

SUTRA 16. All things considered, the lover who is dignified and from whom there is likelihood of future gain for the courtesan is highly desirable.

SUTRA 17. If she has to choose between a lover who has been recommended by a friend and a lover from whom monetary gain is to accrue, the old sages are of the opinion that the latter must have preference.

SUTRA 18. Vatsyayana contends that financial gain is likely to come, even after a lapse of time, from a lover who is wealthy, but a friend is likely to get enraged and alienated if he is dissatisfied.

SUTRA 19. However, Vatsyayana maintains that there is this difference between the two: if the friend does not offer to pay her on the very day, he is most likely to do so after some time (when he returns to her).

SUTRA 20. In these circumstances, she should pacify her friend that a certain job needs to be urgently carried out, and that she promises to look after him the next day; so saying she should accept the offer which her friend makes, in spite of the fact that it has come after some time.

SUTRA 21. If a courtesan must choose between the act of obtaining wealth or that of warding off any danger, she should choose the first, so say the old sages.

SUTRA 22. But Vatsyayana differs from them in as much as money can be measured as a definite quantity, whereas unhappiness when once it befalls the courtesan, will breed uncertainty; there is no knowing where it will end.

SUTRA 23. However, misery can also be great or small, and a courtesan must exercise her judgment in this respect.

SUTRA 24. This is why Vatsyayana explains that the act of avoiding danger and misery is to be chosen in preference to the act of gaining money, whose worth after all is temporary.

The money gained by courtesans should, in part, defray the expenses for the following:

SUTRA 25. Constructing temples, tanks, gardens, groves, bridges, mud huts (providing them with perfumes, rich and valuable offerings to the god of fire), giving thousands of cows through someone to the Brahmins, providing for the worship of deities and for other religious gifts, collecting funds for their maintenance, and so forth. These are the beneficent acts which the best courtesans must carry out after they acquire wealth. (These courtesans are named Ganikas.)

SUTRA 26. The gains of other courtesans whose livelihood depends upon their physical charms, should be spent in bedecking themselves with ornaments, jewels and all manner of fineries; in decorating and furnishing the house, equipping it with costly vessels and maintaining a number of servants. This will demonstrate her wealth. (This is the Rupajiva type of courtesan.)

SUTRA 27. Finally the courtesans who are Kumbhadasis, show the acquisition of wealth by always wearing white garments. They have sufficient food to overcome hunger, and confine their make-up to the daily use of perfumes, betel leaves and few golden ornaments, usually gilded.

SUTRA 28. The old sages maintain that these are the three types of courtesans (the Ganika, Rupajiva and Kumbhadasi), and their respective income groups.

SUTRA 29. Vatsyayana is of the opinion, however, that the acquisition of wealth by these three classes is not always commensurate with their social status. It depends on the various factors such as the province, the time, the financial position of the lover, her own ability, and the nature of the people in the particular province.

SUTRA 30. Courtesans are advised to accept even small gains from their lovers. Their actions are guided by various circumstances: for instance, one courtesan may desire to prevent her lover from going to another; or she may desire to snatch a lover who is already attached to another; or she may desire to deprive her rival of her profits. She should always consider her position, prosperity, dignity, sex appeal, and so forth, and guide her actions accordingly in attaching herself to any particular lover. She may desire to assist him in avoiding any calamity; or she may consider helping him with little kindnesses which one of her former lovers has done to her but who has since become attached to another courtesan. In this way, she can either desire him out of love, or discard him by finding fault with him, or actually court for herself a totally new lover.

SUTRA 31. If a courtesan desires to gain prestige and dignity in the future, and if she, at the same time, wishes to ward off some troubles, she should curse her lover, upbraid him, and should not take anything from him (as her fee).

SUTRA 32. She should obtain her dues from her lover only in the following instances:
- When she desires to leave him and wishes to court another.
- When the lover is likely to leave her and get married.

- When her lover has a mind to squander his wealth.
- When her lover is going to seek the help of his father or guardian after becoming penniless.
- When her lover is likely to lose his present high position, or when he is found to be fickle-minded.

SUTRA 33. The following instances are mentioned when a courtesan may with advantage copy all the activities of his wife for ensuring benefits:

- When her lover is likely to be rewarded by the king.
- When her lover is likely to be appointed an officer in a high position.
- When the time has come for her lover to count his profits.
- When his carts of grain and other produce are likely to arrive.
- When he is likely to have a good crop.
- When she thinks that any good turn done to him is not likely to go unrewarded.
- Or when she is certain he will not go back on his word.

In this context there are some verses:

SUTRA 34 (verse). A courtesan should avoid temporary or permanent relationship with persons who have acquired wealth with great difficulty, persons who are perpetually in the king's favour, and persons who are by nature devoid of kindness. She must always keep at a distance from these persons (as she is likely to have some trouble sometime if she associates with them).

SUTRA 35 (verse). She should make every endeavour to unite herself with prosperous and well-placed persons, and with those whom it is dangerous to avoid or to slight in any way. The courtesan should attach herself, even by incurring some expense to herself, to those ambitious, capable and brave persons who, on being pleased even with a small act on her part, will reward her very handsomely.

CHAPTER VI

ON PECUNIARY GAINS AND OTHER CONSIDERATIONS; ON THE DIFFERENT TYPES OF COURTESANS

SUTRA 1. When a courtesan seeks financial gain and actual payment, it often happens that troubles crop up, which bring along greater troubles.

SUTRA 2. The causes for these are:
- ◆ Weakness of intellect and want of discrimination.
- ◆ Excessive passion.
- ◆ Uncontrolled vanity.
- ◆ Excessive hypocrisy.
- ◆ Extreme straightforwardness.
- ◆ Overwhelming confidence.
- ◆ Excessive anger.
- ◆ Thoughtlessness.
- ◆ Adventurousness.
- ◆ Influence of an evil genius.

SUTRA 3. These faults usually result in:
- Expenditure on futile things.
- Loss of prestige and future good fortune.
- Drying up of the likely source of income.
- Ending of the present income.
- Lesser ability to gain new lovers because of decreasing sex appeal.
- Physical injury or death.
- Cutting off the locks of her hair.
- Being tied with ropes and then being beaten.
- Disfiguring of limbs (such as ears, nose, arms and so forth).

SUTRA 4. The courtesan should, therefore, shun the company of persons who influence her adversely in this way, even at the cost of financial gain.

SUTRA 5. Now Artha or gain is threefold: that of wealth, that of religious merit, and that of physical pleasure. Anartha, or loss of gain, is similarly threefold: evil fortune, loss of religious merit, and loss of physical pleasure.

SUTRA 6. When either of these paths is chosen and acted upon, the resulting effects are bound to follow in quick succession.

SUTRA 7. When gain, in terms of money, becomes doubtful, the doubt of its being a gain is called a simple (Shuddha) doubt.

SUTRA 8. But a mixed doubt (Sarnkirna) arises when there is no certainty about anything – such as whether this may be or may not be, or that may also be or may not be.

SUTRA 9. If two things result from one act while it is being accomplished, it is named Ubhayatah Yoga (that is, producing two results).

SUTRA 10. If there are various results from one act while it is being accomplished, it is called Samantatah Yoga. These definitions will be illustrated later in this chapter.

SUTRAS 11-12. After having explained the nature of Artha, and the opposite threefold Anartha, we come to the ancillary advantages which a courtesan may expect after she gets direct monetary gains by courting a lover of the highest class: her being considered fit for approach by other lovers, future prestige and position, and generally being sought after (Arthanubandha).

SUTRA 13. However, a courtesan may become attached to the person from whom she may derive financial gain alone. In this case, Artha is said to be unattended by ancillary benefits (Niranubandha).

SUTRA 14. In the following instances gain is usually followed by undesirable consequences (Anarthabandha): When the money accepted by the courtesan happens to be given by the lover after he has himself usurped it from somebody else. The lover's loss of prestige or social position (if he is of low caste) results in the courtesan's fee being taken away by, the state officer along with the forfeiture of her own private wealth. If she courts a lover of a low caste she risks the loss of dignity and a good name. The same applies to a lover who is unpopular.

SUTRA 15. But troubles sometimes bring good results in their wake (Arthanubandha): Courting a brave man or a minister or a miser, even at her own expense, may sometimes be fruitless, it is true, but sometimes it is fruitful in warding off some possible trouble. This procedure is recommended for counteracting the causes of loss of money and is quite likely to bring prestige.

SUTRA 16. When a courtesan, at her own expense, courts either a miser, or one who considers himself very fortunate, or one who is ungrateful to her, or one who is given to cheating, her efforts are usually fruitless, since there are no benefits to reap (Niranubandha).

SUTRA 17. If she courts a person favoured by the king, or one who has great influence, or one who is very cruel, her efforts once again are in vain, since discarding of such a lover causes great trouble for her. This becomes a case of loss of money followed by various troubles (Anarthanubandha).

SUTRAS 18-19. Thus, cases where Dharma and Kama are involved are followed by troubles, and other troubles resulting from these troubles (Dharma, Artha, Adharma, Anartha) are followed by attendant troubles.

Now we come to cases of simple doubt. There are six types:

SUTRA 20. First, comes the case where Artha is involved: when the lover, though fully pleased, does not inspire certainty about his payment to the courtesan.

SUTRA 21. Second, it is the case where Dharma is involved: when a lover from whom the courtesan has squeezed money and whom she has subsequently discarded as a useless lover, refrains from giving her any more money.

SUTRA 22. Third, the case where Kama is involved: when the courtesan secures a lover whom she favours, but, in spite of that, goes to another servant or a person belonging to a low caste.

SUTRA 23. Fourth, where Anartha is involved: where she finds a powerful or influential lover, who, however, is of low birth and whom she does not really like, she doubts whether he will create trouble or not.

SUTRA 24. Fifth, the case where Adharma is involved: where her lover is totally unsuccessful but is still attached to her until she discards him; when, after this, he may perhaps go to the world of Pitris after death.

SUTRA 25. Sixth, where Dvesha is involved: when she expects her passion to be satisfied, but is unable to secure the right person and consequently becomes averse to her profession.

SUTRA 26. Now follows a description of mixed doubts. (First, the mixed doubt arising from Dharma or Adharma.)

SUTRA 27. When the courtesan approaches a lover from another province whose conduct is unknown to her, or she approaches a person who is a dependant of her present lover or she attracts a person of importance or one who is a guest, it gives rise to a mixed doubt in her mind.

SUTRA 28. When the courtesan approaches a man because of a friend's recommendations, or out of compassion in the case of a learned Brahmin, or a celibate, or one observing certain vows, or one who has taken to a religious order, or who gets a passionate desire on seeing her, or one who desires to die, the case engenders a mixed doubt. A mixed doubt arising from Artha or Anartha (source of monetary gain and source of trouble respectively).

SUTRA 29. Finally, the mixed doubt arising from Kama or Dvesha (love and dislike respectively). When a courtesan approaches a person about whom she has merely heard, without verifying the details about his other necessary qualities and status, it becomes a case of mixed doubt.

SUTRA 30. In short, mixed doubt arises when several alternative factors bear together on a problem.

SUTRA 31. It is a case of dual gain when a courtesan courts a new lover and earns money, while simultaneously obtaining money from a rival lover who is already attached to her.

SUTRA 32. It becomes a case of financial loss when a courtesan approaches a new lover at her own cost, but the efforts prove fruitless. Her previous lover, who is already attached to her at the time, is enraged at her courting another lover and takes back whatever gifts he has made to her.

SUTRA 33. It becomes a case of doubtful gain on both sides when a courtesan wonders whether courting a new lover will bring her gain or not, while still being attached to her erstwhile lover, but uncertain whether the latter will give her any money.

SUTRA 34. It is a case of monetary loss on both sides when a courtesan at her own expense; courts a new lover, but is doubtful whether he will pay or not, and at the same time, wonders whether her erstwhile lover would be enraged or not, whether he would be opposed to her going to a new lover, whether from anger he would harm her or from jealousy he would take back the money he has given her.

These cases have been cited according to the opinion of Auddalaki.

SUTRA 35. The following are according to the opinion of Babhravya: It is a case of the monetary gain from both sides when a courtesan, upon courting a new lover, obtains money from him while continuing to obtain money from her present lover without actually courting him.

SUTRA 36. It is a case of financial loss from both sides when a courtesan at her own expense approaches a new lover, but in vain, and the present lover, who is attached to her but not approached by her, asks back the money that he has given her.

SUTRA 37. It becomes a case of doubtful gain from both sides when a courtesan, without incurring any expense, approaches a new lover and wonders whether he will give her money or not. Also, when a courtesan, not courting an attachment, doubts whether her lover will give her more money or continue to give her what he had in the past.

SUTRA 38. It is a case of doubtful gain from both sides when a courtesan, at her own expense, courts a new lover but wonders whether she will secure the powerful and rival lover. She fears that if she courts the lover who is already attached to her, her new lover may from anger, cause her some harm or prevent gains from accruing to her.

SUTRA 39. By combining the above-mentioned, the following six kinds of mixed results are produced: Gain from one and loss from the other.

SUTRA 40. Gain from one and doubtful gain from the other.

SUTRA 41. Gain from one and doubtful loss from the other.

SUTRA 42. Loss from one and doubtful gain from the other.

SUTRA 43. Loss from one and doubtful loss from the other.

SUTRA 44. Doubtful gain from one and doubtful loss from the other.

All these are Samkirna Yogas.

SUTRA 45. In such cases the courtesan should confer with her friends who can help her, whether she should proceed with her courting which may bring her much wealth, even though there is a doubt or danger of averting the possibility of great misfortune.

SUTRA 46. In the same way, cases where Dharma and Karma are involved should be solved by her. These cases may be taken together or separately. These are the various Ubhayatah Yogas. (Shuddha, Samkirna and Vyatishakta.)

SUTRA 47. When Vitas combine together to keep a courtesan, it is called Goshti-Parigrahat – that is, 'maintained by a group'.

SUTRA 48. The courtesan who is courted by a number of persons without any rule or regulations regarding time fixtures, should create rivalry among them and thus extract money from each of them.

SUTRA 49. She should let her mother inform them that during festivals like Suvasantaka, her daughter (that is the courtesan), would approach him so that he may please her and fulfil her particular desire.

SUTRA 50. She should always be vigilant about her gains when rivalry exists among her various lovers.

SUTRA 51. The combinations of gains and losses on all sides are: gain from one, gains from all, loss from one, losses from all, gains from half of them, gains from all of them, losses from half of them, and losses from all of them. These are the Samantatah Yogas.

SUTRA 52. The doubtful gain and doubtful loss should be considered in the way previously explained, and considered to be mixed when they occur in combinations.

SUTRA 53. Similarly, cases where Dharma and Kama are involved should also be considered in the same way.

SUTRA 54. The courtesan may be of the following different types:
- A woman who does menial work (Kumbhadasi).
- One who attends on her master (Paricharika).
- One who is a debauch, and goes to another's house for physical pleasure with another man because she fears her husband (Kulata).
- One who is disgusted with her husband and therefore seeks physical pleasure with another man, either in her own or in the other person's house (Svairini).
- A dancing girl or an actress (Nati).
- The wife of an artisan (Shilpakarika).
- One who, during her husband's life or after his death, is kept as a concubine, and who openly indulges in physical pleasure with other men (Prakashavinashta).
- A woman living on her beauty (numbers two and seven are included in this category) (Rupajiva).
- The regular courtesan, well behaved, and following her profession with fitting dignity (Ganika).

SUTRA 55. The manner in which courtesans may operate consists of eight stages:

- Choosing the proper type of person for courting.
- Keeping contact with her helpers.

- Practising in the artifices of pleasing the lover.
- Practising ways and means of acquiring money from the lover.
- Practising ways of discarding a lover.
- Practising ways of reconciling herself with a lover.
- Considering particular gains and incidental ones.
- Adopting clear thinking regarding financial gains, loss and doubtful gains and losses.

SUTRA 56 (verse). Men hanker after physical pleasure: women, too, crave for them. The sacred books impart instructions regarding the motive for these cravings, and since women can fulfil them, they should also study the science of sex and love.

SUTRA 57. (verse). There are women who are extremely passionate; there are others who go exclusively after money or material wealth; we have already described the nature of passion in an earlier chapter, and we have already dilated upon the artifices which courtesans may resort to in the practice of their profession.

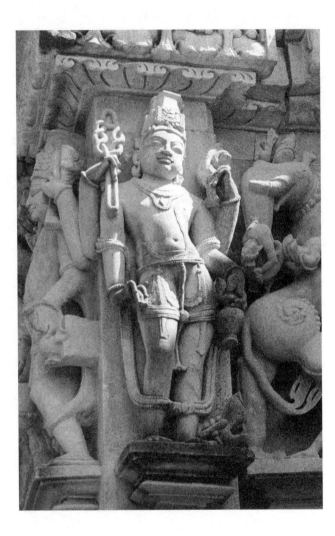

PART VII

ON WAYS OF MAKING ONESELF ATTRACTIVE TO OTHERS;

ON SECRET RECIPES AND EXPERIMENTS

CHAPTER I

ON ADORNING ONESELF AND ON ATTRACTING OTHERS; ON TONIC MEDICINES

SUTRA 1. Kama Sutra (Tantra and Avapa) has already been explained.

SUTRA 2. When a person is unable to fulfil his physical passions by the ways and means described before, he should then have recourse to other ways of attracting others to himself (the ways described herein are in relation to secret recipes, mysterious charms, aphrodisiacs, etc.).

SUTRA 3. The attraction that a man has for others depends on several contributory factors, such as physical beauty, accomplishment, youthfulness and liberality. (But in the absence of these, artificial means have to be resorted to, and the following are some recipes which may be found useful.)

SUTRA 4. Smearing the body all over with paste made of leaves of Tagara, Kushtha and Talisa, helps a great deal in increasing physical beauty.

SUTRA 5. Collyrium, prepared in a human skull, containing oil of Aksha and a cotton wick smeared with a paste made of finely-powdered ingredients (when applied to the eye-lashes, adds to the appearance).

SUTRA 6. Oil made from leaves of Punarnava, Sahadevi, Sariva, Kurantaka and Utpala (when applied, also enhances beauty).

SUTRA 7. The same applies to a wreath of flowers sprinkled with powder made with the ingredients mentioned above.

SUTRA 8. A man regains virility by using the powder of dried lotus, blue lotus and Nagakesara (Kesaras of all these flowers are indicated), in combination with honey and ghee. (This recipe brings results within a month.)

SUTRA 9. Also, applying the powder of these flowers, mixed with the powder from leaves of Tagara, Talisa, and Tamala Patra, adds to a person's beauty.

SUTRA 10. The eye of a peacock or a Tarakshu, covered in a golden amulet and worn on the right wrist or upper arm, is also efficacious in beautifying oneself. (The amulet should be of pure gold and sealed at an auspicious moment. The peacock's eye may be either the right or the left, as both are equally effective.)

SUTRA 11. A person should wear the stone of the Badara fruit and a conch, consecrated with Dharana Yogas mentioned in the Atharva Veda. (The conch should be covered with gold and worn on the head.)

SUTRA 12. The master should keep away his maidservant for the length of one year from the company of young men, by using certain mantras (inscribed on a Bhurja leaf and tying the amulet on the wrist of the maiden). He should then permit her to court one or other persons whom he considers fit for the purpose. These persons who have been rendered more passionate by being kept away from being courted by her, will be now anxious to win her over. The lucky person will give her the largest gift in terms of money, to prevent his rival from getting the better of him. This is a recognised means of increasing the maid's good fortune, the attributes of attractiveness and loving nature.

SUTRA 13. The elderly courtesan should protect her young daughter by inviting young men who are eligible, having the same standard of knowledge conduct and good looks; she should finally declare that whichever young man could give her daughter a certain specified amount, would get her daughter in marriage.

SUTRA 14. The daughter on the other hand, without the knowledge of her mother, should on her own court the wealthy sons of leading citizens.

SUTRA 15. She should meet them at the music school where they are being taught the arts, or in the house of a beggar woman where she might possibly see them. (Other suitable places are temples dedicated to Saraswati and gardens.)

SUTRA 16. The mother should always honour her declaration to young men and give her daughter in marriage to the most suitable young man.

SUTRA 17. However, if before the marriage she is unable to obtain the amount fixed, she should give part of her own money and declare to her daughter that her suitor has given her that specified amount.

SUTRA 18. After her marriage (by the Daiva form) the maid should allow herself to be deflowered.

SUTRA 19. She should declare this fact to the officers of law and justice after having privately united with them, but pretending ignorance of the same.

(The following practices are observed in the various provinces where no man is found coming forward for deflowering the maiden.)

SUTRA 20. Among the people of the Eastern provinces the elderly courtesans seek the help of a woman friend of the girl or of a maiden in artificially deflowering the girl; the young courtesans must, however, possess the qualities of youth, attractiveness, and a loving nature, and must be proficient in all the arts of love.

SUTRA 21. The young courtesan must remain with the person who has accepted her hand in marriage for a period of at least one year, thereafter she may behave as she pleases.

SUTRA 22. If, after the period of one year, she is again invited by her husband to go to him for one night, she should leave aside the thought of gain and return to him. These procedures, and the ceremony of the marriage, increase the Saubhagya (good fortune) of the courtesan, and enhance her attractiveness and lovableness in the eyes of other men.

SUTRA 23. These same rules apply to the daughters of dancers and actors, and the same procedure may also be followed in their case.

SUTRA 24. The only difference is that when the suitable husband is sought, he should be the one most likely to be of greatest help in her own profession of dancing and acting.

SUTRA 25. When a man smears his phallus with the powders of Dhatturaka, Maricha and Pippali, mixed with honey, before engaging in physical union, he succeeds in sexually satisfying the woman completely (Vashikaran).

SUTRA 26. Similar results are achieved when a man (with his left hand) removes the leaves and garlands from a dead body and mixes them with powdered bones of a Jivanjivaka bird, and applies them (to the woman's forehead and on his own feet) (Vashikarana).

SUTRA 27. Similarly, if a man smears his body before taking bath with the mixture of honey, powdered Amalaka and powdered bones of a she-vulture who has died a natural death, he can attract any woman to himself (Vashikarana).

SUTRA 28. Again, a man may win over a woman completely if he coats his phallus with a mixture of honey and powders of Vajrashnuhi, Manahshila Gaudha and Pashana after they have been dried seven different times 'Vashikarana'.

SUTRA 29. If all these ingredients are put in a fire and allowed to smoke, and if the woman is made to see the moon through the screen of this smoke, the woman imagines the moon to be golden.

SUTRA 30. A man captures a maiden for himself when he sprinkles on her head the mixture of these powdered ingredients mixed with a monkey's excreta. (The monkey must be red-faced.)

SUTRA 31. Pieces of Vacha smeared with mango juice and preserved for six months in the crevices of a Sinshapa tree trunk, exude a divine fragrance (liked by Devas), and may be used as scent in winning over women (Vashikarana).

SUTRA 32. The same recipe is used by Gandharvas for the same purpose, but pieces of Khadirasara are used instead.

SUTRA 33. The Nagas vary this recipe by using Priyangu flowers mixed with Tagara and preserve them in mango juice in the trunk of a Naga tree.

SUTRA 34. An ointment made from a camel bone treated with the juice of Bhringaraja and burnt, and then placed in a hollow camel bone after being mixed with Strotoanjana, when applied with a camel bone, they say, is not only auspicious but most potent for arousing a woman's passion (Vashikarana).

SUTRA 35. Collyriums made with bones of Shyena (hawk), Bhasa (vulture), Mayura (peacock), may also be similarly treated for similar results.

Now follow recipes for increasing virility (Vrishya Yogas):

SUTRA 36. The roots of Uchchata, Chavya, and Yashtimadhuka,

powdered and mixed with sugar and milk and then drunk makes a man as virile as a bull.

SUTRA 37. Also drinking the juice obtained by boiling the testicles of a sheep and goat and mixing sugar with that boiled water, results in a man becoming as virile as a bull.

SUTRA 38. The same result is obtained by drinking milk boiled with (a root of) Vidari, seeds of Kshirika, (a root of) Svayamgupta. (Each of these is enough for the purpose.)

SUTRA 39. Similarly, seeds of Priyala and Morata (root of sugar cane) and Vidari (boiled and taken) with milk, bring a man a bull-like virility.

SUTRA 40. The old sages say that a man can enjoy several women without losing his virility if he eats as much as is required of (1) the mixture of Shringataka, Kasheruka and Madhulika, Kshira Kakoli, after it is heated together with sugar, milk and ghee.

SUTRA 41. (2) The mixture of Masha Kamalini, after being washed and softened with warm ghee, and boiled in cow's milk (the cow must have a grown-up calf), then drinking this Payasa with honey and more ghee.

SUTRA 42. (3) The cake of wheat flour with powdered Vidari and Svayamgupta, sugar, honey and ghee.

SUTRA 43. (4) The mixture of rice grains soaked in the fluid of sparrow's eggs and boiled with milk, to which honey and ghee are subsequently added.

SUTRA 44. (5) The mixture of cleaned Sesamum seeds soaked in the fluid of sparrow's eggs, the powder of seeds of Shringataka, Kasheruka, Svayamgupta, wheat flour and Masha, to which sugar is added, and which is then boiled with milk and ghee.

SUTRA 45. The old sages declare that the following tonics bring virility and longevity to a man, besides being very tasty.

(1) The mixture of two Palas (measures) of ghee, honey, sugar and Madhuka, one Karsha of Madhurasa, one Prastha of milk. This mixture actually tastes like nectar.

SUTRA 46. (2) Powdered Pippali and Madhuka ground to a paste and put into the Kashaya (liquid made with jaggery) of Shatavari and Shvadamshtra, and boiled in the milk of a cow or in the ghee of goat's milk till it becomes a thick fluid. This, if taken daily in the required quantity in the spring, is a very effective tonic.

SUTRA 47. (3) The mixture of powders of Shatavari, Shvadamshtra and Shriparni, fruits, with four times the quantity of water added to it, and the whole boiled till the mixture thickens. This should be taken from the beginning of spring, according to the state of one's health.

SUTRA 48. (4) The mixture of two Palas of barley and an equal proportion of powdered Shvadamshtra. This should be taken daily upon rising.

SUTRA 49 (verse). A person who wishes to avail of such recipes in the conduct of his love affairs should study them from the Ayurveda, the (Atharva) Veda and the Tantric Texts, or otherwise from persons who are acquainted with the practice of these Tantras.

SUTRA 50 (verse). Recipes about which the user has the slightest doubt (regarding the exact measures and so forth), or which cause physical harm, or which require the killing of some living animal, or which recommend the use of impure ingredients, must be avoided.

SUTRA 51 (verse). Only those practices found effective after long trial approved of by cultured people and blessed by Brahmins and friends, should be resorted to.

CHAPTER II

ON REGAINING LOST VIRILITY; OTHER MISCELLANEOUS EXPERIMENTS

There are various degrees of loss of virility, and they are treated severally as follows:

SUTRA 1. When a man (suffers from loss of virility and therefore) is unable to satisfy the passion of the woman he may resort to the various means suggested below (after properly considering his own case).

SUTRA 2. The case of slow rise of passion and with weak effect: Before he engages in the final union with the woman, he should at the beginning excite his own passion by manually effecting erection. In this way he will activate his own passion and also be able to satisfy the woman.

SUTRA 3. The case of slow rise of passion, having no ultimate effect: When a man suffers from very weak passion, either from old age, or extreme corpulence or tiredness after a union, he may resort to oral union, which usually regenerates his passion.

SUTRA 4. The case of slow rise of passion, with little or virtually no ultimate effect: In this instance, the man may resort to an artificial phallus, or to similar mechanical devices. Artificial aids to the phallus may be either Aviddha (unperforated) or Viddha (perforated):

SUTRA 5. The Aviddha phalli may be made of gold or silver or copper or iron or ivory, horn, etc.

SUTRA 6. Babhravya maintains, however, that those made of zinc and lead are soft, cool to the touch and permit several rubbings.

SUTRA 7. Vatsyayana is of the opinion that aids to the phallus should be chosen according to the preference shown by the women, and in some cases, may also be wooden.

SUTRA 8. These artificial phallus-aids should be of the size of the phallus, rough on the outer side, and pierced with holes only at the tip. (They should fit the phallus like a ring or glove.)

SUTRA 9. When this is made up of two pieces, it is named Sanghati.

SUTRA 10. When there are three, four or more component parts, it is called Chudaka.

SUTRA 11. If only one strip (of lead) is wound around the phallus, it is called Ekachudaka.

SUTRA 12. When it has large and rough sockets like testicles, and when it fits both the phallus and the testicles when tied around the waist, it is called Kanchuka or Jalaka. (There are various similar kinds, such as Khara Kanchuka and Ardha Kanchuka, Utkirna Jalaka and Math Jalaka.)

SUTRA 13. If any of these aids are not available, a person should improvise one by using the pipe-like portion of the Alabu or the Venu branch, smear it with some oily substance, and tie it with a thread around the waist. Alternatively, he may mount wooden beads on a stem of Alabu, threading them like a necklace, and wind it around the phallus.

These are the various unperforated aids for the phallus.

SUTRAS 14-15. However, some people argue that it is impossible to derive the maximum pleasure from a union without perforating the phallus, and accordingly, among the people of the Southern provinces, it is the practice for young men to perforate their phalli, somewhat as a child's ears are perforated in childhood.

The method for perforating the phallus is now described:

SUTRA 16. After a young man perforates his phallus with a sharp instrument from one end to the other, he should stand in water as long as the blood continues to flow. (Standing in water will ultimately stop the bleeding.)

SUTRA 17. Then at night, the young man should freely cohabit several times, so that the perforation (made during the day), may not contract again or get sealed up.

SUTRAS 18-20. Thereafter, on alternate days, he should wash the hole with (fine) Kashayas, and with Yashtimadhuka, mixed with honey. (This helps to heal the wound.)

SUTRAS 21-22. After that, he should try to widen the perforation with a Karnika of Shishapatra after smearing both with the oil of Bhallataka. (This makes the insertion easier.)

These are the various stages of perforating the phallus.

SUTRA 23. Through this perforation, a man may insert mechanical aids of various shapes and sizes.

SUTRA 24. They may be tubular; or rounded at one end like a wooden mortar; or like a flower having thorns; or like a crow's skeleton; or like the proboscis of an elephant; eight-sided; like a top (or a disc on a pin); or like a Shringataka (triangular) and so forth. These aids may be rough or smooth, and are usually chosen by the lovers according to their own preferences, and according to their needs and to the enduring qualities of the aids themselves.

Now the ways of enlarging the phallus (both in length and thickness) will be related:

SUTRA 25. By rubbing the phallus on all sides with bristles of (Kandalika) insects born on a tree (and caught by a pair of tongs), and massaging it thereafter with oil for ten nights, a man can enlarge his phallus.[1] He should repeat this process until it becomes swollen to the required size, and then he should lie on a cot and cause it to hang down, through a hole in the cot.

SUTRA 26. He should then anoint it with cool concoctions to allay the pain (otherwise the pain and swelling will continue).

SUTRA 27. This enlarging of the phallus can be made to continue throughout a lifetime and the Vitas call it 'Shukashopha'.

SUTRA 28. It can be enlarged for the space of one month if it is anointed with the juice of Ashvagandha, or the root of Shabara, or Jalashuka or the fruit of Brihati, or butter made from buffalo's milk or juice of Hastikarna and Vajravalli.

SUTRA 29. The enlargement can be made to last for six months if the Kashayas or any of the above mentioned plants are boiled in oil, and the resulting fluid is massaged on the phallus.

SUTRA 30. Similar results are obtained if the seeds of pomegranate or Trapusha or a piece of Valuka (Edavaluka) or the fruit of Brihati are slowly boiled in oil, and the resulting fluid used for massaging or giving a hot bath to the phallus. (This will also make the enlargement last for six months.)

SUTRA 31. Other recipes for obtaining similar results may be learnt from experts who have made a thorough study of the Kamashastra.

We now enumerate the miscellaneous experiments and recipes (Chitra Yogas):

SUTRA 32. When a man sprinkles on a woman's head the powdered mixture of Snuhikantaka, Punartiava, the excreta of a monkey and the Langalika root, that woman cannot love any other man.

SUTRA 33. A man's vigorous passion cools down if he unites with a woman whose vagina is smeared with a paste made from the juice of Vyadhighataka leaves and Jambu fruits, to which is added the powder of Somalata, Avalguja, Bhringa and the iron from ants making ant hills.

SUTRA 34. Similarly, a man's passion is diminished if he unites with a woman who has bathed in the curds of buffalo milk mixed with the powders of Gopalika, Bahupadika and Jihvika.

SUTRA 35. If a woman applies the paste made from Nipa, Amrataka and Jambu flowers, or wears a garland of these flowers, she brings misfortune upon herself.

SUTRA 36. Smearing the vagina of a woman belonging to the Cow-elephant type with the juice of the (white) Kokilaksha fruits results in the contraction of the organ within one night.

SUTRA 37. On the other hand, the vagina of the Deer-type of woman can be made to expand within one night if it is treated with the paste made from powdered Padma (white), Utpala (blue), Sarjaka, Sugandha and honey.

SUTRA 38. Hair can be made white if it is treated with the mixture of the milk of Snuhi, Soma and Arka, with the powders of the Amalaka and the Avalguja fruit.

SUTRA 39. Bathing hair in the extract of roots of Madayantika, Kutaja, Anjanika, Girikarnika and Shlakshnaparni, to which water is added, restores original dark colour thereof.

SUTRA 40. If, however, oil is extracted from the Kashaya of all these above-mentioned roots, and applied to hair, its dark colour will be restored in slow stages.

SUTRA 41. Red lips become white if Alaktaka, mixed seven times with the sweat from the testicles of a white horse, is applied to them.

SUTRA 42. Lips can be made to become red if treated with Madayantika and other herbal ingredients.

SUTRA 43. A woman who hears a man playing on a flute dipped in the liquid lotion of Bahupadika, Kushtha, Tagara, Talisa, Devadaru and Vajrakanda, is enslaved by him.

SUTRA 44. Consuming Dhattura fruit (or its diluted juice) causes intoxication.

SUTRA 45. Jaggery which has been preserved for a long time restores steadiness of mind, if consumed.

SUTRA 46. If, after smearing his palm with the excreta of the peacock who has partaken of Haritala and Manahshila, a person touches any object, he makes it invisible.

SUTRA 47. If water is mixed with oil and the ashes of Angara Truna, it looks like milk.

SUTRA 48. Iron vessels become oxidized if (the leaves of) Haritaka and Amrataka and the (fruit of) Shravana Priyanguka (Joytishmati) are powdered together and made into a paste and applied to them.

SUTRA 49. If a lamp is lit with the oil of Shravana Priyanguka, and its wick made of pure muslin and the discarded thin outer skin of a serpent, and if then wooden sticks are placed over it, the sticks will appear long and serpentine.

SUTRA 50. Drinking milk of a white cow who has given birth to a white calf is auspicious and brings longevity.

SUTRA 51. (Similarly) the blessings of learned Brahmins bring health, wealth and happiness.

Finally, some hints about studying and practising the Kama Sutra in life.

SUTRA 52. Although the Kama Sutra has been composed as a brief work, a great deal of study has gone into it – especially earlier works have been studied, selected from and condensed into the present work.

SUTRA 53. A person who has really studied this science of love well will inevitably pay due regard to Dharma, Artha and Kama, and to the practices which he observes among the common people. He is not likely to act simply from his own desires and passions.

SUTRA 54. The ways and means which have been enumerated earlier for the purpose of increasing a man's passion are to be practised only by those who are absolutely in need of them. They are emphatically forbidden to those who do not need to use them.

SUTRA 55. It is not to be understood that simply because this work mentions certain artifices and expedients, that they have to be used by all and sundry. While the science is certainly meant to be studied by everybody, the practice of these expedients should be restricted to particular persons who need them.

SUTRA 56. Vatsyayana composed this Kama Sutra after exhaustively studying the Sutras, and expending a great deal of his own thinking on the subject.

SUTRA 57. Let it be known that Vatsyayana composed it after observing strict celibacy. It has therefore not been marred by any passionate motive. Deep thinking has gone into it and its one purpose is that of merely guiding other men.

SUTRA 58. A person who has mastered the essence of this science of love will eventually be able to control all his senses, and guide his own life with true regard to Dharma, Artha and Kama.

SUTRA 59. If he commands deep and expert knowledge of this science, does not allow excessive passion to cloud his actions as a lover, and always keeps the other two attainments of Dharma and Artha in mind, he will be acclaimed through the world as an example to be followed by one and all.

NOTES

[1] Similar practice is noticed by P. Mantegazza, ibid., p. 73.

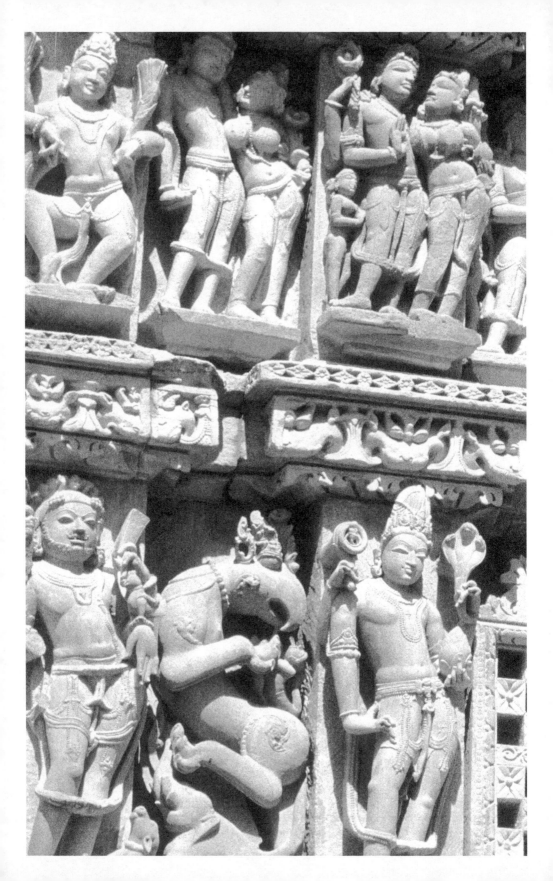

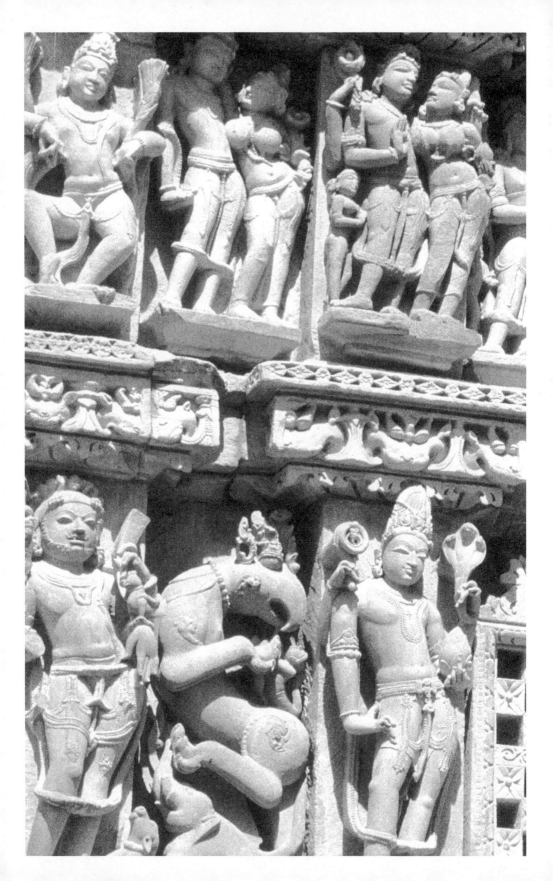

APPENDICES
GLOSSARY AND
BIBLIOGRAPHY

APPENDIX I

PANCHALIKI CHATUHSHASHTI

64 Erotic Acts According to Babhravya Panchalika

I. *Upaguhana*
(The Embrace)
1. Sprishtaka
2. Viddhaka
3. Udghrishtaka
4. Piditaka
5. Lataveshtitaka
6. Vrikshadhirudha
7. Tilatandulaka
8. Kshiraniraka

II. *Chumbana*
(The Kiss)
1. Nimitaka
2. Sphuritaka
3. Ghattitaka
4. Sama
5. Tiryag
6. Udbhranta
7. Avapiditaka
8. Akrishta

III. *Nakhachchhedya*
(The Nail-marks)
1. Achchhuritaka
2. Arddhachandra
3. Mandala
4. Rekha
5. Vyaghranakha
6. Mayurapadaka
7. Shashaplutaka
8. Utpalapatra

IV. *Dashanachchhedya*
(The Teeth-marks)
1. Gudhaka
2. Uchchhunaka
3. Bindu
4. Bindumala
5. Pravalamani
6. Manimala
7. Khadnabhraka
8. Varahacharvitaka

V. *Samveshana*
(The Coital Posture)
1. Jrimbhitaka
2. Utpiditaka
3. Venudarita
4. Shulachita
5. Karkata
6. Piditaka
7. Padmasana
8. Paravrittaka

VI. *Sitkrita*
(The Sounds of Joy)
1. Himkara
2. Stanita
3. Kujita
4. Rudita
5. Sutkrita
6. Dutkrita
7. Phutkrita
8. Ambartha Shabdas

VII. *Purushayita*
(Abhyantara)
1. Nivivishleshana
2. Kapola chumbana
3. Parisparshana
4. Ghattana
5. Avalambana
   Purushayita
   (Bahya)
6. Sandamsha
7. Bhramaraka
8. Premkholita.

VIII. *Auparishtaka*
(Cunnilingus, Fellatio, etc.)
1. Nimita
2. Parshvato-dashta
3. Bahih-Samdamsha
4. Antah-Samdamsha
5. Chumbitaka
6. Parimrishtaka
7. Amrachushitaka
8. Samgara

APPENDIX II

SAMPRAYOGA–AMGA (TUMESCENCE AND DETUMESCENCE)–20

SAMPRAYOGA—AMGA (Tumescence and Detumescence)—20

	Alingana	Chumbana	Nakhach-chhedya / Nakhakshata	Dashanach-chhedya	Samveshana	Sitkrita	Purushayita	Auparishtika K.S. 2-2-5	According to
Babhraviyah	Alingana	Chumbana	Nakhach-chhedya Nakhakshata	Dashanach-chhedya	Samveshana	Sitkrita	Purushayita	Auparishtika K.S. 2-2-5	—
Bharata	Ashlesha	"	"	—	—	—	—	Jihva-pra-vesha	Kumbha's Comm. on G.G. 2-6-6
Bharata	"	"	"	—	—	—	—	—	Shankara Mishra and Kumbha's Comm. on G.G. 5-11-5
Vatsyayana-Shastra									Shankara Mishra. Do. 2-6-6
Vatsyayana	Alingana	(including Jihva-Yud-dha)	Nakhach-chhedya	Dashanach-chhedya	Samveshana	Sitkrita (viruta)	Purushayita	Auparishtika K.S. 2-2-6, etc.	
?	"	Chumbana	Nakha-kshata	Dantakarma	"	Sitkrita	Narayita	Auparishta	Yashodhara on K.S. 2-2-4
Vatsyayana	Ashlesha	"	"	Dantakshata	Surata	—	—	—	Mallinatha on Kirata 9-47; but not found in K.S. 2-2
Damodara	Pariram-bhana	Jihva-Yud-dha	Nakavile-khana	Damsha	"	Sitkrita	Viparita	—	
Kokkoka	Alingana	Chumbana	Nakhach-chheda	Dashana-karma	"	Viruta	Purushayita	—	
Padmashri	"	Sashabda Nihshabda Chumbana	Nakhapada	Dashana-pada	Karana	Sashabda Chumbana	—	—	
Jyotirisha	"	Chumbana	Nakhaghata	Dashana-ghata	Bandha	Sitkrita	Purushayita	Auparishtaka	
Devaraya	"	"	Nakha-kshata	Danta-kshata	Surata	"	"	"	
Kalyanamalla	"	"	Nakhadana	Dashana-vidhana	Bandha	"	Viparita	Auparishtaka	

APPENDIX II—Continued

	Tadana	Mardana	Hastayojana	Rasana-grahana / Nabhi(dif?) Kshobha	Sitkrita (Grahana)	Purushayita (Anguli-rata / Purusho-pasripta, including Karikara)	Karikara-krida	Chitra-yantra / Chitrarata	Keshagra-hana Nipidana (According to)
Babhraviya	Tadana	Sammar-dana	—	—	—	—	—	—	—
Bharata	—	—	—	—	—	—	—	—	—
Bharata	Praharana Prahanana	Mardana	Hastayo-jana	—	—	—	—	—	—
Vatsyayana-Shastra									
Vatsyayana	—	—	—	—	—	—	—	—	—
Damodara	Tadana	Mardana (Kucha)	Hastayo-jana	Rasana-grahana	—	Anguli-rata	—	—	Keshagra-hana Nipidana
Kokkoka	"	Mardana (Kucha) Mardana	Hastayo-jana	Jihvarana Nabhi(dif?) Kshobha	Grahana	Karikara-krida pravesha	Kshepana Purusho-pasripta (including Karikara)	Karikara-krida Chitra-yantra Chitrarata	Keshakar-shana
Padmashri	"	Chushana Mardana	Jihvapra-vesha	"	"	"	Chitra-sambhoga	Chitra-karma	"
Jyotirisha	Santadita	Mardana (Kucha)	—	—	—	—	—	—	—
Devaraya	Praharana	Mardana	—	"	Grahana	Karikara-krida	Chitrarata	Chitra-karma	Keshagri-hana
Kalyanamalla	Kara-tadana	Mardana (Kucha)	—	Rasaurana Nadiksho-bha	—	—	—	—	—

APPENDIX III

KAMASTHANA (Erogenous Zones)—19

	Angustha	Pada	Gulpha	Janu	Jaghana	Nabbi	Vakshah	Stana	Kaksha	Kantha	Kapola	Dantavasana
R.R. 2-2	Angustha	—	—		Guhya	,,	Vaksha-sthala	Vaksho-ruh	Kaksha	Kantha	Kapola	Dantavasana
R.R. 2-5/6	—	—	—	Uru	Yoni	,,		Kucha	Kukshi	Kantha	Kapola	Adhara
N.S. 17-4/6	Angustha-mula / Angustha	Charana		{Jungha / Uru / Janu / Jangha / Janu}	Nilaya / Nitamba	,,	Vakshah	—	Kaksha	,,	,,	,,
P.S. 2-11					Smara-mandira							
R.R.P. 1-28/35	,,		Gulpha		Varanga	,,	,,	Stana	Bahumula	,,	,,	Danta-vasana / Adhara
A.R. 2-1	Angustha-ka	Pada	,,		,,		Vaksha-sthala	Kucha	Kaksha	Galaka	,,	,,
R.K.K. 5-13/18	,,	Charana	,,		Bhaga	,,	Vakshah	Vakshasi-ja	Bahu-kupara	Kantha	,,	Dantach-chhadana

APPENDIX III—Continued

	Netra	Alika	Murddha	Kara	Katiprishtha	Shroni			
R.R. 2-1	Netra	Alika	Murddha	Kara	Katiprishtha	Shroni	—	—	According to Nandishvara
R.R. 2-5/6	Netra / Karna	Lalata	,,	,,	Jathara	—	—	—	According to Gonisuta
N.S. 17-4/6			Shikhashraya				—		
P.S. 2-11	Nayana / Akshi	Lalata	Mauli				—		
R.R.P. 1-20/35		Phala (Bhala?)	Shirah				—		According to Gonisuta.
A.R. 2-1	Lochana		Simanta				—		
R.K.K. 5-13/18			Kesha / Murddha				—		

APPENDIX IV

NAYAKA—LINGA—AYAMA (Classification According to Size)—5

	Shasha	Barkara	Vrisha	Vrishabha	Ashva	Rasabha	
K.S. 2-1-1	Shasha (6)		Vrisha (9)		Ashva (12)		
R.R. 3-1	,, (6)		,, (9)		,, (12)		
N.S. 14	,, (6)		,, (9)		Turaga (12)		
P.S. 2-1	,, (6)		,, (9)		Ashva (12)		
R.R.P. 2-1/32	Mriga (6)	Barkara (8)		Vrishabha (9)	Ashva (12)		
A.R. 3-1			Vrisha (10)		Turaga (12)		
Anye			Vrisha (10)			Rasabha (14)	According to Madhava in his Ayurvedaprakasha
R.R.K. 6-4/6	Shasha (6)		Vrisha (9)	Ashva (12)		Bhadra (12)	
S.D.	Panchala (6)			Dattn (10)	Bhadra (12)		
R.S.D.	Shasha (6)		Vrisha (9)	Vrishabha (10)	Haya (12)		

346

APPENDIX V

NAYIKA—YONI—PARINAHA (Classification According to Depth)—5

	(6)	(8)/(9)	(9)/(10)	(12)	(12)	(14)	According to Madhava in his Ayurvedaprakasha
K.S. 2-1-2	Mrigi (6)	Vadava	—	Hastini	—	—	
R.R. 3-1	Harini (6)	—	—	„ (12)	—	—	
N.S. 14-1	„ (6)	„ (9)	—	Ibhika (12)	—	—	
P.S. 2-1	Mrigi (6)	Ashva (9)	—	Karini (12)	—	—	
R.R.P. 2-1/32	„ (6)	Vadava (9)	—	Hastini (12)	—	—	
A.R. 3-1	„ (6)	Ashva (9)	—	Hastini (12)	—	—	
Anye	Harini (6)	—	Vadava (10)	Dviradamgana (12)	Karini (12)	Karabbi (14)	According to Madhava in his Ayurvedaprakasha
S.D.	Padmini (6)	Chhagi (8)	Chitrini (10)	—	Hastini (12)	—	
R.S.D.	„ (6)	Sankhini (8)	Shankhini (10)	—	Hastini (12)	—	
R.K.K. 6-4/6	Mrigi (6)	Chitrini (8)	Hayi (9)	—	Karini (12)	—	

APPENDIX VI

UPAGUHANA (The Embrace)—14

	Sprish-taka	Viddha-ka	Udghri-shtaka	Pidita-ka	Latavesh-titaka	Vriksha-dhiru-dhaka	Tilatandu-laka	Kshirani-raka	Ekamgo-pagu-hana	Urupa-guhana	Jaghano-paguhana	Stana-lingana	Lalatika Samva-hana
K.S. 2-2-1/25	Sprishtaka	Viddhaka	Udghrishtaka	Piditaka	Lataveshtitaka	Vrikshadhirudhaka	Tilatandulaka	Kshiraniraka	Ekamgopaguhana	Urupaguhana paguhana	Jaghanopaguhana	Stanalingana	Lalatika Samvahana
R.R. 6-1/12	„	„	—	„	Lataveshtita	Vrikshadhirudha	Tilatandula	Kshiranira	—	Urupagudha	Jaghanopashlesha	„	—
N.S. 24-1/9	„	—	—	Pidita	Lataveshtitaka	Vrikshadhirudha	Tilatandula	Dugdhajala	—	—	Jaghanopaguha	Kuchopagudha Jaghana	„
P.S. 4-31/40	—	Viddhaka	—	—	Lataveshtita	Vriksharudha	—	Kshiranira	—	—	Jaghana	„	„
R.R.P. 3-4/27	Sprishtaka	„	Udghrishtaka	Pidita	Lataveshtanaka	Vrikshadhirudha	„	„	—	—	Janghopaguhaka Jaghana	Stanaguhaka lingana	„
A.R. 9-1/10	„	„	„	„	Vallariveshtita	„	„	„	—	—	Jaghana	„	„
K.M.													

Damodara has mentioned in Kattanimata 581, embraces of Chakra, Hamsa, Nakula, and Paravata. In Shabda Kalpadruma, seven others are mentioned, such as, Amoda, Mudita, Prema, Ananda, Ruchi, Madana, and Vinoda.

APPENDIX VII

CHUMBANA (The Kiss)—23

	Nimitaka	Sphuritaka	Ghattitaka	Sama	Tiryag	Udbhranta	Avapidi-taka	Avapidi-taka	Uttara	Samputaka	Antarmu-kha
K.S. 2-3-1/33	Nimitaka	Sphuritaka	Ghattitaka	Sama	Tiryag	Udbhranta	Avapidi-taka	Avapidi-taka	Uttara	Samputaka	Antarmu-kha
R.R. 7-1/8	,,	Sphurita	Ghattita	—	,,	Bhranta	Pidita	Vighatita	,,	Samputa	Anuvadana
N.S. 25-1/5	,,	,,	—	Natagan-da	Vaikrita-ka	Bhramita	Nipidita	—	—	Samhatau-shtha	—
P.S. 4-41/48	Nimita		Ghrishta	—	—	—	Pidita	—	—	Samputa	Samau-shtha
R.R.P. 3-28/48	,,	,,	Ghattita	Sama	Tiryag	Bhranta	Avapidita	Dvijagra-hana	—	,,	Jihvayud-dha
A.R. 9-11/21	Milita (Nimita?)	,,	,,	—	,,	—	Pidita	—	Uttara	,,	Samau-shtha

APPENDIX VII—*Continued*

	Sama	Pidita	Anchita	Mridu	Ragadi-pana	Chalitaka	Pratibodhika	Chhaya Samkranta	Hastam-guli	Padamguli	Uru Chumbana
K.S. 2-3-1/33	Sama	Pidita	Anchita	Mridu	Ragadi-pana	Chalitaka	Pratibodhika	Chhaya Samkranta	Hastam-guli	Padamguli	Uru Chumbana
R.R. 7-1/8	,,	Avapidita	Abhyarthita?	,,	—	—	Pratibodha	Chhayika Samkranta	—	—	—
N.S. 25-1/5	—	—	—	—	—	—	—	—	—	—	—
P.S. 4-41/48	—	—	—	—	—	—	—	—	—	—	—
R.R.P. 3-28/48	—	—	—	—	—	—	Bodhita	Chhaya Samkranta	—	—	—
A.R. 9-11/21	—	—	—	—	—	—	Pratibodha	—	—	—	—

According to Gaunisuta (quoted by Tripathi in his Commentary on K.M. 581) there are Padma Chumbana, Venudarita Chumbana, etc. Tripathi in his Commentary on N.S. (Appendix p. 119) has quoted ten Chumbanas done on Bhala, Netra, Kapola, Rasana, Oshtha, Chibuka Kandhara, Kucha, Nabhi and Guhya.

APPENDIX VIII

NAKHACHCHHEDYA (The Nail Marks)—9

	Achchhuritaka	Ardha-Chandraka	Mandala	Rekha	Vyaghra-nakhaka	Mayurapadaka	Shashapluta	Utpalapatra	Smaraniyaka	
K.S. 2 4-1/22										Vatsyayan (2-4-4) mentions eight but describes the ninth also
R.R. 8-1/6	Uchchhurita	„	„	„	—	„	„	Utpaladala	Smaranartha	
N.S. 22-1/5		„	„	„	Vyaghrapada	„	„	Utpalapatra	—	
P.S. 4-49/58	Chchhurita	Arddhendu	„	„	„	„	„	Pamkaja-patra	Darduraka	
R.R.P. 3-49/62	Chchhuritaka	Ardhachandra	„	„	Vyaghrapada	„	„	Utpalapatra	Smaraka	
A.R. 9-22/29	Chchhurita	„	„	„	—	„	„	„	Smaranartha	

APPENDIX IX

DANTACHHEDYA (The Teeth Marks)—8

	Gudhaka	Uchchhunaka	Bindu	Bindumala	Pravalamani	Manimala	Khandabhraka	
K.S. 2-5-1/17	Gudhaka	Uchchhunaka	Bindu	Bindumala	Pravalamani	Manimala	Khandabhraka	Varahacharvita
R.R. 9-1/4	„	„	„	„	„	„	„	Kolacharvita
N.S. 23-1/4	„	„	„	—	„	„	Gandaka	Varahacharvita
P.S. 4-59/63	—	—	—	—	Vidruma	—	Khandabhraka	Kolacharva
R.R.P. 3-63/75	Gudhaka	Uchchhunaka	Bindu	Bindumala	Pravalamani	Manimala	„	Kroda (Kola?)-charvita
A.R. 9-30/36	„	„	„	„	„	—	„	Kolacharva

APPENDIX X

NADIKSHOBHANA

R. R. 10-6/9	N. S. 18-1/8	P. S. 5-1/4	R. R. P. 4-35/39	A. R. 4-32/35
Kamatapatra	Madanatapatra	Madanatapatra	Kamatapatra	Manmathachhatra
Madanagamana-dola	Shadmadanadika	Samirana	Madanagaradola	Kamankushasama
Purnachandra	..	Chandramasi	Purnachandra	Purnachandra
..	..	Gauri	..	..
Dvyamgulaksho-bhana	Linga and Anguli	(?) Kshobhana	Dvyamgulaksho-bhana	Lingakshobhana

APPENDIX XI

GAJAHASTA-AMGULIPRAVESHA (TITILLATION)

K.S. 2-8-10	R. R. 10-8	N. S. 36-1/2	R. R. P. 4
Gaja	Karikara	Karana	Karihasta
..	Phanibhoga	Kanaka	Phanindrabhoga
..	Arddhendu	Vikana	Arddha-chandarka
..	Kamankusha	Pataka	Smarankusha
..	..	Trisula	..
..	..	Shanibhoga (Phani ?)	

APPENDIX XII

PRAHANANA—11

	Apahastaka	Prasritaka	Mushti	Samata-laka	Kila	Kartari	Bhadra-Kartari	Yamala-Kartari	Shabda-Kartari	Viddha	Samdashika
K.S. 2-7-3	Apahastaka	Prasritaka	Mushti	Samata-laka	Kila	—	Bhadra-Kartari	Yamala-Kartari	Shabda-Kartari	Viddha	Samdashika
R.S. 10-52/60	,,	,,	,,	,,	—	Kartari	—	—	Shabda-Kartari	—	—
N.S. 33-1/2	—	—	,,	,,	—	Kartari	—	—	—	Viddhaka	—
R.R.P. 6-55/56 7-1/18	Apahastaka	Prasritaka	,,	,,	—	Kartari	Bhadra-Kartari	Yamala-Kartari	,,	Viddha	Samdamshika
A.R. 10-39/41	,,	,,	,,	,,	—	—	—	—	—	—	—

APPENDIX XIII

SITKARA (Done by Females)—10

	Himkara	Stanita	Kujita	Rudia	Sutkrita	Dutkrita	Phutkrita	Shvasita	Shabdah	Kakaruta
K.S. 2-7-4/20	Himkara	Stanita	Kujita	Rudia	Sutkrita	Dutkrita	Phutkrita	Shvasita	Shabdah	Kakaruta
R.R. 10-52/63	Himkrita	,,	,,	Rodana	Sitkrita	Utkrita	,,	,,	,,	—
N.S. 20-1/4	Himkrita	,,	,,	—	,,	Dutkrita	Phutkara	,,	—	—
P.S. 5-29/30	—	,,	,,	—	,,	—	—	—	—	—
R.R.P. 7-2/56	Himkrita	,,	Kujita	Rudita	,,	Dutkrita	Phutkrita	Shvasita	Shabdah	—
A.R. 10-45/50	,,	,,	—	—	,,	Utkrita	,,	—	—	Kakaruta

Appendix XIV
GRAHANA

N.S.
35-1/2
1. Baddhamushti
2. Veshtitaka
3. Kritagranthika
4. Samakrishti

Appendix XVIII
CHUSHANA

N.S.
27-1/2
1. Oshthavimrishtha
2. Vichumbitaka
3. Ardrachumbita
4. Samputaka

Appendix XV
KESHAKARSHANA

P. S. 4-64/68		A. R. 9-37/41	
1. Sama-hasta		1. Sama-hasta	
2. Taranga-ramga		2. Taranga-ramga	
3. Kamava-tamsa		3. Kamava-tamsa	
4. Bhujam-gavalli		4. Bhujam-gavalli	

Appendix XIX
RASAPANA

S. D.
1. Payodhara
2. Oshtha
3. Asya
4. Jihva
5. Kuchagra

These are quoted by Tripathi in his Commentary on N. S. 36-2

Appendix XVI
MARDANA

N. S.
34-1/2
1. Adipita
2. Sprishtaka
3. Kampitaka
4. Samakrama

Appendix XVII
JIHVAPRAVESHA

N. S.
26-1

1. Suchi
2. Pratata
3. Kari (Vakali ?)

Appendix XX
SANTADITA (Done by the Female)

P. S. 5-26/28		A. R. 10-42/44	
1. Santadita		1. Santadita	
2. Pataka		2. Pataka	
3. Kundala		3. Kuntala (Kundala?)	
4. Bindumala		4. Bindumala	

APPENDIX XXI

UTTANA BANDHA (Coital Postures)—52

K.S. 2-6-7/31	—	Arddha-piditaka	—	Indrani	Uipiditaka	Utphullaka	Bhugnaka	—	—
R.R. 10-14/28	Arddha-pad-masana	Arddha-ni-pidita	—	Indranika	—	,,	Bhugna	Urddhva-gatoruyuga	Urahsphu-tana
N.S. 28-1/13	,,	Arddhapin-dita	Ayata	Indrani	—	—	Udbhugna	—	—
P.S. 5-5/13	—	—	Avadarita	—	—	—	—	—	—
R.R.P. 4-51/55; 5-1/17	Arddha-pad-masana	Arddham-ganipidita	—	Indrani	—	Utphullaka	Udbhugnaka	—	—
A.R. 10-4/14	Kamal-arddha	—	Avidarita	Aindra	—	Utphullaka	—	Urddhvaga	Sphutana
R.K.K. 8-11/43		Amgarddha-nipidita	—	—	—	—	—	—	Urahsphota-naka

APPENDIX XXI—Continued

K.S. 2-6-7/31	Padmasana	Karkataka	*Krodha	—	—	—	Jrumbhi-taka	Vijrimbhi-taka	—
R.R. 10-14/28	,,	Ma (Ka?)-arkata	—	Kaurma	Gramya	—	Jrimbhaka	Jrimbhita	—
N.S. 28-1/13	Ekpada	,,	—	,,	,,	Chatukelika	Jrimbhita	—	Traivikrama
P.S. 5-5/13									
R.R.P. 4-51/55; 5-1/17	Padmasana	Kauliraka	—	Kaurma	Gramya	—	Jrimbhaka	Jrimbhhita	Jrimbhhitaka
A.R. 10-4/14								Jrimbhhita	—
R.K.K. 8-11/43	Kamalasana	Karkata	—	Kaurma	—	—	—	Jrimbhhitaka	Traivikrama

*Attributed to Vatsyayana, but not found in K.S.

APPENDIX XXI—Continued

K.S. 2-6-7/31	—	—	—	Piditaka	Piditaka	—	—	—	—
R.R. 10-14/28	Phanipasha	Nagaraka	Parivartita	Pidia	Pidita	Pindita	—	—	Sarita
N.S. 28-1/13	—	Nagaraka	—	—	—	—	—	—	Prasarita
P.S. 5-5/13	—	Nagara	—	—	—	—	—	—	—
R.R.P. 4-5 1/55, 5-1/17	Phanabhrit-pasha	Nagarika	—	—	—	—	—	—	Prasarita
A.R. 10-4/14	—	Nagara	—	—	—	—	—	—	—
R.K.K. 8-11/42	Phanipasha	Nagaraka	Vartitaka	Piditaka	Piditaka	—	Kamajaya	Praveshtita	Prasarita

Appendix XXI—*Continued*

K.S. 2-6-7/13	—	—	—	—	—	—	Vadavaka	Venudarita
R.R. 10-14/28	Premkha	—	—	—	—	—	"	Venuvida-rana
N.S. 28-1/13	Premkhana	—	Manduka	Markata	—	—	—	—
P.S. 5-5/13	—	Pritikara	—	—	—	Vyomapada	Vadava	—
R.R.P. 4-5 1/55; 5-1/17	Premkha	—	—	—	—	—	—	Venudari-taka
A.R. 10-4/14	—	—	—	—	—	Vyomapada	—	Venuvida-rita
R.K.K. 8-11/43	Premkha-naka	Pritikara	Mahashula-chita	—	Minake-tana	Ratantaka	"	Vadavaka	"

Appendix XXI—*Continued*

K.S. 2-6-7/13	Veshtita-ka	Shulachita	—	Samputa	Samyama-na	—	—	—
R.R. 10-14/28	Veshtita	"	Swastika	" (two)	Samyama-na	—	—	Hanupada
N.S. 28-1/13	—	—	—	—	—	Suchi	—	—
P.S. 5-5/13	Veshtita	Shulamka	—	Samputa	Samyama	Samapada	Suchi	—
R.R.P. 4-5 1/55; 5-1/17								
A.R. 10-4/14	"	—	Smara-chakra	—	—	Samapada	—	Saumya
R.K.K. 8-11/43	Veshtitaka	Shulachita	—	Samputa	Samyama-na Samvesh-titaka	Sundara	—	—

APPENDIX XXII

PARSHVA BANDHA—12

K.S.	—	—	—	—	—	—	—	—	—	—	—	—
R.R. 10-29/30	—	—	Paravrit-taka	Piditaka	—	—	—	—	—	—	—	—
N.S. 29-1/4	—	—	Parivarta-naka	Pidita	Samudga	—	—	—	—	—	—	—
P.S. 5-14/16	Upavitika	Naga	Paravrit-taka	Piditaka	—	Mudgaka	Yugma-pada	—	Vadavaka	Veshtaka	—	—
R.R.P. 5-19/23	—	—	—	—	Samud-gaka	—	—	—	—	—	—	—
A.R. 10-15/17	Karkata	—	Parivarti-taka	Pidita	—	—	—	—	—	—	—	—
R.K.K. 10-15/17	—	—	—	Bhavuka	Samudga	—	—	Ratavalla-bha	—	—	—	Vinika

APPENDIX XXIII

ASITAKA BANDHA—13

K.S.	—	—	—	—	—	—	—
R.R. 10-31/32	—	—	Kirti	—	—	Vimardi-taka	Marka-taka
N.S. 30-1/2	Asina	—	—	Padmasa-na	—	—	—
P.S. 5-17/18	Asina	—	Kirti	Padmasa-na	Parivar-tita	Phanipa-sha	Bandhu-rita
R.R.P. 5-21/23	—	—	—	—	—	Vimar-dita	Markata
A.R. 10-18/24	Upapada	—	Kaur-maka	Padma-sana	Parivar-tita	Vinardita	"
R.K.K. 8-62/70	Amgar-ddhanipi-dita	Richhha-priyaka	—	—	Bhadraka	Marditaka	—

355

APPENDIX XXIV

UTTHITA BANDHA—17

K. S.	R. R.	N. S.	P. S.	R. R. P.	A. R.	R. K. K.
2-6/36	10-33/36	32-1/4	5-21/22	5-23/29	10-25/27	8-71/81
..	..	..	..	..	..	Arddhalasa
..	..	..	..	..	..	Arddhanata
..	Dvitala	Arpita	..	Tala	..	Dvitala
Avalambitaka	Avalambita	Avalambita	..	Lambita	..	Avalambita
..	..	..	..	Ashritaka	..	..
..	..	..	..	..	..	Utthita
..	..	..	..	..	Kirti	..
..	..	..	..	..	..	Kunchita
..	Janukurpara	Kurparajanu	..	Janukurpara	Kurpara	Dhrita
..	..	..	Tripada	..	..	..
..	..	..	..	Traivikrama	..	..
..	..	Dola	..	..	..	..
..	..	..	..	..	..	Natavallabha
..	..	Vyayata	..	..	..	..
..	..	..	Vyayataka	..	..	..
..	..	..	Sammukta	..	..	..
..	Harivikrama	Harivikrama	..	..	Harivikrama	Harivikrama

APPENDIX XXV

ANATA-PASHU-VYANATA BANDHA—21

K. S.	R. R.	N. S.	P. S.	R. R. P.	A. R.	R. K. K.
2-6	10-37/40	21-1/2	5-30/32	5-30/32	10-28/30	8-82/89
..	..	..	..	..	..	Anatalingita
..	..	..	..	..	..	Uruka
Aineya	Aina	..	Harina	Aina	Aina	Aina
Gajopamardita	Aibha	..	..	Aibha	Aibha	Aibha
Gardabhakranta	Gardabhika	..	..	Gardabha	Gardabha	Gardabhaka
Chhagala	..	..	Chhaga	Chhagala	..	..
Turagadhi-rudhaka	..	..	Turangama	Ashva	..	..
Dhainuka	Dhainuka	..	..	Dhainuka	Dhainuka	Dhainuka
..	Vyanata	Pashukarana	..	..	..	Vyanata
Marjaralalitaka	..	..	..	..	..	Marjara
Varahadhrish-taka	..	..	..	..	..	..
Vyaghravaskan-dana	..	Vyaghra-skandana	..	..	..	..
Shauna	Shauna	..	..	..	..	Shauna
..	Sairibha	..	..	Sairabha	..	Sairibha
..	..	..	..	..	Suakara	..
Sanghataka	Sanghataka	..	..	Sanghataka	..	..
..	Sammadopada	..	..	..	..	..
Gauyuthika	..	..	..	Goyutha	..	..
..	..	..	..	Goyutha (1 female & many men)	..	..
Varikriditaka	..	..	..	Varikelita	..	
Adhorata	..					

APPENDIX XXVI

VIPARITA—PURUSHAYITA BANDHA—12

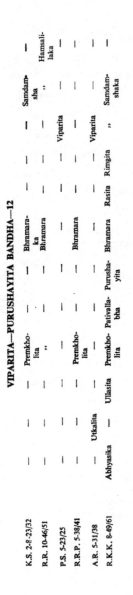

K.S. 2-8-23/32	—	—	—	Premkho-lita	—	—	Bhramara-ka Bhramara	—	—	—	Samdam-sha	—
R.R. 10-46/51	—	—	—	"	—	—	Bhramara	—	—	—	"	Hamsali-laka
P.S. 5-23/25	—	—	—	—	—	—	—	—	—	Viparita	—	—
R.R.P. 5-38/41	—	—	—	Premkho-lita	—	—	Bhramara	—	—	—	—	—
A.R. 5-31/38	—	Utkalita	—	—	—	—	—	—	—	Viparita	—	—
R.K.K. 8-49/61	Abhyasika	—	Ullasita	Premkho-lita	Pativalla-bha	Purusha-yita	Bhramara	Rasita	Rimgita	"	Samdam-shaka	—

APPENDIX XXVII

PLANTS, ROOTS, FLOWERS, SEEDS, LEAVES MENTIONED IN
THE KAMA SUTRA

Sanskrit, *Latin*

Agnimantha, *Clerodendrum phlomidis*
Ahiphena, *Papaver somniferum*
Ajamoda, *Apium graveolens*
Aksha, *Juglans Regia*
Alabu (Tumbi), *Lagenaria siceraria*
Aluka, *Colocasia esculanta or Alocasia Indica*
Amalaka, *Emblica officinalis*
Apamarga, *Achyranthes aspera*
Ardraka, *Zinziber officinalis*
Arjuna, *Terminalia Arjuna*
Aragvadha, *Cassia fistula*
Ashoka, *Saraca Indica*
Ashvagandha, *Withania somnifera*
Atasi, *Linum usitatissimum*
Avalguja, *Vernonia anthelmintica* (cinerea)

Badara, *Ziziphus jujuba*
Bahupadika (Rundika), *Mentha longifolia*
Bhallataka, *Semecarpus anacardium*
Bhrimgaraja, *Eclipta alba*
Brihati, *Terminalia belarica*

Chavya, *Piper Chavya*

Dadiphala, *Cucurbita maxima*
Dadima, *Punica granatum*
Devadaru, *Cedrus Deodara*
Dhanyaka, *Coriandrum sativum*
Dhattura, *Datura innoxia*

Ervaruka (karkatika), *Cucumis melo*

Girikarnika, *Cliporia ternatea*
Godhuma, *Triticum aestivum*
Gokshuraka, *Pedalium murex*
Haritaki, *Terminalia chebula*
Haritala, *Cynodon dactylon*
Hastikarna (Brihat Patra), *Alocasia macrorrhiza*

Ikshu, *Saccharum officinarum*

Japa (Odra Pushpa) *Hibiscus rosasinensis*
Jati, *Grandiflorum Bailey*
Jiraka, *Cuminum cyminum*

Kadali, *Musa paradisiaca*
Kadamba, *Anthocephalus Indicus*
Kakajamgha, *Peristophie bicalenlata*
Kapittha, *Feronia limonia*
Karkatika, *Cucumis sativas*
Karpasa, *Gossypium arboreum*
Kasheruka, *Scripus Kysoor*
Ketaki, *Pandanus tectorius*
Khadira, *Acacia catechu*
Kokliksha, *Asteracentha longifolia*
Kshiraka, *Bambusa arundinaceae*
Kurantaka, *Barleria prionitis*
Kushmanda, *Benincasa hespida*
Kustha, *Saussurea lappa*
Kutaja, *Sterculia urens*

Lamgalika, *Gloriosa superba*
Lashuna, *Allium sativum*

Madayantika, *Lawsonia inermis*
Madhuka, *Madhuca Indica*
Mallika, *Jasminium sambae*
Maricha, *Caspicum annum*
Maruvaka, *Sansevieria roxburghiana*
Masha, *Phaseolus radiatus*
Matulumga, *Citrus medica*
Mulaka, *Raphnus sativus*

Nagavalli, *Piper Betle*
Nandyavarta, *Anthocephalus Indicus* (Kadamba)
Nipa, *Barringtonia racemosa*

Palandu, *Allium capa*
Pashanabheda, *Coleus aromaticus*
Palasha, *Butea monosperma*
Patalika (kedara), *Cocculus hirsutus*
Pippali, *Piper longum*
Priyala, *Buchanania Iatifolia*
Priyamgu, *Panicum Italicum*

Punarnava, *Boerhaavia diffusa*

Sahadevi, *Vernonia cinerea*
Sariva, *Ichnocarpus frutesceus*
Sarshapa, *Brassica campestris*
Shabarakanda, *Symplocos racemosa*
Shana, *Crotalaria juncea*
Shatapushpa, *Anethum sowa*
Shatavari, *Asperagus rasemosus*
Shimshapa, *Dalbergia sissoo*
Shlakshaparni, *Costus speciosus*
Shravana priyamgu, *Cardiospermum halicaecabum*
Shringataka, *Trapa bispinosa*
Shriparni, *Gmelina arborea*
Shukanasa *(Sarvatobhadra)*, ...
Shvadamshtra, (Gokshuraka), *Pedalium murex*
Snuhi, *Euphorbia hirta*
Somalata, *Ruta greveolens*
Surana (Kanda), *Amorphophalus campanulatus*
Svayamgupta, *Mucuna prurita*

Tagara (Pinditagara), *Eryatamia coronaria*
Tala, *Borassus flabellifer*
Talisa, *Abbis Webbiana*
Tilaparnika (Kashmiri), ...
Tamala, *Cinnamomum tamala*
Tambula, *Piper betle*
Tandula, *Amaranthus polygamus*
Tila, *Sesamum Indicum*
Tilaparnika, *Gynandropsis gynandra*

Ushiraka, *Vetiveria zizenioides*
Utpala, *Nelumbium speciosum*

Vacha, *Acorus calamus*
Vajrakanda, *Euphorbia antiquorum*
Vajrasnuhi, *Euphorbia neriifolia*
Valuka, *Vetiveria zizanioides*
Vartaka, *Solanum melongena*
Vidari, *Ipomoea paniculata*
Vyadhighataka, *Cathartocarpus fistula*

Yashtimadhuka, *Glycyrrhiza glabra*
Yava, *Hordeum vulgare*

APPENDIX XXVIII
A List of Medicinal Plants used as Aphrodisiacs

Arbus Precatorius, Chanothi
Abutilon Indicum, Atibala
Acorus Calamus, Vacha, Ghoda vaj
Alhagi Mauorrum, Durlabha, Jawasa
Allium Sativum, Lasan
Alpina Galanga, Barakalinjan
Amaranthus Polygamus, Chola bhaji, Tanduliya
Areca Catechu, Supari
Bambusa Arundinaceae, Bans
Butea Monosperma, Palas
Cannabis Sativa, Bhang
Ceiba Pentandra, Safed semal, Shalmali
Coriandrum Sativam, Dhania, Kothmir
Crocus Sativus, Kesar
Datura Metel, Dhatoora
Datura Innoxia, Dhatoora
Gossypium Herbaceum, Kapas
Juglans Regia, Akhrot
Lepidium Sativum, Asaliya, Asalio

Moringa Oleifera, Sainga, Saragvo
Mucuna Prurita, Kavatch, Atmagupta
Musa Paradisiaca, Kela
Pedalium Murex, Gokharu
Peganum Harmala, Harmara, Hurmal
Phoenix Dactylifera, Khajur
Piper Betle, Pan
Psoralea Cornlifolia, Bavachi
Randia Dumetorum, Madana, Mindhala
Salamia Malabarica, Semal, Shalmali
Saussurea Lappa, Kust, Kashmiraja
Shorea Robusta, Sal, Ral
Sida Cordifolia, Bala, Kungyi Vishatinduka
Strychnos Nux-vomica, Kanchaka, Jherkachola
Tinospora Cordifolia, Ambervel Gaduchi
Tribulus Terrestris, Gokharu
Trigomella Fornum, Methi
Withania Somnifera, Ashvagandha

GLOSSARY

Abhiyoga. According to Yashodhara it means a way of kissing with the ultimate object of the sex relation in view.

Abhukta. The Nayika who is not deflowered according to Kanchinatha.

Abhyantara-rata. Detumescence.

Abhyasika. Kind of *Purushayita* according to Pandita Mathura Prasada.

Achandavega. A person whose sex urge is not powerful.

Achchhuritaka. A nail-mark made with the nails of all the fingers.

Adharagrahana. A kiss involving the gripping of the lips.

Adharapana. According to Yashodara, it is the same as *Chushana*, mentioned by Vatsyayana.

Adhikarana. A division of a work such as Part I, etc.

Adhorata. Sodomy (*Anata* type).

Adhyaya. Chapter.

Adhihata. Rubbing with the fists.

Aharya. Rata wherein there is love subsequently.

Aibha. Coital posture of the *Anata* type. See *Gajopamardita.*

Aineya. Coital posture of the *Anata* type, resembling that of the deer.

Ajatasmara. The love-play of the couple between whom love has not grown.

Akarsha. A game of dice.

Akarshaphalaka. The board on which the dice game is played.

Akarshana. Attracting another person.

Alaktaka. The red resin of certain trees used by women for applying to their feet for decoration.

Alingana. The Embrace.

Amavasya. The last day of the dark half of a month.

Amoda. Joy, pleasure.

Amrachushitaka. A kind of *Auparishtaka* wherein the phallus is sucked like a mango fruit.

Amgarddha-nipidita. Coital posture of the *Asitaka* type.

Anamika. The ring finger.

Ananda. Happiness, joy.

Ananga-sthiti. The (dormant) passion of love.

Anata. Coital posture with the woman bending and the man standing at her back.

Anatalingita. Coital posture of the *Anata* type, according to Pandita Mathura Prasada.

Anchita. A slanting kiss.

Angulipravesha. See *Angulirata.*

Angulirata. Titillation with the fingers.

Angushtha. The toe.

Antah-Sandansha. A kind of *Auparishtaka* wherein pressing inside is done.

Antarakala. Subsidiary arts.

Antar-bahya. A kind of *Bahyrarata, viz, Angulirata*, according to Kanchinatha.

Antarmukha. A kind of kiss made with the help of the tongue, according to Yashodhara.

Anvartha. A kiss according to Kanchinatha,

Apadravya. Mechanical aid to congress, such as objects made of metal, wood, bone, etc., resembling the phallus.

Apahastaka. Thumping on the space between the breasts with the palm, keeping the fingers apart.

Apravartaka. The condition of the sexual urge for which oral union is recommended by Vatsyayana.

Arddhachandraka. A nail-mark resembling the crescent.

Arddhachumbita. Biting the lip and sucking, according to Padmashri.

Arddhakanchuka. An artificial phallus covering only the tip of the male organ.

Arddhalasa. Coital posture of the *Utthita* type, according to Pandit Mathura Prasada.

Arddhanata. Coital posture of the *Utthita* type, according to Pandit Mathura Prasada.

Arddhapadmasana. Coital posture of the *Uttana* type

Arddhapiditaka. Coital posture of the *Uttana* type.

Ardhendu. A kind of movement with the fingers arranged in a particular way, according to Kokkoka.

Arsha. Form of marriage.

Arpita. Coital posture of the *Utthita* type, according to Padmashri.

Artha. The material Wealth, the second Aim of Life.

Arupavat. Nail-mark which is ugly.

Asadharanatva. The characteristic of a thing in being quite distinct from another thing.

Asana. Posture for congress.

Ashritaka. Coital posture of the *Utthita* type, according to Devaraya.

Ashva. Horse.

Asina. Coital posture of the *Asitaka* type

Asitaka. Coital posture with both the persons sitting.

Asura. Form of marriage.

Asya. The month.

Atinicha. The Lowest type of coitus.

Atyuchcha. The Best type of coitus.

Aupanishadika. The part of Kama Sutra which gives recipes for making one's self more attractive, secret charms, herbal medicines, aphrodisiacs and artificial aids to congress.

Auparishtaka. The oral union.

Avadarita. Coital posture of the *Uttana* type.

Avalambitaka. Coital posture of the *Utthita* type, according to Vatsyayana.

Avamardana. A kind of *Upasripta* wherein rubbing is done.

Avapa. The ways and means by which the Nayaka and Nayika are united. These are described in four parts of the Kama Sutra.

Avapiditaka. A kiss indulged in by adult lovers, according to some writers.

Avaroha. Downward position of *Kamala* in *Vyanatarata.*

Aviddha. The artificial aid to congress without any holes.

Ayama. The size of the male sex organs.

Ayantrita. A *Rata* of unfettered love.

Ayata. Coital posture of the *Uttana* type.

Baddhamushti. Catching and holding tightly some of the limbs of the body.

Buhih-Sandansha. A kind of *Auparishtaka* wherein male organ is drawn in and then released.

Bahirbahya. A kind of *Bahya-rata* – love-play including the embrace, according to Kanchinatha.

Bahumula. The armpit.

Bahya-rata. Tumescence.

Baja. A maiden below the age of sixteen, according to Kokkoka.

Bandha. See *Asana.*

Bandhurita. Coital posture of the *Asitaka* type, according to Kalyanamalla.

Bhadra. A kind of Nayaka, according to Harihara.

Bhadraka. Coital posture of the *Asitaka* type, according to Pandit Mathura Prasada.

Bhadrakartari. A blow given with the palm, with the fingers straight and separate.

Bhaga. The female sex organ.

Bhakshya. Food to be masticated.

Bharyaduti. Wife acting as a messenger

for her own husband.

Bhavuka. Coital posture of the *Parshva* type.

Bhojya. Food to be chewed.

Bhramaraka. A kind of *Purushayita* wherein the woman makes circular movements.

Bhugnaka. Coital posture of the *Uttana* type.

Bhujangavalli. Entwining the man's fingers in the hair of the woman, according to Jyotirisha.

Bindu. A teeth-mark small as a point.

Bindumala. A number of point-like teeth-marks made in a line.

Bindumala. Giving blows to the man with her thumb when the woman is having sex relation in the inverse position, according to Jyotirisha.

Brahma. Form of marriage.

Buddha. Learned.

Chakrahva. The bird whose love for its mate is well known.

Chalitaka. A kiss given to the lover when he is not sober, engaged in arguments or sleeping with his face turned away.

Chanda. Sexual urge of the highest type (forceful).

Chandavega. A person whose sexual urge is forceful.

Chandrakala. The passion of love.

Chandramasi. A *Nadi*, according to Jyotirisha.

Charshani. Woman who does the chores in the house.

Chatakavilasita. A kind of *Upasripta* wherein the sport of a sparrow is imitated.

Chatukelika. Coital posture of the *Uttana* type.

Chhagala. Coital posture of the *Anata* type resembling that of the goat.

Chhaya. A kiss given to the shadow on a wall in a lighted room, or a reflection in a mirror or water.

Chimta. A pinch.

Chira. Coitus in which the man discharges after prolonged intromission. The excellent type.

Chitra-rata. See *Chitrasambhoga.*

Chitrasambhoga. Vatsyayana refers to sex relations in the standing posture, etc., by the term *Chitra.* Kokkoka refers to the male strokes by this word.

Chitrini. Type of Nayika.

Chudaka. A kind of artificial phallus.

Chumbana. The kiss.

Chumbada-dyuta-kalaha. Quarrel arising out of misleading acts of one of the persons indulging in kissing according to a wager.

Chumbitaka. Sucking the tip of the tongue hurriedly, according to Padmashri.

Chumbitaka. A kind of *Auparishtaka* where the male organ is kissed.

Chunti. A pinch.

Chushana. Sucking.

Daiva. Form of Marriage.

Dakshina. Things given by a pupil to his teacher on leaving him.

Dantachchhedya. The Teeth-Marks.

Dantakshata. A teeth-mark.

Darduraka. A nail-mark serving as a memento, according to Jyotirisha.

Dashana. A kind of kiss wherein the tongue of the man touches the teeth of the woman, according to Yashodhara.

Datta. A kind of Nayaka, according to Harihara.

Dhainuka. Coital posture of the *Anata* type, resembling that of the bull.

Dharma. The prescribed course of conduct. The first Aim of Life.

Dhrita. Coital posture of the *Utthita* type.

Dola. Coital posture of the *Utthita* type, according to Padmashri.

Duta. A messenger (male).

Duti. A messenger (female).

Dutkrit. A kiss given with a sound like that produced by a falling pearl, according to Padmashri.

Dutkrita. A sound resembling the splitting of a bamboo, made by a woman.

Dvitala. Coital posture of the *Utthita* type, according to Kokkoka.

Dyutashraya. Arts in the practice of which the element of wagering enters.

Ekacharini. Wife who is devoted to (one person) the husband only.

Ekachuda. A kind of attificial phallus.

Ekapada. Coital posture of the *Uttana* type.

Ekapadika. Name of a game.

Gajopamardita. Coital posture of the *Anata* type, resembling that of the elephant.

Galaka. The neck.

Gandharva. Form of marriage.

Garika. A courtesan who is liberal, pious and devoted.

Garbha. Embryo.

Gardabhakranta. Coital posture of the *Anata* type, resembling that of the donkey.

Gauri. A *Nadi,* according to Jyotirisha.

Gauyuthika. Coitus of a woman with many men, resembling that of the cow.

Ghattitaka. A kiss indulged in by a maiden, according to Vatsyayana.

Goshthi. A gathering of citizens of similar age, wealth, learning, etc.

Ghona. A maiden who is 'Kapila'— whose colour of the skin is grey.

Grahana. Catching, holding fast.

Gramya. Coital posture of the *Uttana* type.

Griva. The neck.

Gudhaka. A teeth-mark with the molar in the front generally done on the lower lip.

Guhya. The female sex organ.

Gulpha. Leg from knee to ankle.

Guna. The inherent quality of a thing.

Hakara. A sound produced by a woman when experiencing sexual pleasure.

Hansa. The swan.

Hamsalilaka. Kind of *Purushayita,* according to Kokkoka.

Hanupada. Coital posture of the *Uttana* type.

Harini. Deer (female).

Harivikrama. Coital posture of the *Utthita* type.

Hastakshobhalila. See *Angulirata.*

Hastashakhavimarda. See *Angulirata.*

Hastini. Cow-elephant.

Hastini. Type of Nayika.

Hikkrit. A kiss with a sound like 'Hik' when the breath is controlled, according to Padmashri.

Hinkrita. A sound produced by the throat and nose, according to Kokkoka.

Hrid. The bosom.

Hula. A kind of *Upasripta,* wherein piercing movements are made.

Hunkara. A sound resembling 'Hun'.

Indrani. Coital posture of the *Uttana* type.

Jaghana. The uppermost part of the thigh.

Jaghanopaguhana. An embrace, according to Suvarnanabha.

Jalaka. An artificial phallus covering the whole of the male organ.

Jangha. The thigh.

Janu. The knee.

Janukurpara. Coital posture of the *Utthita* type.

Jastasmara. The love-play of the couple between whom love has already developed.

Jihva. A kind of kiss wherein the tongues combat with each other, according to Yashodhara.

Jihvapravesha. Love-play with the help of the tongue while kissing according to Padmashri.

Jihvayuddha. Love-quarrel wherein each person makes use of the tongue.

Jrimohitaka. Coital posture of the *Uttana* type.

Jyeshtha. The second finger.

Kachagraha. Catching the forelocks on the man's head before kissing his raised face, according to Vatsyayana.

Kakaruta. A cow-like sound produced by a woman.

Kakundara. The cavities of the loins.

Kala. The arts.

Kalabheda. Difference in time.

Kama. The third Aim of Life: sexual pleasure.

Kamajaya. Coital posture of the *Uttana* type.

Kamalarddha. See *Arddhapadmasana.*

Kamankusha. The spiked goad of love, the male organ.

Kamankusha. A kind of movement with the fingers arranged in the particular way according to Kokkoka.

Kamashastra. The science of love. Treatises dealing with the subject.

Kamasthana. Erogenous zone.

Kamatapatra. See *Madanachhatra.*

Kamavatansa. Pulling the hair near the ear of a woman by a man, according to Jyotirisha.

Kamodaya. The rise of the passion of love.

Kampitaka. Rubbing with a quivering hand.

Kanaka. Titillation with the second finger with the index finger kept behind it, according to Padmashri.

Kanchuka. A kind of artificial aid to congress with rough globules on the outer surface.

Kanda. Bulbous roots; vegetable growing underground, such as Surana.

Kantha. The neck.

Kanthopagrahana. The embrace of the neck.

Kanyasamprayukta. That part of the Kama Sutra which deals with the selection of the bride, marriage, etc.

Kapata-dyuta. Misleading acts of one of the persons while indulging in love-play, according to a wager.

Kapola. The cheek.

Karana See *Asana.*

Karana. Titillation with the index finger, according to Padmashri.

Karashakhabhimardana. See *Angulirata.*

Karashakhayoga. See *Angulirata.*

Karatadana. Beating with the hand.

Kari. Quivering the tongue after insertion in the mouth, according to Padmashri.

Karikarakrida. Keeping three fingers joined and resembling the proboscis of an elephant for manipulating in the female organ.

Karkataka. Coital posture of the *Uttana* type.

Karkata. Coital posture of the *Parshva* type, according to Kalyanamalla.

Karmashraya. Arts which require the use of technical skill.

Karnapatra. Ornamental designs made of ivory, conch shell, etc.

Karnapura. An ear ornament.

Kartari. A kind of blow with palm.

Katiprishtha. The waist, that is, the part below the ribs and above the hips.

Kauliraka. Coital posture of the *Uttana* type.

Kaurma. Coital posture of the *Uttana* type.

Kaurmaka. Coital posture of the *Asitaka* type, according to Kalyanamalla.

Kavacha. A eulogistic poem consisting

of prayers for self-preservation.

Kavi. Poet.

Keshakarshana. Catching the forelock.

Khala. A *Rata* which is degrading.

Khandabhraka. A teeth-mark made by broad, medium and small teeth together on the breast of the woman and the chest of the man, according to Yashodhara.

Kharvata. Small village.

Kila. A blow given with the palm folded into a fist and the index and middle fingers out.

Kirti. Coital posture of the *Asitaka* type, according to Jyotirisha.

Kirti. Coital posture of the *Utthita* type, according to Kalyanamalla.

Kolacharvita. See *Varahacharvita.*

Krishna-paksha. The dark half of a month.

Kritagranthika. Gripping in such a way as to entwine the woman's fingers.

Kritakadhvaja. Artificial phallus.

Kritrima. A *Rata* based on artificial love.

Kritrima. Arrangement of three fingers resembling the proboscis of an elephant.

Kritrlma linga. See *Kritakadhvaja.*

Kshiranira. An embrace, according to the school of Babhravya.

Kshobhana Mantra. Secret incantations for production of sexual excitement.

Kuchagra. The nipple.

Kuchamardana. Rubbing and twisting the breasts.

Kuchimara. A kind of Nayaka, according to Harihara.

Kujita. A kiss with a sound like that of a bird in a joyous mood, according to Padmashri.

Kumbhadasi. Courtesan whose aim is the acquisition of wealth, physical comfort and an easy life.

Kunchita. Coital posture of the *Utthita* type, according to Pandita Mathura Prasada.

Kundala. Giving of blows to the man with the thumb and the middle finger when the woman is experiencing sex relations in the inverse position, according to Jyotirisha.

Kuntala. Giving of blows to the man when the woman is experiencing sex relations in the inverse position, according to Kalyanamalla.

Kurpara. Coital posture of the *Utthita* type.

Kurparajanu. Coital posture of the *Utthita* type.

Laghu. Coitus in which the man discharges prematurely. The low type.

Lalatika. An embrace, according to Suvarnanabha.

Lambita. Coital posture of the *Utthita* type, according to Devaraya.

Lataveshtitaka. An embrace, according to the school of Babhravya.

Lavaka. Name of a bird. A quail.

Lavanavithika. Name of a game.

Laya. See *Asana*

Lehya. Food to be licked.

Linga. The male organ of reproduction.

Lokayatika. A follower of the materialistic school.

Madana. Love. Sexual love.

Madanabhumi. Erogenous zone.

Madanachhatra. Name of a part of the female sex organ.

Madanadika. The clitoris and the adjoining parts which under the stress of sexual emotion receive and transmit the stimulatory voluptuous sensation imparted by friction with the man's organ.

Madanagamanadola. Literally, the seat of love. Name for the clitoris.

Madanalaya. The female sex organ.

Madanasadana. Literally, the abode of love – the female sex organ.

Madhu. A beverage.

Madhya. Coitus in which the man discharges some time after intromission. The medium type.

Madhyama. The middle (long) finger.

Mahashulachita. Coital posture of the *Uttana* type.

Mallika. Portable seat made from a staff and small plank.

Manasijasthiti. See *Anangasthiti.*

Manda. Low type of sexual urge.

Mandala. A nail-mark which is circular in appearance.

Mandavega. A person whose sexual urge is slow.

Manduka. Coital posture of the *Uttana* type.

Mandukika. Name of a game.

Manijalaka. See *Valaya.*

Manimala. A string of jewels.

Maniraksha. See *Arddhakanchuka.*

Manmathachhatra. See *Madanochhatra.*

Manmathagara-mudrabhanga-krida. See *Angulirata.*

Mantha. The doctrine of resuscitation propounded by Uddalaka in the Brihadaranyaka Upanishad. 2 The sanctified oblation.

Manthana. A kind of *Upasripta* wherein there are 'churning' movements.

Mardana. Rubbing with force.

Marditaka. Coital posture of the *Asitaka* type.

Marjaralalitaka. Coital posture of the *Anata* type resembling that of the cat.

Markata. Coital posture of the *Uttana* type.

Markataka. Coital posture of the *Asitaka* type, according to Kokkoka, Devaraya and Kalyanamalla.

Matangalilayita. Movements resembling the dangling of the proboscis of an elephant. See *Karikara.*

Mauli. The head.

Mayurapadaka. A nail-mark resembling the feet of a peacock.

Minaketana. Coital posture of the *Uttana* type.

Moksha. The Final Emancipation. The last Aim of Life.

Mridu. A kiss of the soft type.

Mudhaduti. Female messenger who befriends the Nayaka's wife, teaches her the arts, makes them quarrel and thus accomplishes her own object.

Mudgaka. Coital posture of the *Parshva* type.

Mudita. Pleasure, happiness.

Mukaduti. Female messenger who is quite innocent or one who is a young girl and is sent often to the Nayika's house.

Mukha. The mouth.

Mukha-Chumbana. The kiss on the mouth.

Mula. Root.

Mulakala Arts of which knowledge is essential.

Mushti. A blow given with the fist.

Nabhi. The navel.

Nabhimula. The lower most part of the trunk. According to Yashodhara, it is synonymous with the female sex organ.

Nadi. Glands secreting odourless mucous in the female sex organ when sexually roused

Nadikshobhana. Erection of the clitoris manually or by rubbing it with the male organ.

Naga. Coital posture of the *Parshva* type, according to Jyotirisha.

Nagara. Coital posture of the *Uttana* type.

Nagaraka. The urban connoisseur and expert in affairs of love.

Nakhachchhedya. Nail-marks.

Nakula. The mongoose.

Nanda. Puja. Adoration.

Nandana. Puja. Adoration.

Nandini. That science which deals with Nanda. It is practised by householders, it brings knowledge, physical loveliness, moral wellbeing, and benefits to women.

Narayita. See *Purushayita.*

Nasika. The nose.

Nashtaraga. A person having very poor sexual urge or none at all.

Natavallabha. Coital posture. of the *Utthita* type, according. to Pandit Mathura Prasada.

Nayaka. The male (lover).

Nayika. The female (beloved).

Netra. The eyes.

Nicha. Low (coitus).

Nih-shabda. A kiss in which there is no accompanying sound, according to Padmashri.

Nimita. A kind of *Auparishtaka* quite nominal.

Nimitaka. A kiss indulged in by a maiden, according to Vatsyayana.

Nighata. A kind of *Upasripta* wherein movements are made as if giving blows.

Nirjiva. Those arts in which inanimate objects are played with.

Nisrishtartha. Female messenger who accomplishes the mission by means of her own intelligence.

Nivivishleshana. Untying the knot of the lower garment, petticoat.

Oshtha. The lip.

Ostha-vimrishtha. Sucking the tip of the tongue, according to Padmashri.

Padangushitha (chumbana). A kiss indulged in by the masseuse while the lover is asleep.

Padmasana. Coital posture of the *Uttana* type.

Padmasana. Coital posture of the *Asitaka* type, according to Jyotirisha and Kalyanamalla.

Padmini. The first type of Nayika.

Paishacha. Form of marriage.

Panchala. A kind of Nayaka, according to Harihara.

Panch-bhutas. Five elements: earth, water, light, wind, and atmosphere.

Panchasamaya. Name of a game in which there is some wagering.

Paradarika. The part of Kama Sutra which deals with extramarital relations of a person.

Parakiya. Name of a class of Nayikas consisting of widows, recluses, etc.

Paravata. The pigeon.

Paravrittaka. Coital posture of the *Parshva* type.

Parisparshava. Touching all over the body with the hand.

Parivartita. Coital posture of the *Uttana* type.

Parivartita. Coital posture of the *Asitaka* type, according to Pandita Mathura Prasada.

Parashvadvaya. The two sides.

Pataka. Titillation with the first two fingers joined and outstretched, according to Padmashri.

Parimitartha. Female messenger who executes particular duties.

Parimrishtaka. A kind of *Auparishtaka* wherein the male organ is kissed all over.

Parinaha. The size (depth) of the female sex passage.

Pashu. Coital posture similar to the one of quadrupeds.

Parshva. Coital posture with both the persons in the lateral position.

Parsvatah. A kind of *Auparishtaka* wherein the biting is done on the side.

Pataka. Giving blows with the open palm on the man's chest by the woman while experiencing sex relations in the inverse position, according to Jyotirisha.

Patala. The nethermost region.

Pativallabha. Kind of *Purushayita,* according to Pandita Mathura Prasada.

Patrahari. Female messenger who

carries letters.

Pattana. Town.

Payodhara. The breasts.

Peya. Food which is to be drunk.

Phalabheda. Difference in result.

Phala. Fruit.

Phalini. Maiden who is dumb.

Phanibhoga. A kind of movement with fingers arranged in a particular way, according to Kokkoka.

Phanipasha. Coital posture of the *Asitaka* type, according to Kalyanamalla.

Phanipasha. Coital posture of the *Uttana* type.

Phenaka. Foam-producing and cleansing substance.

Phutkrita. A sound resembling that which is produced by a berry falling in water.

Padita. Coital posture of the *Uttana* type.

Piditaka. An embrace, according to the school of Babhravya.

Piditaka. Coital posture of the *Uttana* type.

Paditaka. Coital posture of the *Parshva* type.

Piditaka. A kind of *Upasripta* wherein pressing movenents are made.

Pindita. Coital posture of the *Uttana* type.

Pithamarda. One well versed in the arts, of good family, possessing little or no money, carrying 'Mallika', the wooden seat and 'Phenaka', mediating between lovers.

Pota. A *Rata* wherein the woman is not the man's equal.

Pradipana-vidhi, The ways and means of exciting the passion of love.

Pradeshini. The first or index finger.

Pradipana-vidhi. The ways and means of exciting the passion of love.

Prahanana. Sadistic acts.

Prahastaka. Beating on the head with the palm with the fingers slightly bent.

Prajapatya. Form of marriage.

Prakarana. Portion or part of a book, a chapter, wherein the subject matter is dealt with.

Praksuri. Teachers who flourished previously.

Pramana. Size.

Prasarita. Coital posture of the *Uttana* type.

Prasrita. A kind of blow which makes a woman give out *Kujita* and *Phutkrita* sounds.

Pratata. Broadening of the tonguc after insertion in the mouth, according to Padmashri.

Pratibodhika. A kiss for awakening the sleeping lover.

Pravalamani. Teeth-mark resembling coral made on the cheek.

Pravartaka. The low condition of the sexual urge for which manual manipulation and other similar means are prescribed.

Praveshtita. Coital posture of the *Uttana* type.

Prema. Love. Affection.

Premkha. Coital posture of the *Uttana* type.

Prenkholita. A kind of *Purushayita* wherein the woman adopts swinging positions.

Prishata. Maiden having white spots on the body.

Pritikara. Coital posture of the *Uttana* type.

Punarbhu. A woman married and then deserted or widowed.

Purana. The general name for ancient semi-historical chronicles. Eighteen such Puranas are well known.

Purnachandra. A *Nadi,* according to Kalyanamalla. According to Kokkoka, it is full of odourless mucous.

Purnima. The last day of the bright half of a month.

Purushayita. The sex posture in which the woman is on the top with the man lying on his back.

Purushayita. Kind of *Viparita* posture, according to Pandita Mathura Prasada.

Purvasuri. Sec *Praksuri.*

Pushpapida. A cluster of flowers arranged in the hair for adornment.

Putkara. A kiss with a sound like 'Put' when the lips are gripped, according to Padmashri.

Radana-kalaha. Love-quarrel wherein the persons indulge in biting.

Ragadipana. A kiss for arousing the passion of love

Ragavasanakala. The time when the passion of love begins to wane after the sex act.

Ragavat. *Rata* which is of a loving type.

Rajadanta. The teeth in the front.

Raka. Maiden who is menstruating.

Rakshasa. Form of marriage.

Rasana-rana. Sec *Jihva-yuddha.*

Rasapana. Sucking (drinking the juice, as it were), according to Harihara.

Rasita. Kind of *Purushayita*, according to Pandita Mathura Prasada.

Rata. Coitus, the sex act.

Ratantaka. Coital posture of the *Uttana* type.

Ratavallabha. Coital posture of the *Parshva* type, according to Pandita Mathura Prasada.

Ratikala. See *Chandrakala.*

Ratipradipana. Rousing of sexual passion.

Ratisangara. The battle of love.

Ratitithi. Day on which the passion of love rises in a particular part of the body.

Rekha. A short nail-mark.

Richchhapriya. Coital posture of the *Asitaka* type

Rimgita. Kind of *Purushayita*, according to Pandita Mathura Prasada

Rishabha. Maiden who is masculine in appearance.

Romancha. Horripilation.

Ruchi. Desire. Pleasure.

Rudita. A kind of sound like that given out by a woman at the end of sexual relations.

Rupajiva. A courtesan who considers her physical charms as the sole means of her livelihood.

Rupavat. Nail-mark with a pleasant appearance.

Sadharana. General. A part of a book wherein miscellaneous subjects are dealt with.

Sairibha. Coital posture of the *Anata* type, resembling that of the buffalo.

Sajiva. Those arts in which the wagering relates to animate things, such as, birds, animals, etc.

Sama. Coitus of partners equal as regards the size of their sex organs.

Sama. A kiss indulged in by adult lovers, according to some writers.

Samahasta. Pulling the hair of a woman by a man with both hands, according to Jyotirisha.

Samakrama. Rubbing here and there with pressure.

Samakrishti. Pinching on the neck and breasts with the thumb and index finger kept together.

Samapada. Coital posture of the *Uttana* type.

Samatalaka. A blow given steadily with the palm.

Samaushtha. A kiss in which the woman with her tongue and lips presses the lips of the man, according to Kalyanamalla.

Sambadh. The female sex organ.

Sambhogavastha. The different stages in the act of coitus.

Samdamsha. A kind of *Purushayita* wherein the woman maintains the grip on the male organ as if with tongs.

Samdamshika. A type of blow with the fist with either the index finger and thumb or index and second fingers kept out.

Samgara. A kind of *Auparishtaka* wherein the male organ is taken deep inside till the man discharges.

Samirana. A *Nadi,* according to Jyotirisha.

Samkirna. Coitus of the mixed type.

Samkrantaka. A kiss given to an image of a person,made of clay, stone or wood, or to a child playing on the lap.

Sammukta. Coital posture of the *Utthita* type, according to Jyotirisha.

Samprayoga. Tumescence and Detumescence.

Samprayukta Viddhi. See *Asana.*

Samputa. Coital posture of the *Uttana* type.

Samputa. A kind of *Upasripta* wherein both the persons remain united after intromission.

Samputaka. A kiss with a sound indulged in by the female or the male who has not grown a moustache

Samputaka. Sucking the lips of each other, according to Padmashri.

Samudga. Coital posture o the *Parshva* type.

Samvahana. I. An embrace, according to some writers, 2. Shampooing.

Samveshana. See *Asana.*

Samveshtitaka. Coital posture of the *Uttana* type.

Samyamana. Coital posture of the *Uttana* type.

Sanghataka. Coitus of a woman with two men simultaneously.

Sankara. Coital posture of the *Anata* type.

Santadita. Giving blows on the chest of a man when the woman is experiencing sex relations in the inverse

position, according to Jyotirisha.

Santanika. Giving blows to the man when the woman is experiencing sex relations in the inverse position according to Kalyanamalla.

Sarita. Coital posture of the. *Uttana* type.

Sa-shabda. A kiss in which there is a sound, according to Padmashri.

Sasitkritam. A kiss in which the female gives out a shriek or cry according to Vatsyayana.

Saumya. Coital posture of the *Uttana* type.

Sayaka. A chapter of the work of Jyotirisha.

Shabdakartana. A blow given on the head with the fingers bent.

Shabdakartari. A blow given by keeping the index finger on the thumb.

Shanibhoga. See *Phanibhoga.*

Shankhini. Type of Nayika.

Shasha. Hare.

Shashaplutaka. A nail-mark resembling the feet of a hare.

Shastra. Science. Scientific treatise.

Shauna. Coital posture of the *Anata* type, resembling that of the dog.

Shayanopacharika. Bedroom arts.

Shikhashraya. See *Mauli.*

Shitopachara. Prescription for allaying heat, etc.

Shringara. The sentiment of love synonymous with *Rati, Kama,* etc.

Shroni. The posteriors.

Shuddha. Coitus of the clear type.

Shukla-paksha. The bright half of a month.

Shulachita. Coital posture of the *Uttana* type.

Shulamka. Coital posture of the *Uttana* type.

Shvasita. Kiss with a sound like a sigh, according to Padmashri.

Shvasita. Sound produced by a woman on reaching the acme of sexual pleasure, according to Padmashri.

Sitkara. Kiss with a sound with the help of the teeth and lips while exhaling, according to Padmashri.

Sitkrita. Cries of joy, pain, etc., made in love-play.

Slatha. Sluggish.

Smarachakra. Coital posture of the *Uttana* type.

Samaradasha. The different stages of one's mind when one is deeply in love with another person.

Samrajala. The odourless mucous which bathes as it were all the parts of the female sex organ around the entrance to the vagina, when the woman is sexually roused.

Smaraka. See *Smaraniyaka.*

Smaraniyaka. A nail-mark made as a memento by the man before going on a journey.

Smriti. The general name for old texts enjoining certain rules of conduct, etc.

Sphuritaka. Kiss indulged in by a maiden, according to Vatsyayana.

Sphutana. Coital posture of the *Uttana* type.

Sprishtaka. An embrace, according to the school of Babhravya.

Sprishtaka. Rubbing with the palm held straight.

Stanalingana. An embrace, according to Suvarnanabha.

Stanayugma. The breasts.

Stanita. Kiss with a guttural sound, like thundering in the clouds, according to Padmashri.

Suchi. Coital posture of the *Uttana* type.

Suchi. Insertion of the contracted and twisted tongue into the mouth of the other person, according to Padmashri.

Sundara. Coital posture of the *Uttana* type.

Surata. Coitus.

Sutra. Short and pithy writing.

Svara-matrika-nyasa. Diagram having certain letters of the alphabet for invocation of supernatural aid for one's benefit.

Svayamduti. Female messenger undertaking to do the work from selfish motives.

Tadana. Beating.

Tala. Coital posture of the *Utthita* type, according to Devaraya.

Talu. A kind of kiss wherein the tongue of a person is rubbed against the palate of the other person.

Tantra. The ways and means by which sexual love is heightened. The part of the Kama Sutra dealing with these is *Samprayogika.*

Taragaranga. Pulling the hair of a woman by a man with one hand, according to Jyotirisha.

Tarjani. The index finger.

Tilatandula. An embrace, according to the school of Babhravya.

Tiryag. A kiss indulged in by adult lovers, according to some writers.

Tithi. A day of the month.

Traivikrama. Coital posture of *Uttana* type, according to Devaraya.

Trapa. Feeling of bashfulness.

Tripada. Coital posture of the *Utthita* type, according to Jyotirisha.

Trishula. Titillation with the first three fingers, according to Padmashri.

Tritiya Prakriti. A eunuch.

Turagadhirudhaka. Coital posture of the *Anata* type, resembling that of the horse.

Uchcha. Excellent (coitus).

Uchchhunaka. A teeth-mark more forceful than the *Gudhaka.*

Udbhranta. A kiss indulged in by adult lovers, according to some writers.

Udbhugnaka. Coital posture of the *Uttana* type.

Udghrishtaka. An embrace, according to

the school of Babhravya.

Udyanayatra. Picnic in sylvan groves.

Uha. Guessing the meaning before using the word.

Ullasita. Kind of *Purushayita,* according to Pandita Mathura Prasada.

Upabhukta. The Nayika who is already deflowered, according to Kanchinatha.

Upaguhana. See *Alingana.*

Upapada. Coital posture of the *Asitaka* type, according to Kalyanamalla.

Upani Rata. See *Purushayita.*

Upasripta. Movements of the male organ after intromission.

Upavitika. Coital posture of the *Parshva* type.

Urahsphutana. Coital posture of the *Uttana* type.

Urddhvaga. Coital posture of the *Uttana* type.

Uru (chumbana). A kiss indulged in by the masseuse while the lover is asleep.

Uruka. Coital posture of the *Anata* type, according to Pandita Mathura Prasada.

Urumula. See *Urusandhi.*

Urupaguhana. An embrace, according to Suvarnanabha.

Urusandhi. The uppermost part of the thighs.

Utkalita. Kind of *Purushayita,* according to Kalyanamalla.

Utpala. A blue lotus.

Utpala-patraka. A nail-mark resembling the leaf of the blue lotus.

Utpalapatrika. See *Shabdakartari.*

Utphullaka. Coital posture of the *Uttana* type.

Uttana. Coital posture with the woman supine.

Utpiditaka. Coital posture of the *Uttana* type.

Uttarakala. Those arts which are to be practised last.

Utthita. Coital posture with both the persons standing.

Utthita. Coital posture of the *Utthita* type, according to Pandita Mathura Prasada.

Vadana. The mouth.

Vadava. Mare.

Vadavaka. Coital posture of the *Uttana* type.

Vadavaka. Coital posture of the *Parshva* type, according to Padmashri.

Vaishika. The part of the Kama Sutra which deals with relations with courtesans, their life, etc.

Valaya. An artificial phallus having many holes.

Vankshana. See *Urusandhi.*

Varahachrvita. A teeth-mark resembling the bite of a boar made by a person with a powerful sexual urge.

Varahadhrishtaka. Coital posture of the *Anata* type, resembling that of the boar.

Varahaghata. A kind of *Upasripta* wherein rubbing is done on one side only.

Varana. The act of selection of the bride.

Varanga. See *Guhya.*

Varikriditaka. Sexual act in a pool of water, resembling that of the elephant.

Varshakari. A maiden who perspires profusely.

Varttitaka. Coital posture of the *Uttana* type.

Vashikarana. The art of enticing a person.

Vataduti. Female messenger who delivers the message in a code unintelligible to others.

Vega. Force of sexual urge.

Venudarita. Coital posture of the *Uttana* type.

Veshtitaka. Catching of the forelocks.

Veshtitaka. Coital posture of the *Parshva* type, according to Padmashri.

Vicheshitita. Peculiar movements of limbs made by a person when teeth-marks are being made, according to Jyotirisha.

Veshtitaka. Coital posture of the *Uttana* type.

Viddha. A blow given with the fist with the thumb kept between the index and middle fingers or between the middle and ring fingers.

Viddhaka. An embrace, according to the school of Babhravya.

Vidushaka. Vaihasika whose aim is to provoke laughter knowing some arts, enjoying the confidence of all, mainly indulging in jests and pranks.

Vigna. See *Buddha.*

Vijati. Females of bipeds and quadrupeds.

Vikana. Titillation by changing the position of the first two fingers, according to Padmashri.

Vikata. Maiden whose thighs are held apart while walking.

Vimarditaka. Coital posture of the *Asitaka* type.

Vimunda. Maiden having a broad forehead.

Vinata. Maiden who is bent from the shoulders.

Vinika. Coital posture of the *Parshva* type, according to Kalyanamalla.

Vinoda. Pleasure. Gratification.

Viparita. Kind of *Purushayita,* according to Jyotirisha and Kalyanamalla.

Virayita. See *Purushayita.*

Viruta. Generally denoting sounds made by a woman with whom the man is engaged in sadistic acts.

Vishama. Coitus of persons of mixed type.

Visheshaka. A mark made on the forehead by a woman with Bhurja leaf.

Vita. Married person, honoured by citizens and courtesans, having very artistic nature, depending upon courtesans for livelihood

Viyoni. Place other than the female sex organs, such as armpit.

Vrikshadhirudha. An embrace, according to the school of Babhravya.

Vrisha. Bull.

Vrishaghata. A kind of *Upasripta* wherein movements are done like the onslaught of a bull.

Vyaghranakha. A nail-mark resembling a tiger-claw.

Vyaghravaskandana. Coital posture of the *Anata* type, resembling that of the tiger.

Vyanata. Coital posture. See *Anata.*

Vyanata. Coital posture of the *Anata* type.

Vyavahita. A *Rata* based on transferred love.

Vyayata. Coital posture of the *Utthita* type, according to Padmashri.

Vyayataka. Coital posture of the *Utthita* type, according to Jyotirisha.

Vyomapada. Coital posture of the *Uttana* type.

Yama. One of the eight divisions of day and night combined, i.e. duration of three hours.

Yamalakartari. A blow given by two palms joined together.

Yantra-yoga. The sexual union.

Yoni. See *Guhya.*

Yugmapada. Coital posture of the *Parshva* type.

BIBLIOGRAPHY

A. SANSKRIT
  1) Vedic
   Atharva Veda
   Rig Veda
   Taittiriya Samhita
   Brihadaranyaka Upanishad

  2) Epic
   Mahabharata
   Ramayana

  3) Purana
   Agni
   Bhavishya
   Devi Bhagavata
   Garuda
   Harivamsha
   Skanda
   Shrimad Bhagavata
   Vishnudharmottara

  4) Smriti
   Amgira
   Apastamba
   Atri
   Atri Samhita
   Brihadyama
   Daksha
   Manu
   Narada
   Prajapati
   Shankha
   Vasishtha
   Vriddaharita
   Vishnu
   Yagnavalkya

  5) Vyakarana
   Mahabhashya

  6) Artha, Ayurveda, etc.
   Arthashastra
   Ayurvedaprakasha
   Brihatsamhita

Charakasamhita
Sushrutasamhita

  7) Kavya
   Buddhacharita
   Chaurapanchashika
   Gitagovinda
   Janakiharana
   Kiratarjuniya
   Kumarasambhava
   Meghaduta
   Naishadhiya
   Raghuvamsha
   Shishupalavadha

  8) Nataka
   Abhignana Shakuntala
   Malatimadhava
   Ratnavali
   Uttararama Charita

  9) Prabandha
   Dashakumaracharita
   Kadambari

  10) Kamashastra
   Anangaranga
   Haramekhala
   Kamasamuha Mss.
   Kamasutra
   Kandarpachudamani
   Kuitanimata
   Nagarasarvasva
   Panchasayaka
   Ratikelikutuhala
   Ratiratnapradipika
   Ratimanjari
   Ratirahasya
   Ratishastra
   Smaradipika
   Shiringaramanjari
   Uddishatantra
   Varnaratnakara

11) Prakirna
Adharashataka
Amarukashataka
Aryasaptashati
Deshopadeshamala
Jarajatashataka
Kalavilasa
Samayamatrika
Shringarashataka
Subhashitaratnakara

12) Bhana etc.
Dhurtasamagama
Latakamelaka
Mukundananda
Rasasadana
Shringarabhushana
Shringarasarvasva
Shringaratilaka

B. PRAKRIT
Dhurtakhyana
Paumachariya

C. GUJARATI
Chumbana mimansa
Forbes Sabha Mahotsava Grantha
Kalavilasa (Trans.)
Kamasutra (Trans.)
Kokashastra (*Narbudacharya*)

D. MARATHI
Anangaranga (Trans.)
Bhavartha Ramayana
Kamapurushartha
Kamasutra, Pt. I (Trans.)
Prachinacharitra Kosha
Vatsyayana-Kalina-Samaja
Vyavastha (Trans.)

E. HINDI
Asali Kokashastra
Kamasutra, 2 Vols. (Trans.)

F. FRENCH
Le Livre, d'amour de l'*Orient:*
1) *Anangaranga* (Trans.)
2) *Les Kamasutra* (Trans.)
3) *Le Breviaire de la Courtisane* (Trans.)

G. GERMAN
Das Kamasutram (Trans.)
Rati Rahasyam (Trans.)
Beitrage zur Indischen der Erotic
Sechzig Upanishada des Veda (Trans.)
Shukasaptati
Kamasutram, das Indische Lehrbuch der Liebe.

H. ENGLISH
Agrawala – *India as Known to Panini*
Barua – *History of Pre-Buddhistic Indian Philosophy*
Basu – 1. *A Manual for Husband and Wife*, 2 Vols.
2. *Sexual Side of Love*
3. *The Art of Love in the Orient.*
Bloomfield – *Atharvaveda*
Chakladhar – *Social Life in Ancient India*
Dastur – 1. *Useful Plants of India and Pakistan*
2. *Medicinal Plants of india and Pakistan*
3. *Everybody's Guide to Ayurvedic Medicine*
Davis – *Factors in the Sex Life of 2200 women*
De – *Ancient Indian Erotics and Erotic Literature*

Ellis 1. *Studies in the Psychology of Sex*, 2 Vols.
2. *Sex and Marriage*
3. *Psychology of Sex*
4. *On Life and Sex*
Ghosh – *Urban Morals in Ancient India*
Gode – *Studies in Indian Literary History*, 3 Vols.
Havil – *The Technique of Sex*
Iyengar – *Kama Sutra* (Trans.)
Keith – *History of Sanskrit Literature*
Keith – *Sanskrit Drama*
Kieffer – *Sexual Life in Ancient Rome* (Trans.)
Krafft-Ebing – *Psychopathia Sexualis* (Trans.)
Leeson – Kama Shilpa
Lewinsohn – *A History of Sexual Customs* (Trans.)
Licht – *Sexual life in Ancient Greece* (Trans.)
Macdonell – *Vedic Mythology*
Major – *India in the 15th Century*
Majumdar – 'Plants in Erotics,' *Indian Culture.*
Malinowski – *Sexual Life of Savages*
Mantegazza – *Sexual Relations of Mankind* (Trans.)
Max Muller – *Vedic Hymns* (S.B.E. XLIL) (Trans.)
Mazumdar – 1. *Vedic Age,*
2. *Classical Age,*
3. *Age of Imperial Unity,*
4. *Age of Imperial Kanauja,*
5. *Struggle for Empire*
Mehta – *1001 Ways of kissing*
Meyer – *Sexual Life in Ancient India* (Trans.)
M.R.A.S. – Sex Life in India
Pillay – The *Art of Love and Sane Sex Living*
Puri – *India in the Time of Patanjali*

Rapson – *Cambridge History of India*, Vol. 1
Shastri – *Mauryas and Satavahanas*
Shende – *Studies in Atharvaveda*
Sutor – *The Psychology of Love*
Thomas – *Kama Kalpa*
Vecki – *Mechanism of Love*
Velde – *Ideal Marriage, its Physiology and Technique*
Watt – *Dictionary of the Economic Products of India*, 10 Vols.
Winternitz – *History of Indian Literature*, Vol. 1 (Trans.)
Y.D.T.J. – 1. *Kokkokam* (Trans.)
2. *Love in Ancient India*
3. *Physiology of Love*

Sculpture, Painting, etc.
Anand – *Homage to Khajuraho*
Bachhoffer – *Early Indian Sculpture*, 2 Vols.
Burnier – *Hindu Mediaeval Sculpture*
Coomaraswamy – 1. *Vishvakarma*
2. *Catalogue of the Indian Collections*, Vols. 1, 2, 4, 6
Fouchet – *Erotic Sculpture of India*
Goswami – 1. *Orissan Sculpture and Architecture*
2. *Designs from Orissan Temples*
3. *The Art of the Chandelas*
4. *The Art of the Pallavas*
5. *The Art of the Rashtrakutas*
Department of Archaeology *Khajuraho*
Khandalavala – *Indian Sculpture and Painting*
Kramrisch – 1. *The Hindu Temple*, 2 Vols.
2. *The Art of India through the Ages*
Mookerjea – *The Art of India*
Motichandra – *Jaina Miniature Paintings from W. India*
Nawab – *Jaina Chitrakalpadruma*
Zannas – *Khajuraho*